HERBS, SPICES, AND MEDICINAL PLANTS FOR HUMAN GASTROINTESTINAL DISORDERS

Health Benefits and Safety

HERBS, SPICES, AND MEDICINAL PLANTS FOR HUMAN GASTROINTESTINAL DISORDERS

Health Benefits and Safety

Edited by

Megh R. Goyal, PhD
Preeti Birwal, PhD
Durgesh Nandini Chauhan, MPharm

AAP APPLE
ACADEMIC
PRESS

First edition published 2023

Apple Academic Press Inc.
1265 Goldenrod Circle, NE,
Palm Bay, FL 32905 USA

4164 Lakeshore Road, Burlington,
ON, L7L 1A4 Canada

CRC Press
6000 Broken Sound Parkway NW,
Suite 300, Boca Raton, FL 33487-2742 USA

2 Park Square, Milton Park,
Abingdon, Oxon, OX14 4RN UK

Library and Archives Canada Cataloguing in Publication

Title: Herbs, spices, and medicinal plants for human gastrointestinal disorders : health benefits and safety / edited by Megh R. Goyal, PhD, Preeti Birwal, PhD, Durgesh Nandini Chauhan, MPharm.
Names: Goyal, Megh R., editor. | Birwal, Preeti, editor. | Chauhan, Durgesh Nandini, editor.
Series: Innovations in plant science for better health.
Description: First edition. | Series statement: Innovations in plant science for better health: from soil to fork | Includes bibliographical references and index.
Identifiers: Canadiana (print) 20220175187 | Canadiana (ebook) 20220175306 | ISBN 9781774637142 (hardcover) | ISBN 9781774638019 (softcover) | ISBN 9781003189749 (ebook)
Subjects: LCSH: Gastrointestinal system—Diseases—Alternative treatment. | LCSH: Herbs—Therapeutic use. | LCSH: Spices—Therapeutic use. | LCSH: Phytochemicals—Therapeutic use. | LCSH: Medicinal plants.
Classification: LCC RM666.H33 H49 2022 | DDC 615.3/21—dc23

Library of Congress Cataloging-in-Publication Data

Names: Goyal, Megh R., editor. | Birwal, Preeti, editor. | Chauhan, Durgesh Nandini, editor.
Title: Herbs, spices, and medicinal plants for human gastrointestinal disorders : health benefits and safety / Megh R. Goyal, Preeti Birwal, Durgesh Nandini Chauhan.
Other titles: Innovations in plant science for better health.
Description: First edition. | Palm Bay, FL, USA : Apple Academic Press, [2023] | Series: Innovations in plant science for better health: from soil to fork | Includes bibliographical references and index. | Summary: "Herbs, Spices, and Medicinal Plants for Human Gastrointestinal Disorders: Health Benefits and Safety presents valuable information for exploring the health claims of plant-based phytochemicals for the treatment and prevention of gastrointestinal disorders. It details the healing benefits of specific spices and herb plant-based remedies, such as garlic, onion, black pepper, aloe vera, Indian gooseberry, chamomile, and dandelion for the treatment of colorectal cancer and hemorrhoids, irritable bowel syndrome, gallstones, celiac disease, peptic ulcers, etc. It also discusses the therapeutic properties of fermented foods and beverages and the healing benefits of lectins in the management of gastrointestinal disorders. The abundance of research presented in this volume will be valuable for researchers, scientists, growers, students, processors, traders, industries, and others in the development of plant-based therapeutics for gastrointestinal diseases"-- Provided by publisher.
Identifiers: LCCN 2022007969 (print) | LCCN 2022007970 (ebook) | ISBN 9781774637142 (hardback) | ISBN 9781774638019 (paperback) | ISBN 9781003189749 (ebook)
Subjects: LCSH: Materia medica. | Herbs--Therapeutic use. | Medicinal plants. | Gastrointestinal system--Diseases.
Classification: LCC RS431.M37 H47 2023 (print) | LCC RS431.M37 (ebook) | DDC 615.3/21--dc23/eng/20220223
LC record available at https://lccn.loc.gov/2022007969
LC ebook record available at https://lccn.loc.gov/2022007970

ISBN: 978-1-77463-714-2 (hbk)
ISBN: 978-1-77463-801-9 (pbk)
ISBN: 978-1-00318-974-9 (ebk)

Other Books on Plant Science for Better Health by Apple Academic Press, Inc.

- **Phytochemicals from Medicinal Plants: Scope, Applications, and Potential Health Claims**
  Editors: Hafiz Ansar Rasul Suleria, PhD, Megh R. Goyal, PhD, and Masood Sadiq Butt, PhD

- **Plant- and Marine-Based Phytochemicals for Human Health: Attributes, Potential, and Use**
  Editors: Megh R. Goyal, PhD, and Durgesh Nandini Chauhan, MPharm

- **Plant-Based Functional Foods and Phytochemicals: From Traditional Knowledge to Present Innovation**
  Editors: Megh R. Goyal, PhD, Arijit Nath, PhD, and Hafiz Ansar Rasul Suleria, PhD

- **Plant Secondary Metabolites for Human Health: Extraction of Bioactive Compounds**
  Editors: Megh R. Goyal, PhD, P. P. Joy, PhD, and Hafiz Ansar Rasul Suleria, PhD

- **The Role of Phytoconstitutents in Healthcare: Biocompounds in Medicinal Plants**
  Editors: Megh R. Goyal, PhD, Hafiz Ansar Rasul Suleria, PhD, and Ramasamy Harikrishnan, PhD

- **The Therapeutic Properties of Medicinal Plants: Health-Rejuvenating Bioactive Compounds of Native Flora**
  Editors: Megh R. Goyal, PhD, PE, Hafiz Ansar Rasul Suleria, PhD, Ademola Olabode Ayeleso, PhD, T. Jesse Joel, and Sujogya Kumar Panda

About the Senior Editor-in-Chief

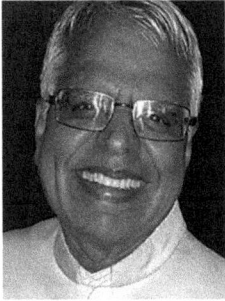

Megh R. Goyal, PhD, PE, is a Retired Professor in Agricultural and Biomedical Engineering from the General Engineering Department in the College of Engineering at the University of Puerto Rico–Mayaguez Campus; and Senior Acquisitions Editor and Senior Technical Editor-in-Chief in Agriculture and Biomedical Engineering for Apple Academic Press, Inc. He has worked as a Soil Conservation Inspector and as a Research Assistant at Haryana Agricultural University and Ohio State University.

During his professional career of 52 years, Dr. Goyal has received many prestigious awards and honors. He was the first agricultural engineer to receive the professional license in Agricultural Engineering in 1986 from the College of Engineers and Surveyors of Puerto Rico. In 2005, he was proclaimed as "Father of Irrigation Engineering in Puerto Rico for the Twentieth Century" by the American Society of Agricultural and Biological Engineers (ASABE), Puerto Rico Section, for his pioneering work on micro irrigation, evapotranspiration, agroclimatology, and soil and water engineering. The Water Technology Centre of Tamil Nadu Agricultural University in Coimbatore, India, recognized Dr. Goyal as one of the experts "who rendered meritorious service for the development of micro irrigation sector in India" by bestowing the Award of Outstanding Contribution in Micro Irrigation. This award was presented to Dr. Goyal during the inaugural session of the National Congress on "New Challenges and Advances in Sustainable Micro Irrigation" held at Tamil Nadu Agricultural University.

Dr. Goyal received the Netafim Award for Advancements in Microirrigation: 2018 from the American Society of Agricultural Engineers at the ASABE International Meeting in August 2018. VDGOOD Professional Association of India awarded Lifetime Achievement Award at 12th Annual Meeting on Engineering, Science and Medicine that was held on 20–21 of November of 2020 in Visakhapatnam, India. A prolific author and editor, he has written more than 200 journal articles and textbooks and has edited over 100 books. He is the editor of three book series published by Apple Academic Press: Innovations in Agricultural & Biological Engineering, Innovations and Challenges in Micro Irrigation, and Research Advances in Sustainable Micro Irrigation. He is also instrumental in the development of the new book series Innovations in Plant Science for Better Health: From Soil to Fork.

Dr. Goyal received his BSc degree in engineering from Punjab Agricultural University, Ludhiana, India; his MSc and PhD degrees from Ohio State University, Columbus; and his Master of Divinity degree from Puerto Rico Evangelical Seminary, Hato Rey, Puerto Rico, USA.

About the Editor

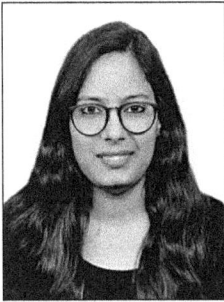

Preeti Birwal, PhD
Scientist (Processing and Food Engineering),
Department of Processing and Food Engineering,
College of Agricultural Engineering and Technology,
Punjab Agricultural University, Ludhiana, Punjab, India

Preeti Birwal, PhD, is working as a Scientist (processing and food engineering) in the Department of Processing and Food Engineering at the College of Agricultural Engineering and Technology at Punjab Agricultural University, Ludhiana, Punjab, India. She is currently working in the area of nonthermal food preservation, fermented beverages, food packaging, and technology of millet-based beer. She has served at Jain Deemed to be University, Bangalore, as a member of the board of examiners and placements. She has participated at several national and international conferences and seminars and has delivered lectures as a resource person on doubling farmers' income through dairy technology in training sponsored by the directorate of Extension, Ministry of Agriculture and Farmers Welfare, Government of India. Dr. Birwal has published research papers, an edited book, book chapters, popular articles, conference papers, abstracts, and editorial opinions. She is advising several MTech scholars in food technology and has successfully guided five postgraduate students for their dissertation work. She also serves as an external examiner for various Indian state agricultural universities and as an editor and reviewer of several journals. Dr. Birwal has been named outstanding reviewer of the month by the online journal *Current Research in Nutrition and Food Science*. She has successfully completed AUTOCAD 2D & 3D certification. She is a life member of IDEA. She graduated with a degree in Dairy Technology from ICAR–National Dairy Research Institute, Karnal, India; a master's degree in Food Process Engineering and Management from NIFTEM, Haryana; and PhD (Dairy Engineering) from ICAR–NDRI, Bangalore, India. She has received several fellowships from MHRD, Nestle India, GATE, and UGC-RGNF.

About the Coeditor

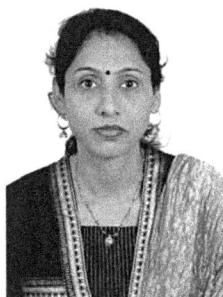

Durgesh Nandini Chauhan, MPharm

Durgesh Nandini Chauhan is working at Ishita Research Organization, Raipur, India, as a freelance writer and is also guiding pharmacy, Ayurvedic, and science students in their research projects. Mrs. Chauhan has 14 years of academic experience at various institutes in India in pharmaceutical sciences. She taught subjects such as pharmaceutics, pharmacognosy, traditional concepts of medicinal plants, drug-delivery phytochemistry, cosmetic technology, pharmaceutical engineering, pharmaceutical packaging, quality assurance, dosage designing, and anatomy and physiology. She is a member of the Association of Pharmaceutical Teachers of India, SILAE: The Scientific Network on Ethnomedicine (Italy), among others. Her previous research work included "Penetration Enhancement Studies on Organogel of Oxytetracycline HCL." She attended an AICTE-sponsored Staff Development Program on "Effects of Teaching and Learning Skills in Pharmacy: Tools for Improvement of Young Pharmacy Teachers" and a workshop on analytical instruments. She is also active as a reviewer for several international scientific journals and an active participant in national and international conferences, such as Bhartiya Vigyan Sammelan and International Convention of Society of Pharmacognosy.

She has written more than 10 publications in national and international journals, 13 book chapters, and two books: *Optimization and Evaluation of an Organogel* and *Plant- and Marine-Based Phytochemicals for Human Health: Attributes, Potential, and Use*. Mrs. Chauhan completed her BPharm degree at the Rajiv Gandhi Proudyogiki Vishwavidyalaya, Bhopal, India, and her MPharm in pharmaceutics from Uttar Pradesh Technical University (currently Dr. A.P.J. Abdul Kalam Technical University), Lucknow, India, in 2006.

Contents

Contributors

Doreen Kwankyewaa Adjei
Department of Pharmaceutics, Faculty of Pharmacy and Pharmaceutical Sciences,
Kwame Nkrumah University of Science and Technology, Kumasi AK 448 0660, Ghana;
E-mail: adjeidoreen18@gmail.com

Christian Agyare
Department of Pharmaceutics, Faculty of Pharmacy and Pharmaceutical Sciences,
Kwame Nkrumah University of Science and Technology, Kumasi AK 448 0660, Ghana;
E-mail: cagyare.pharm@knust.edu.gh

Eugene Kusi Agyei
Department of Pharmaceutics, Faculty of Pharmacy and Pharmaceutical Sciences,
Kwame Nkrumah University of Science and Technology, Kumasi AK 4480660, Ghana;
E-mail: eugenekusiagyei@gmail.com

Richard Agyen
Department of Pharmaceutics, Faculty of Pharmacy and Pharmaceutical Sciences,
Kwame Nkrumah University of Science and Technology, Kumasi AK 448 0660, Ghana;
E-mail: agyenrichard20@gmail.com

Caterina Anania
Policlinico Umberto I Hospital, Department of Pediatrics, Sapienza University of Rome,
12 Francesco Morosini Square, 00136 Rome, Italy; E-mail: caterina.anania@uniroma1.it

Ruchita Balu Bhor
P. E. Society's Modern College of Pharmacy, Yamunanagar, Nigdi, Pune 411044, Maharashtra, India;
E-mail: bhorruchita@gmail.com

Preeti Birwal
Punjab Agricultural University, Ferozpur Road, Ludhiana-141004, India;
E-mail: preetibirwal@gmail.com

Yaw Duah Boakye
Department of Pharmaceutics, Faculty of Pharmacy and Pharmaceutical Sciences,
Kwame Nkrumah University of Science and Technology, Kumasi AK 448 0660, Ghana;
E-mail: ydboakye.pharm@knust.edu.gh; yawduahb@gmail.com

Durgesh Nandini Chauhan
Columbia College of Pharmacy Sarona, Raipur 492010, Chhattisgarh, India;
E-mail: pharmanandini@gmail.com

Pooja Chawla
Department of Pharmaceutical Chemistry and Analysis, ISF College of Pharmacy, Ghal Kalan,
GT Road, Moga, 142001, Punjab, India; E-mail: pvchawla@gmail.com

Viney Chawla
University Institute of Pharmaceutical Sciences and Research, Baba Farid University of Health
Sciences, Sadiq Road, 151203, Faridkot, Punjab, India; E-mail: drvineychawla@gmail.com

Anju Dhiman
Department of Pharmaceutical Sciences, Maharshi Dayanand University, Rohtak 124001, Haryana, India; E-mail: admdudops@gmail.com

Kyle Drinnon
Department of General Surgery, Texas Tech University Health Sciences Center in Lubbock, TX 3601 4th Street, Lubbock, TX 79430, USA; E-mail: kyle.drinnon@ttuhsc.edu

Nandini Dutta
Department of Food Technology, School of Engineering and Technology, JAIN (Deemed-to-be University), 45th km NH-209, Jakkasandra Post, Kanakapura Road, Karnataka 562112, India; E-mail: nandini.dutta11@gmail.com

Hasya Nazlı Ekin
Department of Pharmacognosy, Faculty of Pharmacy, Gazi University, 06330, Ankara, Turkey; E-mail: hasyaekin@gmail.com

Abdul Faruk
Department of Pharmaceutical Sciences, HNB Garhwal University (A Central University) Srinagar, Garhwal 246174, Uttarakhand, India; E-mail: abdul_faruk@yahoo.com

Hugh James Freeman
Professor of Medicine, UBC Hospital, 2211 Wesbrook Mall, Vancouver, BC Canada V6T 1W5; Email: hugfree@shaw.ca

Megh R. Goyal
University of Puerto Rico-Mayaguez, USA; E-mail: goyalmegh@gmail.com

Amrita Milind Kulkarni
P. E. Society's Modern College of Pharmacy, Yamunanagar, Nigdi, Pune 411044, Maharashtra, India; E-mail: amritak0805@gmail.com

Vivek Kumar
Shri Baba Mastnath Institute of Pharmaceutical Sciences and Research, Rohtak 124001, Haryana, India; E-mail: vivek21288@gmail.com

Daniel Obeng Mensah
Department of Pharmaceutics, Faculty of Pharmacy and Pharmaceutical Sciences, Kwame Nkrumah University of Science and Technology, Kumasi AK 4480660, Ghana; E-mail: danny66810@gmail.com

Souvik Mukherjee
Department of Pharmaceutical sciences, Guru Ghasidas Vishwavidyalaya (A Central University), Bilaspur, C.G 495 009, India; E-mail: mukherjees388@gmail.com

Francesca Olivero
IRCCS Policlinico San Matteo, Department of Pediatrics, University of Pavia, 72 Luigi Rizzo Rd, 00136 Rome, Italy; E-mail: francescaol@hotmail.it

Didem Deliorman Orhan
Department of Pharmacognosy, Faculty of Pharmacy, Gazi University, 06330, Ankara, Turkey; E-mail: didemdeliorman@gmail.com, didem@gazi.edu.tr

Dilipkumar Pal
Department of Pharmaceutical sciences, Guru Ghasidas Vishwavidyalaya (A Central University), Bilaspur, C.G 495009, India; E-mail: drdilip2003@yahoo.co.in

Bhushan Prakash Pimple
P. E. Society's Modern College of Pharmacy, Yamunanagar, Nigdi, Pune 411044, Maharashtra, India;
E-mail: bhushanppimple@rediffmail.com

Yana Puckett
PGY-5, Department of General Surgery, Texas Tech University Health Sciences Center in Lubbock,
TX 3601 4th Street, Lubbock, TX 79430, USA; E-mail: puckettyana@gmail.com

Supriyo Saha
School of Pharmaceutical Sciences & Technology, Sardar Bhagwan Singh University,
Dehradun 248161; Uttarakhand, India; E-mail: supriyo9@gmail.com

Mrinmoy Sarkar
Department of Pharmaceutical Chemistry and Analysis, ISF College of Pharmacy, Ghal Kalan,
GT Road, Moga,142001, Punjab, India; E-mail: mrinmoy102sarkar@gmail.com

Gurpreet Singh
Department of Pharmaceutical Sciences, Guru Nanak Dev University, Amritsar, Punjab 143005,
India; E-mail: gurpreet_pharma85@yahoo.com

S. Supreetha
Department of Food Technology, School of Engineering and Technology,
JAIN (Deemed-to-be University), 45th km NH-209, Jakkasandra Post, Kanakapura Road,
Karnataka 562112, India; E-mail: supreethasrini@gmail.com

Abbreviations

AA	amino acid
ACA	ascorbic acid
ACALD	aloeride
ACE	angiotensin-converting enzyme
ADME	absorption, distribution, metabolism, and excretion
AEMOD	aloe-emodin
AKT	protein kinase B
AlAt	alanine aminotransferase
ALP	alkaline phosphatase
AP	alkaline phosphatase
APCs	antigen presenting cells
APG	aigenin-7-glucoside
APOB	apolipoproteins B
APOE	apolipoproteins E
AR	adequate relief
AsAt	aspartate aminotransferase
AUC	area under curve
b.i.d.	twice a day
BSS	bowel symptom score
BW	bowel
CAGR	compound annual growth rate
CAM	complementary and alternative medicine
cAMP	cyclic adenosine 3', 5' monophosphate
CarO	*Carum carvi* essential oil poultice
Cat	catalase
CCAD	chebulic acid
CCK	cholecystokinase
CCKAR	cholecystokinin A receptor
CCl_4	carbon tetrachloride
CD	celiac disease
CD	Crohn's disease
CDCA	chenodeoxycholic acid
CETP	cholesterol ester transporting proteins

CGA	chlorogenic acid
CGI	Clinical Global Impression
CHD	coronary heart disease
CK	cytokinin
CLA	conjugated linoleic acid
CLS	cells
CN	corilagin
COX	cyclooxygnease
COX-1	cyclooxygenase-1
COX-2	cyclooxygenase-2
CU-FEO	curcumin and fennel essential oil
CVD	cardiovascular disease
DADS	diallyl disulfide
DAS	diallyl sulfur
DATS	diallyl trisulfide
D-GalN	D-galactosamine
DNA	deoxyribose nucleic acid
DSS	dextran sulfate sodium
DU	deodenal ulcer
E-7-O-G	Eriodicytol-7-0-glucoside
EA	ellagic acid
EGCG	epigallocatechin gallate
EO	*Embilica officinalis*
EPOCG	ethnopharmacology
EQ-5D	The EuroQol Questionnaire
ERK	extracellular signal-regulated kinases
ESWL	extracorporeal shock wave lithotripsy
FIT	fecal immunochemical test
G6PD	glucose-6-phosphate dehydrogenase
GA	gallic acid
GABA	gamma amino butyric acid
GB	gall bladder
GFD	gluten-free diet
GI	gastro intestinal
GPX	glutathione peroxidase
GR	glutathione reductase
GSRS	Gastrointestinal Symptoms Rating Scale
GST	glutathione S-transferase

GU	gastric ulcer
GV	governing vessel
HADS	Hospital Anxiety and Depression Scale
HCl	hydrochloride
HDL	high density cholesterol
HDL	high density lipids
HDPE	high density polyethylene
HIF-1a	hypoxia-inducible factor 1-alpha
HIPS	high intensity polystyrene
HMG CoA	β-hydroxy β-methylglutaryl-CoA
HUVECs	human umbilical vein endothelial cells
i.p.	intraperitoneal
IBD	inflammatory bowel disease
IBS	irritable bowel syndrome
IBSQOL	Irritable Bowel Syndrome Quality of Life Questionnaire
IBS-SSS	IBS-Symptom Severity Scale
IC_{50}	half-maximal inhibitory concentration
IFL	inflammation
IGD	inflammatory gut disease
IL	interleukin
IMS	immune system
JNK	c-Jun N-terminal kinases
L-4-O-G	luteolin-4-O-glucoside
LAB	lactic acid bactria
LDL	low density cholesterol
LDL	low density lipids
LDLR	low density lipoprotein receptor
LDPE	low density polyethylene
LOX	lipoxygenase
LPS	lipopolysaccharide
MALDI	matrix-assisted laser desorption/ionization
MAO-A	monoamine oxidase
MAP	modified atmosphere packaging
MAPK	mitogen-activated protein kinase
MAPKS	mitogen-activated protein kinase
MBC	minimum bactericidal concentration
MEO	mace essential oil
Mg^{+2}	magnesium (II) ion

$MgSO_4$	magnesium sulphate
MIC	minimum inhibitory concentration
mRNA	messenger RNA
MTBE	methyl-tert-butyl ether
mTOR	mammalian target of rapamycin
MU	mouth ulcer
NCCIH	National Centre for Complementary and Integrative Health
NDI	Nepean Dyspepsia Index
Ne-MEO	nano encapsulated mace essential oil
NF	nuclear factor
NO	nitric oxide
NOCT	n octanol
NOS	nitrous oxide systems
NSAIDs	nonsteroidal anti-inflammatory
NVU	neurovascular units
OlivH	hot olive oil poultice
Pagg	pentagalloylglucose
Pdln	pedunculagin
PG	prostaglandin
PGE_2	prostaglandins
PGE2	prostaglandin E2
Phc	phytoconstituent
PHYEM	phyllaemblicin-A, B and C
PI3K	phosphoinositide 3-kinase
Pngn	punigluconin
PPARα	proliferator-activated receptor alpha
Prcs	preclinical study
PTEN	phosphatase and tensin homolog
PTHB	propyl 3,4,5-trihydroxybenzoate
PU	peptic ulcer
PVC	polyvinyl chloride
PXR	pregnane X receptor
PYA	phyllaembilic acid
QOL	quality of life
RAS	renin–angiotensin system
RHT	rheumatic
RNA	ribonucleic acid
ROS	reactive oxygen species

RoS	reactive oxygen species
SEER	Surveillance, Epidemiology, and End Results
SF12	Short Form 12
SGOT	serum glutamic oxaloacetic transaminase
SGPT	serum glutamic pyruvic transaminase
SoD	superoxide dismutase
SPN	saponin
SST	site-specific targeting
SYTLY	synthetically
TAA	thioacetamide
TCAM	traditional medicine/complementary and alternative medicine
TH-1	T helper cell-1
TH-2	T helper cell-2
THP1	Tohoku Hospital Pediatrics-1
TISS	total IBS symptom score
TNF	tissue necrosis factor
TNF-α	tumor necrosis factor-alpha
TNSSFALF	tumor necrosis factor-α:
TOF	time of flight
TRPM8	transient receptor potential cation channel subfamily m (melastatin) member
UC	ulcerative colitis
UDCA	ursodeoxycholic acid
UHT	ultra-high treatment
VAS	visual analogue scale
VEGF	vascular endothelial growth factor
VM	vitamin
w/w	weight by weight

Preface

The digestive system of the human body is one of the most important pillars of the entire human body system, because the food consumed by human beings has either a direct or an indirect side effect on their health, which leads to various diseases. In a world where problems related to stomach and intestine are very common, functional gastrointestinal system diseases are the most commonly found diseases, which occur due to eating habits and erratic lifestyles. When there is a problem in the human body, nature has always provided remedies for it. Plants, especially medicinal plants, herbs, and spices, have unlimited basic and therapeutic importance in conditions such as hypoglycemia. They also exhibit antidiabetic, anticancerous, antithrombic, antihypertensive, anti-inflammatory, and antioxidant activities. Among the therapeutic benefits, a plant-based diet helps in the prevention against gastrointestinal diseases. These plant-based foods can be consumed either in the form of plant extracts, essential oils, or can be directly included in food. Due to several health benefits, the demand for plant-based diets, especially medicinal, herbal, and spices, is growing. Phytomedicine compounds are also important in the prevention and the treatment of gastrointestinal diseases.

This book *Herbs, Spices, and Medicinal Plants for Human Gastrointestinal Disorders: Health Benefits and Safety* attempts to exemplify the health benefits of plant-based phytochemicals and the role of herbs and spices in therapeutic applications. Each chapter covers major features pertaining to health benefits and cures for gastrointestinal diseases through various plant-based foods.

This book is divided into three parts. Part I: Natural Phytochemicals in Gastrointestinal Disorders describes the potential of *Carica papaya*, healing benefits of nutmeg (*Myristica fragrans*), healing benefits of plant-based phytochemicals in the prevention of colorectal cancer, and healing benefits of medicinal plants in the treatment of hemorrhoids. Part II: Role of Spices and Herbs in the Management of Gastrointestinal Disorders covers the healing benefits of garlic (*Allium sativum*), onion (*Allium cepa*), lectins, black pepper, chamomile, and dandelion in the management of gastrointestinal disorders. Part III: Plant-based Remedies in the Treatment of Gastrointestinal Diseases explains the role of *Aloe vera* in the treatment of irritable bowel disease, herbal treatment of irritable bowel syndrome, role of plant-based medicines in the treatment of gall bladder stones, role of pseudocereals in the treatment of celiac disease, role of amla (*Emblica officinalis*) in peptic ulcer, and therapeutic properties of fermented foods and beverages.

This book would serve as a paragon of material and an exceptional reference material for researchers, scientists, growers, students, processors, traders, industries, and others in the development of plant-based diet for gastrointestinal diseases.

This book will aid experts working in the area of food science, technology, and medicine around the world. The book will also act as a reference book for researchers, students, scholars, industries, universities, and research centers.

This book has taken its present shape because of the excellent contribution by the contributing authors, who have been the soul of this compendium. We have mentioned their names in each chapter and also in the list of contributors. We are indeed indebted to them for their knowledge, dedication, and enthusiasm.

We also extend our sincere thanks to Apple Academic Press, Inc.

We hereby appeal to our readers to provide their productive suggestions that may form the basis for improving future editions.

We take this opportunity to thank (1) our families for their motivation, moral support, and blessings in counteracting every obstacle coming in the way; (2) our spouses for their understanding, patience, and encouragement throughout this project; (3) our institutes: PAU, Ludhiana, Punjab; ICAR-NDRI, Karnal, Columbia College of Pharmacy, Chhattisgarh; and UPRM, Mayaguez for their support during the compilation of this publication.

—Editors

PART I

Natural Phytochemicals in Gastrointestinal Disorders

CHAPTER 1

Ethnopharmacology and Therapeutic Potential of *Carica papaya*

GURPREET SINGH, POOJA CHAWLA, ABDUL FARUK, and
VINEY CHAWLA

ABSTRACT

Papaya (*Carica papaya* Linn) has been widely used as traditional herbal
remedy for the prevention and management of several conditions and
diseases. During the past few decades, it has been used in the treatment of
digestive problems, wounds, dengue, and jaundice, etc. Its major bioactive
phytoconstituents are: papain, chymopapain, alkaloids, flavonoids, lycopene, carotenoids, anthraquinones glycoside, antioxidants, and vitamins.
This chapter has highlighted various ethnopharmacological and traditional
uses of different parts of *Carica papaya.*

1.1 INTRODUCTION

Carica papaya is a member of the family *Caricaceae* (a family of dicots
plants with four genera).[56] *Papaya* is a delicious fruit in most tropical and
semitropical countries and is cultivated mostly for its consumption as
fresh fruit, and for use in drinks, jams, salads, and candies.[2] The papaya
plant has been well-documented in the literature for a number of medicinal properties and has been used against diseases, such as gastroenteritis,
urethritis, typhoid fever, wound infection, asthma, rheumatism, fever,
diarrhea, boils, and hypertension, etc.[7,11,37,59,60,67,71] All parts of papaya
(seeds, roots, rinds, and fruits) have beneficial therapeutic and protective
properties (Fig. 1.1). Different parts of the papaya plant have been used in

the food (nutraceuticals), skincare products, leather, and pharmaceutical production.[41] Scientists have reported the activity of papaya for antifertility, anthelmintic, and anti-inflammatoryeffects.[50,53,55,58,97] The latex of unripe fruit is widely used in pharmaceutical and cosmetics products.[18,69,78]

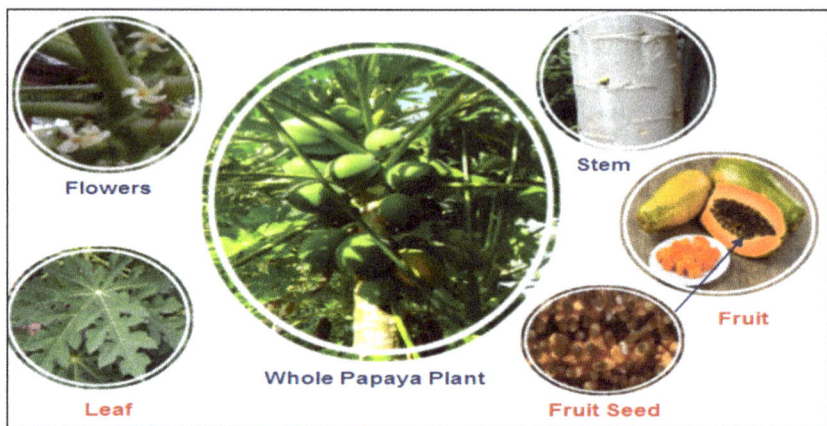

FIGURE 1.1   Major parts of *Carica papaya* plant.

The Spanish chronicler Oviedo indicated the papaya on Panamanian and Colombian coasts in 1526. Due to the high viability of papaya seeds, the fruit was rapidly produced in the tropics.[23] During this century, papaya has been cultivated in tropical regions with fertile soils and heavy rainfall. Then, papaya seeds were introduced to Southeast Asia and India by Spanish and Portuguese mariners. Later, papaya seeds reached Hawaii between 1800 and 1820.[77] In the 20th century, papaya seeds were taken to Barbados, Jamaica, Mexico, and Florida.

1.2   GEOGRAPHICAL DISTRIBUTION

It is local to the tropics of the Americas, however, now it is generally developed all through the world, and is accessible consistently.[3] It is cultivated in different parts of the world and the significant cultivators of papaya plants include India, tropical America, Europe, Australia, Hawaii, and South-East Asia.[30] Papaya is cultivated in all five continents due to its capability of growing in all soil types, but it requires good drainage.[1,73]

The major contribution of its total production[98] comes from Asia, Central America, and other countries as shown in Figure 1.2, and major cultivars of papaya plant are listed in Table 1.1. Different vernacular names of *C. papaya* and the taxonomic hierarchy of *C. papaya* have been illustrated by many investigators.[20,44,73]

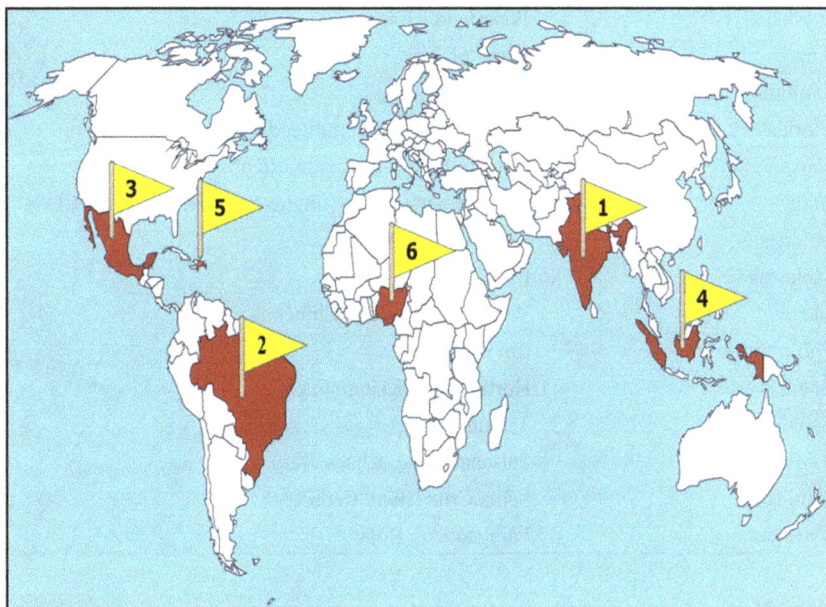

FIGURE 1.2   Major producers of papaya plant: (1) India, (2) Brazil, (3) Mexico, (4) Indonesia, (5) Dominican Republic, and (6) Nigeria.

1.3   MORPHOLOGY

Papaya is a small softwood and unbranched tropical fruit tree of 5–10 m in height with the spirally arranged leaves. The seven lobed leaves are large in diameter of about 50–70 cm, vary in sizes and shapes in different maturity stages. Fruits are commonly green while young and yellow-greenish or orange when ripe with the large ovoid smooth surface.[1,10] The fruit has a hollow berry, which contains small black seeds that constitute about 15% of the total weight and the seeds are lined in five rows to the interior wall of the fruit. Papaya tree starts to bear fruit within 1–2 years.[72] It can be cultivated in either home gardens or outdoors.

TABLE 1.1 Major Cultivars of Papaya in the World.

Country	Variety
Australia	Improved Petersen, Guinea Gold
Barbados	Wakefield, Graeme
Cuba	Maradol
Dominican Republic	Cartagena
Florida	Cariflora, Betty, Homestead
Hawaii	Kapoho Solo, Waimanalo, Rainbow
India	Coorg Honey Dew, Coimbatore Varieties (CO1–CO8)
Indonesia	Semangka, Dampit
Malaysia	Eksotika, Sekaki
Mexico	Verde, Gialla, Cera, Chincona
Philippines	Cavite, Sinta
South Africa	Hortus Gold, Kaapmuiden
Taiwan	Tainung five
Thailand	Sai-nampueng, Khaek Dam
Trinidad	Santa Cruz Giant, Cedro
Venezuela	Paraguanera, Roja

On the basis of reported literature, papaya plant is categorized into three primary sexes (Fig. 1.3), such as male (staminate) (♂), hermaphrodite (bisexual) (⚥), and female (pistillate) (♀). A typical male and female plants bear individual unisexual flowers, while hermaphrodite plant bears a combination of male unisexual and hermaphroditic flowers.[33,54] The typical female flower is mostly large and conical in shape when it is mature with five petals spread from the base. The ovary is large in structure with a circular smooth surface, which produces spherical or ovoid-shaped flowers. Fruit progresses from globular to egg-shaped. In the case of hermaphrodite intermediate type, the flower is undefined and petals may be fused in their length or may be free from the base. Hermaphrodite elongated type of flower has fused petals from one-fourth to three-fourths of their total length with 10 anthers, out of which five are long and five are short. The long ovary contains five or more carpels and forms the fruit which is cylindrical to pear-shaped and is of great commercial value.

The typical male flower has a long and thin corolla. It contains anthers in two series of five; one series is longer than the other. The male flowers have nonfunctional rudimentary pistil.[33,61] Multiple species of papaya have been documented in the scientific literature, which belong to five genera, that is, *Jacaratia, Jarilla, Horovitzia, Carica,* and *Vasconcellea.*[24]

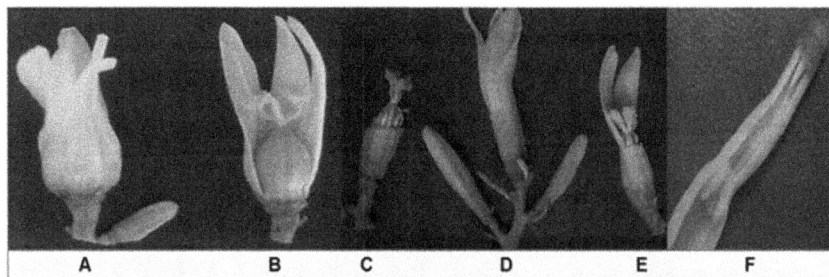

FIGURE 1.3 Six varieties of flowers of papaya plant: Typical female (A, B). Hermaphrodite intermediate (C). Hermaphrodite elongated (D). Hermaphrodite sterile (E). Typical male (F).

1.4 PHYTOCONSTITUENTS

Primary phytoconstituents reported from various parts of the *C. papaya* plant include papain (proteolytic enzyme), lycopene (tetraterpene), carotenoids, alkaloids, monoterpenoids, flavonoids, mineral (potassium, etc.), vitamins (A, C, and E; thiamine, niacin, and riboflavin), malic acid, and glycosides.[1,34,69,74,81,96] Fresh fruit juice contains flavonoids, tannins, and anthocyanins with antioxidant ability as free radical scavengers.[68] Young leaves of papaya include carpaine, pseudocarpaine, dehydrocarpaine, choline, carposide, and vitamins (C and E). Phytochemical analysis of the different parts of the plant revealed the presence of various bioactive phytochemicals, which have pharmacological importance (Fig. 1.4).

Papaya fruit exhibits wide range of medicinal properties (i.e., antimicrobial, antiviral, anti-inflammatory, healing of wound and dressing aid, anticancer, neurodegenerative, diuretic, abortifacient agent, and contraceptive).[43] It is highly well-known for its nutritional values and it aids in digestion. Extract of the whole fruit contains immunity boosters (i.e., vitamin C, ferulic, caffeic acid, and *p*-coumaric) that protect human cells against oxidative stresses.[13]

Unripe fruit of papaya contains proteolytic enzyme papain (cysteine protease), which acts like pepsin in gastric juice. The papain is more active in green fruit and shows extensive proteolytic activity toward proteins. The extract from the seeds of papaya shows antioxidant and anticancer activities due to the presence of various phenolic compounds, vanillic acid, and vitamin C.[52,62,86]

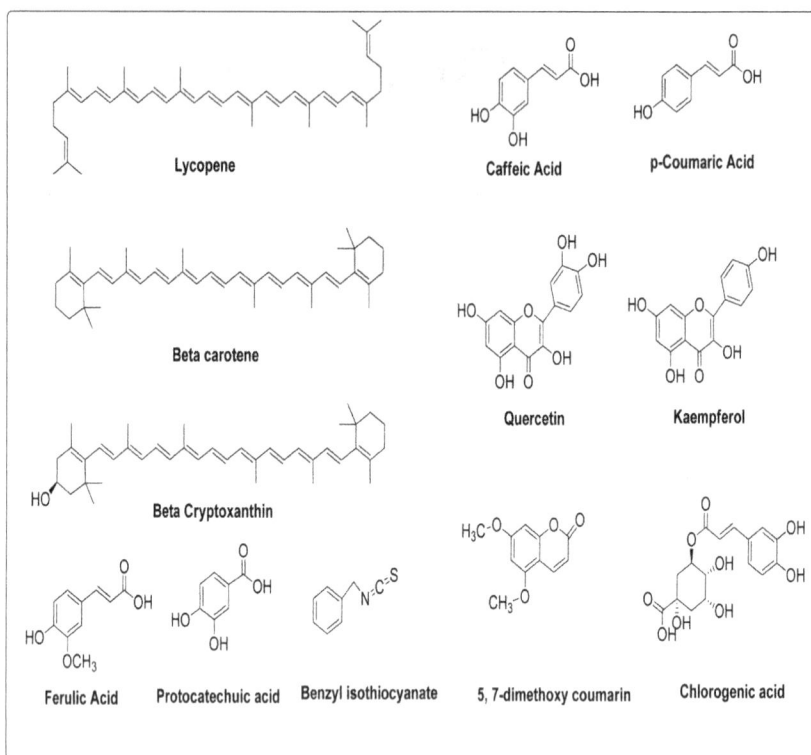

FIGURE 1.4   The structures of some phytoconstituents isolated from *C. papaya*.

Another source of papain is latex, which is harvested by incision on the surface of unripe fruit. After 4–5 days, latex is collected and further processed into dry powder for various uses in pharmaceutical and food industries.[51] The process of isolation of papain from unripe fruit latex is shown in Figure 1.5.

The papaya fruit is suitable for human consumption due to its nutritional and digestive value, with a low caloric content, which provides a favorable cost-benefit to human health.[69] Furthermore, scientific studies report the nutritional content of 100 g of ripe and unripe papaya fruits as summarized in Table 1.2. Results revealed that unripe papaya has the highest concentrations of different vitamins and minerals as compared with ripe fruits.[22,79]

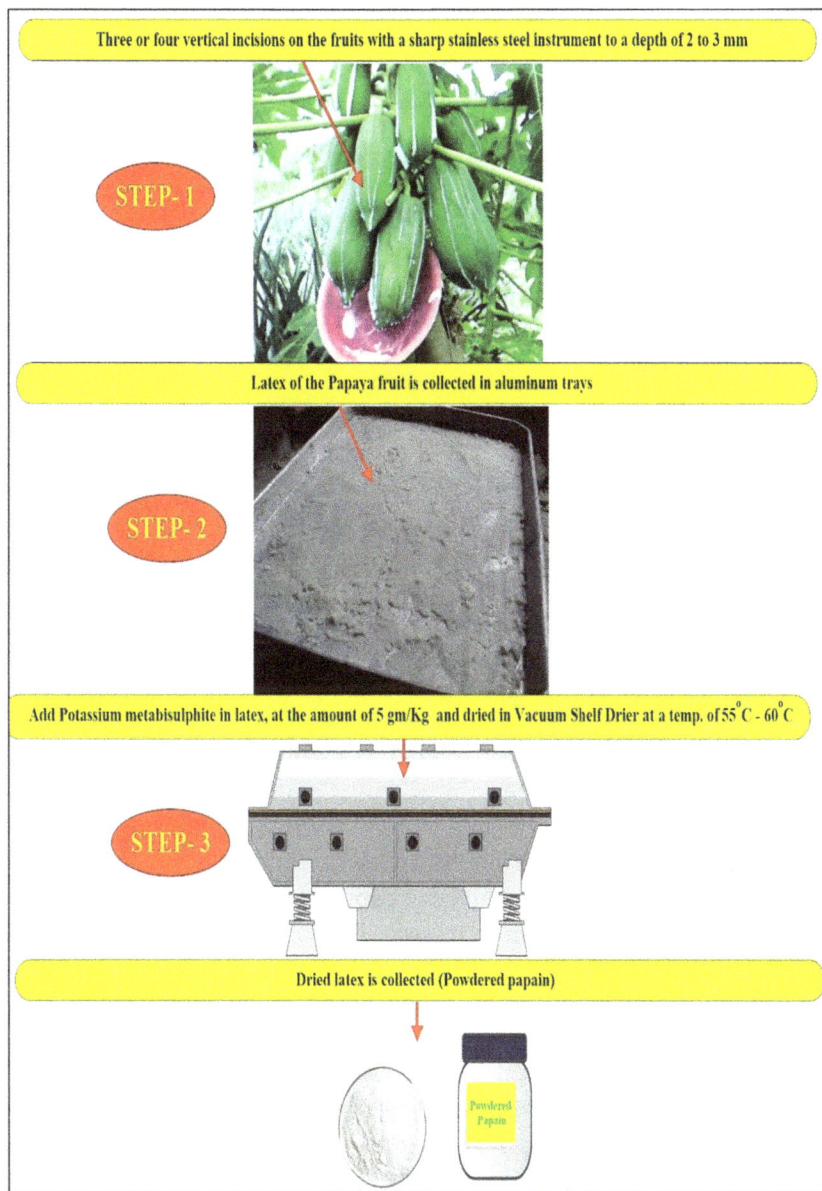

FIGURE 1.5 Isolation of papain powder from the latex from the papaya fruit.

TABLE 1.2   Nutritional Value of a Papaya Fruit.

Constituent	Ripe fruit (g)	Unripe fruit (g)
Water	89.1	92.6
Proteins	8.26	10.8
Total lipid	0.93	1.35
Ash	0.00459	6.76
Carbohydrates	86.2	81.1
Mineral Macronutrients:		
Sodium	0.1284	0.2838
Potassium	1.238	2.743
Magnesium	0.2294	0.6351
Calcium	0.1468	0.4324
Micronutrients:		
Iron	0.01284	0.00811
Copper	0.00018	0.00014
Zinc	0.00092	0
Vitamins:		
Vitamin C	0.5688	0.0003919
Thiamine	0.00028	0.00054
Riboflavin	0.00028	0.026
Niacin	0.0028	0.00405
Carotene	7.807(µg)	0

1.5   PHARMACOLOGICAL ACTIVITIES AND THERAPEUTIC USAGES OF *CARICA PAPAYA*

Every part of papaya plant holds the therapeutic value from leaves to roots.[56,69] The fruits, latex, and juice of papaya plant are the main source of many vitamins, which aid in dyspepsia, intestinal irritation, and habitual constipation.

The main constituent papain plays a vital role to improve the immune system.[9] In traditional veterinary medicine, papaya seeds are used as de-wormers and is also used in tropical folk medicine. The fresh latex is used as a vermifuge.[6] Papain is a proteolytic digestive enzyme that is used in several herbal formulations. Fresh juice of papaya prepared from peeled or unpeeled fruit is also sold as immunity booster drink because of its low cost, easy availability throughout the year and high nutritive value. In certain countries, the latex of the plant is used for tumors of uterus, psoriasis, and ringworm. The root infusion is used against syphilis.[82] Through several scientific studies, the traditional, pharmacological, and biological effects of *C. papaya* have been validated.[10,44,74,78]

1.5.1   Anthelmintic Activity

A wide collection of papaya and their extracts have been used traditionally for the management of helminths (parasites). Papaya contains many biologically active compounds with varying properties in fruit, latex, leaves, and roots that aid in digestion. It has also been employed for treating intestinal worms.[6,16] Papain, which is present in the latex of unripe green fruits of papaya, has been commercialized in various forms. Dried seeds of papaya have shown significant activity in the management of human intestinal parasites, which have increased the stool clearance rate of parasites without any side effects. It is represented as a novel class of antihelminthic due to the efficacy of papaya latex and cysteine proteinases against *Heligmosomoid espolygyrus* (nematode).[89] Shaziya et al. reported the antihelminthic action of papaya leaves on *A. Caninum* nematode infecting mice.[87]

Papain is a protein enzyme with cysteine protease, chymopapain, and lysozyme, which can accelerate the reaction within body cells. During the digestion process, pancreas commonly produces enzymes in the human body, these enzymes break down the foods into micronutrients, which can be used by the body for energy and other functions.[12] Two main proteolytic enzymes (papain and chymopapain) in the latex of the papaya simply break down the proteins into amino acids through cleavage of the peptide bond. These proteins contained peptide bonds and can be easily broken down by enzymatic action into easily digestible micronutrients. It also helps to promote the digestion of wheat protein.[40]

1.5.2   Antioxidant Activity

Antioxidant properties of aqueous extract of papaya leaves were evaluated in alcohol-induced acute gastric damage. The outcomes revealed that gastric ulcer index was significantly better in rats pretreated with the extract of papaya leaf as compared with the alcohol-treated rats. Further, leaf extract also offered reduced blood oxidative stress level in rats via the reduction of lipid peroxide levels in plasma and amplified red blood cell glutathione peroxidase activity.[39]

Another study showed strong in vivo antioxidant actions of ethyl acetate fraction of unripe pulp of papaya on antioxidant enzymes (i.e., glutathione peroxidase (GPX), glutathione S-transferase (GST), glutathione reductase (GR), catalase, and glucose-6-phosphate dehydrogenase (G6PD)) in albino mouse. It has been suggested that it can be used for protection against gastric ulcer and oxidative stress.[64] Natural source of antioxidants may responsible for total antioxidant effect due to the presence of carotenoid, polyphenols, vitamin C, and vitamin E.[57] Several studies showed that the antioxidant property is related to the diminished DNA damage and decreased lipid peroxidation, which maintained the immune function.[46,48]

1.5.3   Antiviral Activity

The published studies on dengue specified that the juice of papaya leaves could help to increase the platelets and white blood cells count in these patients.[15,80] A study in 2012 has reported about in vitro studies of papaya leaf extracts on persons infected with dengue. Papaya leaf extract inhibited the heat- and hypotonicity-induced hemolysis of red blood cells and has membrane-stabilizing properties.[76] In a randomized controlled trial in dengue patients, there was an increment in platelets-related genes like arachidonate 12-lipoxygenase and platelet-activating factor receptor gene and that contributed to the prevention of platelet lysis. In folk medicine, papaya leaves have been used for the management of dengue fever with hemorrhagic symptoms.[91]

1.5.4   Antimicrobial Activity

Osato et al.[65] and Calzada et al.[17] reported the ability of papaya seeds as antimicrobial agent against several Gram-positive and Gram-negative bacteria like *Trichomonas vaginalis* trophozoites, *Bacillus subtilis*, *Escherichia coli* and *Salmonella typhi*.[17,65] The aqueous extract of papaya leaves and roots at different concentrations showed antimicrobial effects against pathogenic bacteria.[8] The pulp and fruits of papaya also showed remarkable antibacterial effect against *B. subtilis, K. pneumonia, P. vulgaris, E. coli, P. aeruginosa, S. typhi, E. cloacae, and S. aureus*.[11]

1.5.5   Antifungal Activity

The papaya leaves and seeds of ripe and unripe fruits were evaluated against phytopathogenic fungi (i.e., *R. stolonifer*, Fusarium spp. and *C. gloeosporioides*), which exhibited good antifungal activity. The antifungal activity was observed to increase in a concentration-dependent manner.[19] The latex of papaya also inhibits the growth of *Candida albicans*. The latex shows antifungal activity due to partial degradation of the outermost layers of fungal cell wall, which lacks polysaccharides.[26] The synergistic effect of latex of papaya with fluconazole in *C. albicans* was also reported.[25]

1.5.6   Anti-Inflammatory Activity

It has been well documented in the literature that the dried papaya leaves are used for the management of inflammation, arthritis, rheumatism, and as wound dressing material. The ethanolic extract of the leaves was examined in rats using a paw edema model with indomethacin-treated control group. The results showed that the extracts significantly reduced edema and amount of granuloma. Similar results were confirmed with other models, that is, cotton pellet granuloma model and formaldehyde-induced arthritis model.[67,92,93]

Papaya leaves are a rich source of carpaine, nicotinic acid, which may be accountable for the anti-inflammatory effect. Ahmed et al.[4] assessed the inflammation at acute, subchronic, and chronic phase using the cotton pellet granuloma model, formaldehyde-induced arthritis and carrageenan-induced paw edema models. They suggested that the anti-inflammatory activity of the ethyl alcohol extract of papaya was due to the inhibition of *prostaglandin-* mediated inflammation.[4] Papaya leaf extract also exhibited anti-arthritic activity by the modulation of inflammatory mediators, such as, cytokines or chemokines, prostaglandins or leukotrienes.[67]

1.5.7   Antifertility Effects

The antifertility activity of papaya fruit was evaluated in adult rat and pregnant rat model. The results revealed that the unripe fruit disturbed the estrous cycle and encouraged the abortion.[27] Seed extract showed anti-fertility activity due to gradual degeneration of Sertoli and Leydig cells, which induced long-term azoospermia.[95] A recent report revealed that seeds possess reversible male contraceptive potential by directly rendered the spermatozoa process.[90] It is further reported that root extract exerts morphological changes in the endometrium of rat uterus[83] and the aqueous extract of seeds has shown miscarriage in female *Sprague Dawley* rats.

The crude extract of papaya bark showed antifertility activity in rats due to its effect on sperm motility; and while the aqueous/petroleum ether/ alcoholic extracts in rabbits inhibited ovulation cycle. Therefore, it can be utilized as an effective contraceptive in animals.[47] It was further reported that the unripe or half-ripe fruits contain a high concentration of the latex, which increased the uterine contraction. Normal consumption of ripe papaya is safe in pregnancy, but unripe papaya is unsafe.[2]

1.5.8   Anticancer Activity

Many studies scientifically validated the anticancer effects of papaya leaves. The aqueous extract of papaya leaves exhibits a dose-dependent significant activity against the cells of breast and lung adenocarcinoma, cervical, hepatocellular and pancreatic epithelial carcinoma, and mesothelioma. These results indicate that extracts may inhibit the growth of different types of cancer cell lines. However, the precise cellular mechanism of action remains unclear.[29,66] Several studies have claimed that mechanisms in the inhibition of proliferation by papain include the production of cytokines by human peripheral blood mononuclear cells, interfering in cancer cell wall and cleavages of proteins into amino acid form.[21]

Leaves of *C. papaya* (which contain a high concentration of tocopherol, lycopene, flavonoid, and benzyl isothiocyanate) potentially contribute to anti-tumor activity.[79] Similarly, fermented product of papaya (FPP®) claimed the immunity booster and antioxidant activity. The role of free radicals in propagating cancer is fully documented. Thus, by acting as an antioxidant, it helps to control cancerous growth.[49]

1.5.9   Antihypertensive Activity

Methanolic extract of papaya elicited the antihypertensive effects due to in vivo inhibition of angiotensin-converting enzyme and it improved the effect on the baroreflex. It was reported that angiotensin-converting enzyme inhibitory activity was similar to those of enalapril and reduced the cardiac hypertrophy.[14]

1.5.10   Antimalarial Activity

Daily consumption of papaya leaves is a common practice in tropical communities for preventing malaria caused by *Plasmodium* genus. In vitro antiplasmodial effect of the leaf extracts was reported to be due to carpaine, which is an alkaloid.[42,94] Petroleum ether extract of the rind of papaya fruit also exhibits antimalarial activity.[99]

1.5.11   Hematological Activity

The study revealed that phytochemicals in seed, leaf, and pulp produced significant effects on certain blood parameters in treated rats. A dose-dependent effect was observed, which could be attributed to the existence of folic acid, vitamin B_{12}, alkaloids, and glycosides. It can be used for the treatment of sickle-cell anemia.[36,38]

1.5.12   Wound Healing Activity

Papaya latex contains papain, which can break down the necrotic tissue contributing to wound healing process. The study showed that the latex of *C. papaya* decreases the oxidative tissue damage thus ensuring the clot formation process during healing and the increase in di-hydroxyproline content.[28] It is also known to be effective in diabetic wound healing by preventing infection due to its antimicrobial activity.[5]

1.5.13   Hepatoprotective Activity

Ethanol and aqueous extracts of papaya fruit hold the hepatoprotective effect against carbon tetrachloride (CCl_4)-induced hepatotoxicity in rats. Results revealed significant hepatoprotection by reduction in biochemical parameters, such as, SGPT (serum glutamic pyruvic transaminase), SGOT (serum glutamic-oxaloacetic transaminase), ALP (alkaline phosphatase), and serum bilirubin, which are indicators of liver damage.[75]

1.5.14   Topical Use

Various topical applications of papaya fruits have been used in developing countries, such as topical ulcer dressings and burn dressing. It is a cost-effective remedy for desloughing necrotic tissue and preventing burn wound infection.[31] It also provides a granulating tissue, which is suitable for the application of skin graft. Now-a-days, papaya is commonly used in children's burns dressing. Papaya fruit is crushed and is daily applied on the infected burns as a layer.[88]

1.6   SUMMARY

Scientists around the globe have focused on papaya plant for its high medicinal value with simple availability in nature. *C. papaya* has the potential of capturing the global market of herbal formulations for therapeutic potential in digestive disorders. However, this needs a clinical validation. The presence of secondary metabolites has been identified, which may help in the planning of such clinical studies, which are needed to understand and explore the exact pharmacological and molecular mechanisms action of *C. papaya* activity. It will also help to establish its toxicity profile along with drug interactions.

KEYWORDS

- abortifacient
- anthelmintic activity
- antifertility
- *Carica papaya*
- caricaceae
- chymopapain
- dengue
- digestion enhancer
- nutraceutical
- papain powder

REFERENCES

1. Abdulazeez, M. A.; Sani, I. Use of Fermented Papaya (*Carica papaya*) Seeds as a Food Condiment, and Effects on Pre- and Post-implantation Embryo Development. In *Nuts and Seeds in Health and Disease Prevention*; Preedy, V. R., Watson, R. R., Patel, V. B., Eds.; Academic Press: San Diego, 2011; pp 855–863.
2. Adebiyi, A.; Adaikan, P. G.; Prasad, R. N. Papaya (*Carica papaya*) Consumption Is Unsafe in Pregnancy: Fact or Fable? Scientific Evaluation of a Common Belief in Some Parts of Asia using a Rat Model. *Br. J. Nutr.* **2002**, *88* (2), 199–203.
3. Adeneye, A. A. The 6-Subchronic and Chronic Toxicities of African Medicinal Plants. In *Toxicological Survey of African Medicinal Plants*; Kuete, V., Ed.; Elsevier, 2014; pp 99–133.
4. Ahmed, M.; Ramabhimalah, S. Anti-Inflammatory Activity of Aqueous Extract of *Carica papaya* Seeds in Albino Rats. *Biomed. Pharmacol. J.* **2012**, *5*, 173–177.
5. Ajani, R.; Ogunbiyi, K. *Carica papaya* Latex Accelerates Wound Healing in Diabetic Wistar Rats. *Eur. J. Med. Plants* **2015**, *9*, 1–12.
6. Ameen, S.; Azeez, O. M.; Baba, Y.; Raji, L. Anthelmintic Potency of *Carica papaya* Seeds Against Gastro-intestinal Helminths in Red Sokoto goat. *Ceylon J. Sci.* **2018**, *47*, 137–143.
7. Amzad-Hossain, M.; Hitam, S.; Hadidja I. A. Pharmacological and Toxicological Activities of the Extracts of papaya Leaves used Traditionally for the Treatment of Diarrhea. *J. King Saud Univ.– Sci.* **2020**, *32* (1), 962–969.
8. Anibijuwon, I.; Augustine, U. Antimicrobial Activity of *Carica papaya* on Some Pathogenic Organisms of Clinical Origin from South-Western Nigeria. *Ethnobot. Leaflets* **2009**, *13*, 850–864.
9. Anjum, V.; Arora, P.; Ansari, S. H.; Najmi, A. K.; Ahmad, S. Antithrombocytopenic and Immunomodulatory Potential of Metabolically Characterized Aqueous Extract of *Carica papaya* Leaves. *Pharm. Biol.* **2017**, *55* (1), 2043–2056.
10. Aravind, G.; Bhowmik, D.; S, D.; Harish, G. Traditional and Medicinal uses of *Carica papaya*. *J. Med. Plants Stud.* **2013**, *1*, 7–15.
11. Asghar, N.; Naqvi, S. A. R.; Hussain, Z. Compositional Difference in Antioxidant and Antibacterial Activity of all Parts of the *Carica papaya* using Different Solvents. *Chem. Central J.* **2016**, *10* (1), 5–9.
12. Azarkan, M.; Moussaoui, A.; Wuytswinkel, D.; Dehon, G.; Looze, Y. Fractionation and Purification of the Enzymes Stored in the Latex of *Carica papaya*. *J. Chromatogr. B Anal. Technol. Biomed. Life Sci.* **2003**, *790*, 229–238.
13. Boshra, V.; Tajul, A. Y. Papaya-an Innovative Raw Material for Food and Pharmaceutical Processing Industry. *Health Environ. J.* **2013**, *4*, 68–75.
14. Brasil, G. A.; Ronchi, S. N.; do Nascimento, A. M. Antihypertensive Effect of *Carica papaya* via a Reduction in ACE Activity and Improved Baroreflex. *Planta Medica* **2014**, *80* (17), 1580–1587.
15. Bsr, D.; Kj, G.; Lakshmiprasad, J. Effect of Papaya Leaf Juice on Platelet and WBC Count in Dengue Fever: A Case Report. *J. Ayurveda Holistic Med.* **2013**, *1*, 44–47.
16. Buttle, D. J.; Behnke, J. M.; Bartley, Y. Oral Dosing with Papaya Latex is an Effective Anthelmintic Treatment for Sheep Infected with *Haemonchus contortus*. *Parasites Vectors* **2011**, *4* (1), 36–40.

17. Calzada, F.; Yepez-Mulia, L.; Tapia-Contreras, A. Effect of Mexican Medicinal Plant Used to Treat Trichomoniasis on Trichomon as vaginal istrophozoites. *J. Ethnopharmacol.* **2007,** *113* (2), 248–251.

18. Chandrasekaran, R.; Seetharaman, P. *Carica papaya* (Papaya) Latex: A New Paradigm to Combat Against Dengue and Filariasis Vectors Aedesaegypti and Culexquinque fasciatus (Diptera: Culicidae). *3 - Biotech* **2018,** *8* (2), 83–91.

19. Chavez-Quintal, P.; Gonzalez-Flores, T.; Rodriguez-Buenfil, I.; Gallegos-Tintore, S. Antifungal Activity in Ethanolic Extracts of *Carica papaya* L. cv. Maradol Leaves and Seeds. *Ind. J. Microbiol.* **2011,** *51* (1), 54–60.

20. Cotruţ, R.; Butcaru, A.; Mihai, C.; Stănică, F. *Carica papaya* L. Cultivated in Greenhouse Conditions. *J. Horticulture Forestry Biotechnol.* **2017,** *21* (3), 130–136.

21. Desser, L.; Rehberger, A.; Paukovits, W. Proteolytic Enzymes and Amylase Induce Cytokine Production in Human Peripheral Blood Mononuclear Cells in vitro. *Cancer Biother.* **1994,** *9* (3), 253–263.

22. Fauziya, S.; Krishnamurthy, R. Papaya (*Carica papaya*): Source Material for Anticancer. *CIB Tech J. Pharma. Sci.* **2013,** *2*, 25–34.

23. Fuentes, G.; Santamaría, J. M. Papaya (*Carica papaya* L.): Origin, Domestication, and Production. In *Genetics and Genomics of Papaya.* Ming, R., Moore, P. H., Eds.; Springer: New York, NY, 2014; pp 3–15.

24. Geetika, S.; Ruqia, M.; Harpreet, K.; Neha, D.; Shruti, K.; Singh, S. P. Genetic Engineering in Papaya. Chapter 7; In *Genetic Engineering of Horticultural Crops*; Rout, G. R., Peter, K. V., Eds.; New York: Academic Press, 2018; pp 137–154.

25. Giordani, R.; Gachon, C.; Moulin-Traffort, J.; Regli, P. Synergistic Effect of *Carica papaya* Latex Sap and Fluconazole on *Candida albicans* Growth. *Mycoses* **1997,** *40* (11–12), 429–437.

26. Giordani, R.; Siepaio, M.; Moulin-Traffort, J.; Regli, P. Antifungal Action of *Carica papaya* Latex: Isolation of Fungal Cell Wall Hydrolyzing Enzymes. *Mycoses* **1991,** *34* (11–12), 469–477.

27. Gopalakrishnan, M.; Rajasekharasetty, M. R. Effect of papaya (*Carica papaya* Linn) on Pregnancy and Estrous Cycle in Albino Rats of Wistar strain. *Ind. J. Physiol. Pharmacol.* **1978,** *22* (1), 66–70.

28. Gurung, S.; Škalko-Basnet, N. Wound Healing Properties of *Carica papaya* latex: In vivo Evaluation in Mice Burn Model. *J. Ethnopharmacol.* **2009,** *121* (2), 338–341.

29. Hadadi, S.; Li, H.; Rafie, R.; Kaseloo, P.; Witiak, S.; Siddiqui, R. Anti-oxidation Properties of Leaves, Skin, Pulp, and Seeds Extracts from Green papaya and Their Anti-cancer Activities in Breast Cancer Cells. *J. Cancer Metastasis Treat.* **2018,** *4*, 25–29.

30. Hewajulige, I.; Wijeratnam, S.; Hutchinson, M. Hexanal Compositions for Enhancing Shelf-life and Quality in Papaya Chapter 9, In *Postharvest Biology and Nanotechnology*; Paliyath, G., Subramanian, J., Lim, L.T., Subramanian, K., Handa, A.K., Mattoo, A.K., Eds.; Wiley: USA, 2018; pp 199–214.

31. Hewitt, H.; Whittle, S.; Lopez, S.; Bailey, E.; Weaver, S. Topical Use of papaya in Chronic Skin Ulcer Therapy in Jamaica. *West Ind. Med. J.* **2000,** *49* (1), 32–3.

32. Hounzangbe-Adote, M. S.; Paolini, V.; Fouraste, I.; Moutairou, K.; Hoste, H. In vitro Effects of Four Tropical Plants on Three Life-cycle Stages of the Parasitic Nematode, Haemonchus contortus. *Res. Veterin. Sci.* **2005,** *78* (2), 155–160.

33. https://www.itfnet.org/v1/2016/05/papaya-name-taxonomy-botany/; Accessed on March 02, 2020.

34. Hussain, S. Z.; Razvi, N.; Ali, S. I.; Hasan, S. M. F. Development of Quality Standard and Phytochemical Analysis of *Carica papaya* Linn leaves. *Pakistan J. Pharma. Sci.* **2018,** *31* (5), 2169–2177.

35. Ianiro, G.; Pecere, S.; Giorgio, V.; Gasbarrini, A.; Cammarota, G. Digestive Enzyme Supplementation in Gastrointestinal Diseases. *Curr. Drug Metabol.* **2016,** *17* (2), 187–193.

36. Ikpeme, E. V.; Ekaluo, U. B.; Kooffreh, M. E.; Udensi, O. Phytochemistry and Hematological Potential of Ethanol Seed Leaf and Pulp Extracts of *Carica papaya* (Linn.). *Pak. J. Biol. Sci.* **2011,** *14* (6), 408–411.

37. Ikram, E. H. K.; Stanley, R.; Netzel, M.; Fanning, K. Phytochemicals of Papaya and Its Traditional Health and Culinary Uses: Review. *J. Food Compos. Anal.* **2015,** *41,* 201–211.

38. Imaga, N.; Gbenle, G.; Okochi, V.; Akanbi, S. Antisickling Property of *Carica papaya* Leaf Extract. *Afr. J. Biochem. Res.* **2009,** *3* (4), 102–106.

39. Indran, M.; Mahmood, A. A.; Kuppusamy, U. R. Protective Effect of *Carica papaya* L Leaf Extract against Alcohol-induced Acute Gastric Damage and Blood Oxidative Stress in Rats. *West Ind. Med. J.* **2008,** *57* (4), 323–326.

40. Islam, R. Isolation, Purification and Modification of Papain Enzyme to Ascertain Industrially Valuable Nature. *Int. J. Bio-Technol. Res.* **2013,** *3,* 11–22.

41. Jagtiani, J.; Chan, H. T.; Sakai, W. S. The 4-Papaya. In *Tropical Fruit Processing*; Jagtiani, J., Chan, H. T., Sakai, W. S., Eds.; Academic Press: New York, 1988; pp 105–147.

42. Julianti, T.; Oufir, M.; Hamburger, M. Quantification of the Antiplasmodial Alkaloid Carpaine in papaya (*Carica papaya*) Leaves. *Planta Medica* **2014,** *80* (13), 1138–1142.

43. Kadiri, O.; Olawoye, B.; Samson, O.; Adalumo, O. Nutraceutical and Antioxidant Properties of the Seeds, Leaves and Fruits of *Carica papaya*: Potential Relevance to Humans Diet, the Food Industry and the Pharmaceutical Industry–A Review. *Turkish J. Agric.—Food Sci. Technol.* **2016,** *4,* 1039–1052.

44. Kaliyaperumal, K.; Kim, H. M.; Jegajeevanram, K.; Xavier, J.; Vijayalakshmi, J. Papaya: Gifted Nutraceutical Plant—Critical Review of Recent Human Health Research. *Int. J. Genuine Trad. Med.* **2014,** *4,* 1–17.

45. Kermanshai, R.; McCarry, B.; Rosenfeld, J.; Summers, P.; Weretilnyk, E.; Sorger, G. Benzyl Isothiocyanate is the Chief or Sole Anthelmintic in papaya seed Extracts. *Phytochemistry* **2001,** *57,* 427–435.

46. Kurutas, E. B. The Importance of Antioxidants Which Play the Role in Cellular Response Against Oxidative/ Nitrosative Stress: Current State. *Nutr. J.* **2016,** *15* (1), 71–77.

47. Kusemiju, O.; Noronha, C.; Okanlawon, A. The Effect of Crude Extract of the Bark of *Carica papaya* on the Seminiferous Tubules of Male Sprague-Dawley Rats. *Nigerian Postgraduate Med. J.* **2002,** *9* (4), 205–209.

48. Lobo, V.; Patil, A.; Phatak, A.; Chandra, N. Free Radicals, Antioxidants and Functional Foods: Impact on Human Health. *Pharmacognosy Rev.* **2010,** *4* (8), 118–126.

49. Logozzi, M.; Di Raimo, R.; Mizzoni, D. Beneficial Effects of Fermented Papaya Preparation (FPP®) Supplementation on Redox Balance and Aging in a Mouse Model. *Antioxidants* **2020,** *9* (2), 144–149.

50. Lohiya, N. K.; Goyal, R. B.; Jayaprakash, D.; Ansari, A. S.; Sharma, S. Antifertility Effects of Aqueous Extract of Carica papaya Seeds in Male Rats. *Planta Medica* **1994,** *60* (5), 400–404.

51. Macalood, J.; Vicente, H.; Boniao, R.; Gorospe, J.; Roa, E. Chemical Analysis of *Carica papaya* L. Crude Latex. *Am. J. Plant Sci.* **2013,** *4*, 1941–1948.

52. Malek, K.; Norazan, M.; Ramaness, P. Cysteine Proteases from *Carica papaya*: An Important Enzyme Group of Many Industrial Applications. *IOSR J. Pharm. Biol. Sci.* **2016,** *11*, 11–16.

53. Manpreet, K.; Naveen C. T.; Seema, S.; Arvind, K.; Elena, E. S. Ethnomedicinal Uses, Phytochemistry and Pharmacology of *Carica papaya* Plant: Review. *Mini-Rev. Org. Chem.* **2019,** *16* (5), 463–480.

54. Ming, R.; Yu, Q.; Moore, P. H. Sex Determination in Papaya. *Semin. Cell Devel. Biol.* **2007,** *18* (3), 401–408.

55. Mohansrinivasan, V.; Janani, S. V. Exploring the Bioactive Potential of *Carica papaya*. *Nat. Prod. J.* **2017,** *7* (4), 291–297.

56. Moy, J. H. Papayas. In *Encyclopedia of Food Sciences and Nutrition*; Caballero, B., Ed., 2nd ed.; Academic Press: Oxford, 2003; pp 4345–4351.

57. Mutalib, M.; Amira, B.; Asmah, R.; Othman, F. Antioxidant Analysis of Different Parts of Carica Papaya. *Int. Food Res. J.* **2013,** *20*, 1043–1048.

58. Nafiu, A. B.; Alli-Oluwafuyi, A. Papaya (*Carica papaya* L., Pawpaw). Chapter 3.32; In *Nonvitamin and Nonmineral Nutritional Supplements*; Nabavi, S. M., Silva, A. S., Eds.; Academic Press: New York, 2019; pp 335–359.

59. O'Hare, T. J.; Williams, D. J. Papaya as a Medicinal Plant. In *Genetics and Genomics of Papaya*; Ming, R., Moore, P. H., Eds; Springer: New York, NY, 2014; pp 391–407.

60. Odoh, U. E.; Uzor, P. F.; Eze, C. L.; Akunne, T. C. Medicinal Plants used by the People of Nsukka Local Government Area, South-eastern Nigeria for the Treatment of Malaria: An Ethnobotanical Survey. *J. Ethnopharmacol.* **2018,** *218*, 1–15.

61. Odu, E. A.; Adedeji, O.; Adebowale, K. Occurrence of Hermaphroditic Plants of *Carica papaya* L. in Southwestern Nigeria. *J. Plant Sci.* **2010,** *5*, 335–344.

62. Ojimelukwe, P.; Eji, C. Chemical Composition of Leaves, Fruit Pulp and Seeds in *Carica papaya* (L) Morphotypes. *Int. J. Med. Arom. Plants* **2012,** *2*, 200–206.

63. Okeniyi, J. A.; Ogunlesi, T. A.; Oyelami, O. A.; Adeyemi, L. A. Effectiveness of Dried *Carica papaya* Seeds Against Human Intestinal Parasitosis: A Pilot Study. *J. Med. Food* **2007,** *10* (1), 194–196.

64. Oloyede, O.; Franco, J.; Roos, D. Antioxidant Properties of Ethyl Acetate Fraction of Unripe Pulp of *Carica papaya* in Mice. *J. Microbiol., Biotechnol. Food Sci.* **2011,** *1*, 409–425.

65. Osato, J. A.; Santiago, L. A.; Remo, G. M.; Cuadra, M. S.; Mori, A. Antimicrobial and Antioxidant Activities of Unripe Papaya. *Life Sci.* **1993,** *53* (17), 1383–1389.

66. Otsuki, N.; Dang, N. H.; Kumagai, E. Aqueous Extract of *Carica papaya* Leaves Exhibits Anti-tumor Activity and Immunomodulatory Effects. *J. Ethnopharmacol.* **2010,** *127* (3), 760–767.

67. Owoyele, B. V.; Adebukola, O. M. Anti-inflammatory Activities of Ethanolic Extract of *Carica papaya* Leaves. *Inflammo Pharmacol.* **2008,** *16* (4), 168–173.

68. Panzarini, E.; Dwikat, M.; Mariano, S.; Vergallo, C.; Dini, L. Administration Dependent Antioxidant Effect of *Carica papaya* Seeds Water Extract. *Evidence-Based Comple. Altern. Med.: eCAM* **2014,** *2014,* article ID: 281508.
69. Parle, M.; Gurditta. Basketful Benefits of Papaya. *Int. Res. J. Pharm.* **2011,** *2,* 6–12.
70. Pavan, R.; Jain, S.; Shraddha; Kumar, A. Properties and Therapeutic Application of Bromelain: A Review. *Biotechnol. Res. Int.* **2012,** *2012,* article ID: 976203.
71. Pendzhiev, A. M. Proteolytic Enzymes of Papaya: Medicinal Applications. *Pharm. Chem. J.* **2002,** *36* (6), 315–317.
72. Plantvillage; https://plantvillage.psu.edu/topics/papaya-pawpaw/infos; Accessed on March 12, 2020.
73. Robert, E. P.; Odilo, D. Papaya. Chapter 11; In *Tropical Fruits., Volume 1*; 2nd ed.; CABI: Wallingford, 2011; pp 389–400.
74. Rajasekhar, P. Nutritional and Medicinal Value of *Carica papaya*. *World J. Pharm. Pharm. Sci.* **2017,** *6* (8), 2559–2578.
75. Rajkapoor, B.; Jayakar, B.; Kavimani, S.; Murugesh, N. Effect of Dried Fruits of *Carica papaya* Linn on Hepatotoxicity. *Biol. Pharm. Bull.* **2002,** *25* (12), 1645–1646.
76. Ranasinghe, P.; Ranasinghe, P.; Abeysekera, W. P. In vitro Erythrocyte Membrane Stabilization Properties of *Carica papaya* Leaf Extracts. *Pharm. Res.* **2012,** *4* (4), 196–202.
77. Richard, M., The Papaya in Hawaii. *HortScience Horts* **2012,** *47* (10), 1399–1404.
78. Saeed, F.; Arshad, M.; Pasha, I.; Naz, R. Nutritional and Phyto-Therapeutic Potential of Papaya: Overview. *Int. J. Food Prop.* **2014,** *17* (7), 1637–1653.
79. Santana, L. F.; Inada, A. C.; Espirito-Santo, B. Nutraceutical Potential of *Carica papaya* in Metabolic Syndrome. *Nutrients* **2019,** *11* (7), 1608–1613.
80. Sarala, N.; Paknikar, S. Papaya Extract to Treat Dengue: Novel Therapeutic Option? *Ann. Med. Health Sci. Res.* **2014,** *4* (3), 320–324.
81. Saran, P. L.; Choudhary, R. Drug Bioavailability and Traditional Medicaments of Commercially Available Papaya-A Review. *Afr. J. Agric. Res.* **2013,** 8, 3216–3223.
82. Saran, P. L.; Choudhary, R.; Solanki, I.; Devi, G. Traditional Medicaments Through Papaya in Northeastern Plains Zone of India. *Ind. J. Trad. Knowledge* **2015,** *14,* 537–543.
83. Sarma, H. N.; Mahanta, H. C. Modulation of Morphological Changes of Endometrial Surface Epithelium by the Administration of Composite Root Extract in Albino Rat. *Contraception* **2000,** *62* (1), 51–54.
84. Satrija, F.; Nansen, P.; Bjorn, H. Effect of Papaya Latex against Ascarissuum in Naturally Infected Pigs. *J. Helminthol.* **1994,** *68* (4), 343–346.
85. Satrija, F.; Nansen, P.; Murtini, S.; He, S. Anthelmintic Activity of Papaya Latex Infections in Mice. *J. Ethnopharmacol.* **1995,** *48* (3), 161–164.
86. Senthilvel, P.; Pandian, L.; Kumar, K. Flavonoid from *Carica papaya* Inhibits NS2B-NS3 Protease and Prevents Dengue-2 viral assembly. *Bioinformation* **2013,** *9,* 889–895.
87. Shaziya, B.; Goyal, P. K. Anthelmintic Effect of Natural Plant (*Carica papaya*) Extract against the Gastrointestinal Nematode, Ancylostoma caninum in Mice. *Int. Res. J. Biol. Sci.* **2012,** *1* (1), 2–6.
88. Starley, I. F.; Mohammed, P.; Schneider, G.; Bickler, S. W. The Treatment of Pediatric Burns using Topical Papaya. *Burns: J. Int. Soc. Burn Inj.* **1999,** *25* (7), 636–639.

89. Stepek, G.; Buttle, D. J.; Duce, I. R.; Lowe, A. Assessment of the Anthelmintic Effect of Natural Plant Cysteine Proteinases Against the Gastrointestinal Nematode, Heligmosomoid espolygyrus, in vitro. *Parasitology* **2005,** *130* (2), 203–211.
90. Stokes, T. Papaya Male Contraceptive. *Trends Plant Sci.* **2001,** *6* (4), 143–148.
91. Subenthiran, S.; Choon, T. C.; Cheong, K. C. *Carica papaya* Leaves Juice Significantly Accelerates the Rate of Increase in Platelet Count among Patients with Dengue Fever and Dengue Hemorrhagic Fever. *Evidence-Based Complem. Altern. Med.: Ecam* **2013,** article ID: 616737.
92. Sultana, A.; Afroz, R.; Yasmeen, O.; Aktar, M.; Yusuf, M. Anti-Inflammatory Effect of Ethanolic Extract of *Carica papaya* Leaves and Indomethacin in Cotton Pellet Induced Granuloma in Animal Model. *J. Curr. Adv. Med. Res.* **2019,** *6*, 2–5.
93. Sultana, A.; Khan, A.; Afroz, R.; Yasmeen, O.; Aktar, M.; Yusuf, M. A. Comparison of Anti-Inflammatory Effect of Ethanolic Extract of *Carica papaya* Leaves and Indo-methacin in Carrageenan Induced Rat Paw Edema Animal Model. *J. Sci. Foundation* **2019,** *16*, 49–53.
94. Teng, W. C.; Chan, W.; Suwanarusk, R. In vitro Antimalarial Evaluations and Cyto-toxicity Investigations of *Carica papaya* Leaves and Carpaine. *Nat. Product Commun.* **2019,** *14* (1), 33–36.
95. Udoh, P.; Essien, I.; Udoh, F., Effects of *Carica papaya* Seeds Extract on the Morphology of Pituitary-gonadal Axis of Male Wistar Rats. *Phytotherapy Res.* **2005,** *19* (12), 1065–1068.
96. Verma, S.; Varma, R.; Singh, S., Medicinal and Pharmacological Parts of *Carica papaya*: A Review. *Ind. J. Drugs* **2017,** *5*, 88–93.
97. Vij, T.; Prashar, Y. Review on Medicinal Properties of *Carica papaya* Linn. *Asian Pacific J. Trop. Dis.* **2015,** *5* (1), 1–6.
98. Wikipedia – Papaya; https://en.wikipedia.org/wiki/List_of_countries_by_papaya_production; Accessed on March 16, 2020.
99. Zeleke, G.; Kebebe, D.; Mulisa, E.; Gashe, F. In Vivo Antimalarial Activity of the Solvent Fractions of Fruit Rind and Root of *Carica papaya* Linn against *Plasmodium berghei* in Mice. *J. Parasitol. Res.* **2017,** *2017*, 1–9.

CHAPTER 2

Therapeutic Activities of Nutmeg (*Myristica fragrans*)

BHUSHAN PRAKASH PIMPLE, AMRITA MILIND KULKARNI, and RUCHITA BALU BHOR

ABSTRACT

Main phytochemicals in nutmeg (*Myristica fragrans* Houtt) are: myristicin, trimyristin, myristic acid, alpha-pinene, beta-pinene, etc. In the traditional system of medicine, nutmeg is preferably used to treat insomnia, depression, intestinal worms, and oligospermia. etc. Nutmeg extract has been scientifically proven to exhibit antimicrobial activity in GI flora thereby suppressing the levels of tumorigenic uremic toxins. Furthermore, methanol extract of nutmeg is effective in *H. pylori*-induced gastritis and DSS-induced colitis. This chapter focuses on the traditional claims and therapeutic benefits related to GI disorder of *Myristica fragrans*.

2.1 INTRODUCTION

Myristica fragrans Houtt (nutmeg) is widely distributed in western India (i.e., Kerala and Konkan) and is also cultivated in Srilanka and Indonesia.[16] The plant reaches up to 15 m of height. The seeds have hard testa lined with thin papery mace.[15] Kernel and mace of the seed are rich in essential oils (Fig. 2.1). Both the mace and kernel are normally used in culinary preparation owing to their aromatic principles. Table 2.1 presents traditional claims of nutmeg in different countries. Phytoconstituents in *M. fragrans* are listed in Table 2.2.

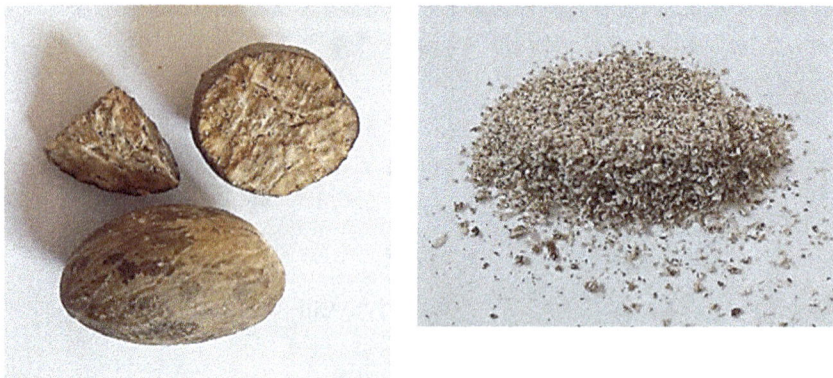

FIGURE 2.1   Seeds of *Myristica fragrans*: Left (seed); right (seed powder).

TABLE 2.1   Traditional Claims for Nutmeg in Various Countries.

Traditional medicine system	Used as a remedy for	Ref.
Iranian medicine	Gastric and liver tonic; peptic ulcer	[12]
Indonesian medicine	Stomach and kidney disorders	[30]
Malayan medicine	Overeating, distended stomach, appetite stimulant, malaria, madness	
Javanese medicine	Calming	

TABLE 2.2   Phytoconstituents in *Myristica fragrans*.

Class of phytoconstituents	Phytoconstituents	Ref.
Terpenes	Sabinene, Pinene, Myrcene Phellandrene, Camphene Limonene, Pcymene, Terpinene	[17]
Fixed oil	Glycerides, Lauric acid Linoleic acid, Myristic acid Palmitic acid, Stearic acid Trimyristin	[11]
Lignans	Erythro-austrobailignan-6 Meso-dihydroguaiaretic acid Nectandrin-B Licarin-A and Licarin-B Myristagenol	[4]
Others	Calcium, Iron, Niacin Phosphorous, Riboflavin, Thiamine	[18]

This chapter has highlighted the traditional claims: phytochemistry, therapeutic benefits (related to GI disorder), drug interactions, toxicities, and traditional marketed formulation aspects of *M. fragrans.*

2.2 DRUG INTERACTIONS OF *MYRISTICA FRAGRANS*

2.2.1 Synergistic Hepatoprotective Effect of Myristica Fragrans, Astragalus Membranaceus and Poriacocos (Map) on Acetaminophen and Carbon Tetrachloride-Induced Hepatotoxicity

Extracts of *M. fragrans*, *Astragalus membranaceus*, and *Poriacocos (MAP)* collectively were able to correct hepatic damage in female mice. Remarkable reduction in serum aspartate amino transferase (AST), serum alkaline phosphatase, serum alanine amino transferase (ALT), total bilirubin, bile acid levels, and hepatocyte necrosis as an effect of induction of antioxidant enzymes, free radical scavenging mechanisms, suppression of TNF-α (tumor necrosis factor: inflammatory marker) produced hepatoprotective effects.[34]

2.2.2 Gastrointestinal Effects of Mebarid: Combined Effect of Holarrhena Antidysenterica, Berberisaristate, Aeglemarmelos, Punicagranatum, Myristica Fragrans, Salmaliamalabarica and Panchamrutparpati

Gastrointestinal effects of Mebarid on diarrhea, ulcer, ileal motility were studied in Wistar rats. Mebarid and loperamide delayed the onset of first defecation and decreased the cumulative fecal weight in castor oil-induced diarrhea dose-dependently. Mebarid inhibited intestinal motility. Mebarid and ranitidine decreased the severity of ulcer.[5]

2.3 TOXICITY STUDIES OF *MYRISTICA FRAGRANS*

The first evidence of nutmeg poisoning dates back to 1576, when a pregnant English woman experienced inebriety after ingestion of 10–12 nutmegs. The Poison Information Centre, Erfurt reported the clinical symptoms due to nutmeg overdose.[29]

Carstairs et al.[8] studied the clinical symptoms due to intentional and unintentional nutmeg exposure. Tachycardia, vomiting, nausea, abdominal pain, dizziness, hallucinations, and agitations were observed. Agitations and tachycardia were significantly experienced by patients with intentional nutmeg exposure than the patients with unintentional nutmeg exposure. The fatality was not observed. However, till date, there are two cases involving nutmeg exposure that led to the death of an 8-year-old boy and a 55-year-old woman due to intervention of other treatment or drugs; but the reason for deaths is unclear.[8]

Adverse effects after nutmeg overdose[7] are listed below:

GIT effects:	CVS effects:	CNS effects:
• Nausea, vomiting	• Hytpotension	• Seizure
• Xerostomia	• Tachycardia	• Incoherent speech
• Burning epigastric pain	• Flushing	• Confusion
• Excessive thrist		• Anxiety
		• Dizziness
		• Hyperactivity
		• Euphoria
Gynecological/ urological effects:	Psychiatric effects:	Peripheral effects:
• Abortifacient	• Depression	• Hypothermia
• Urinary urgency	• Suicidal	• Numbness
	• tendency	• Swelling
		• Miosis

Mbadugha and his colleagues[23] studied the gastric histological changes in rats after the administration of ground nutmeg powder. The 10 g, 15 g, and 20 g ground nutmeg degenerated simple columnar epithelium, longitudinal folds, coil pyloric glands and caused hypertrophy of the surface mucous cells and mucous neck cells in the stomach. They concluded that 10 g or more of nutmeg powder had adverse effects on the stomach upset.[23]

2.4   NANOENCAPSULATION OF MACE ESSENTIAL OIL

Nanoencapsulated mace essential oil (Ne-MEO) was assessed for the antifungal and antioxidant activities, ergosterol content, C-source utilization, and the membrane integrity due to aflatoxin B1 by *Aspergillus flavus* against the mace essential oil (MEO) (Table 2.3). Ne-MEO inhibited evanescence of volatile oil and thereby there was fungal growth and aflatoxin B1 production at a lower concentration than the MEO. Increased concentrations of Ne-MEO decreased the ergosterol content in the plasma membrane of the fungal cell and it also led to the leakage of cellular ions essential for the fungal growth.[31]

TABLE 2.3   Various Effects of Mace Essential Oil (MEO).

Parameter	Ne-MEO	MEO
Aflatoxin B1 production and fungal growth	Inhibition at lower concentration	Inhibition at higher concentration than Ne-MEO
Antioxidant activity	Strong free radical scavenging property	Strong free radical scavenging property
C-source utilization in *Aspergillus flavus*	Impaired	–
Ergosterol content	Decreased ergosterol content on increasing concentration of Ne-MEO	–
Leakage of ions	Ca^{2+}, Mg^{2+}, K^+ leakage observed	–

2.5 PHARMACOLOGY OF *MYRISTICA FRAGRANS*

2.5.1 Antibacterial Activity

Ethyl acetate extract of the flesh and ethanol extract of the mace and seeds of *M. fragrans* exhibited marked antibacterial effect on Gram-positive cariogenic (*Streptococcus mutans, Streptococcus mitis,* and *Streptococcus salivarius*) and Gram-negative periodontopathic bacteria (*Aggregatibacteractino mycetemcomitans, Porphyromonas gingivalis*) due to investigated antibacterial effects of trimyristin and myristicin.[27]

Methanol extract of *M. fragrans* showed in vitro antibacterial effect against *Helicobacter pylori* and thereby depicted its use in chronic gastritis, gastric carcinoma, peptic ulcer disease, and primary gastric B-cell lymphoma.[22]

Antibacterial action on foodborne pathogens (*Staphylococcus aureus, S. epidermidis, Klebsiellapneumoniae, Bacillus cereus, Pseudomonas aeruginosa Escherichia coli,* and *Salmonella typhi*) was produced by the volatile oil fraction and ethanol fraction of *M. fragrans*. The essential oil components permeate the cell membrane of the microbe and can affect the cellular functions and promote the death of the microbe.[25]

Chung et al.[10] studied the anticariogenic effect of mace lignans from the methanol extract of *M. fragrans* against *S. mutans* (oral pathogen) and *Lactobacillus* spp.

2.5.2   Hepatoprotective Effect

In vivo suppression of TNF-α (tumor necrosis factor, inflammatory marker) and DNA fragmentation induced by lipopolysaccharide (LPS) plus D-galactosamine (D-GalN) by myristicin proved its hepatoprotective effect. Inhibition of TNF-α may be due to suppressed release from macrophages by myristicin.[24]

Peroxisome proliferator-activated receptor alpha (PPARα) mediated hepatoprotective activity in thioacetamide (TAA)-induced acute liver injury mice model. Regulation of liver health biomarkers and suppression of proinflammatory cytokines was observed.[33]

2.5.3   Activation of Transient Receptor Potential Melastatin 8 (TRPM 8) Ion Channel

Agonists of TRPM 8 ion channel produced the cooling sensation (<28°C). Neolignan isolated from *M. fragrans* seeds produced the cooling effect by the activation of TRPM 8 ion channel. The additive cooling effect was observed with l-(-) menthol and neolignan from the seeds of nutmeg. Activation of TRPM 8 ion channel was able to ameliorate pain, inflammation due to the cooling effect.[28]

2.5.4   Inhibition of CYP3A4, CYP2C9 and CYP1A2 (Drug Metabolizing Enzymes) by Nutmeg and Mace

Phytoconstituents extracted from mace inhibited 6-β-hydroxylation of testosterone by CYP3A4 and 4'-hydroxylation of diclofenac by CYP2C9.[20] Yang et al.[33] studied the mechanism-based inhibition (MBI) of CYP1A2 (metabolizing enzyme) by myristicin and its reactive metabolites.[32]

2.5.5   Induction of CYP3A4 via Pregnane-X-receptor (PXR)

Bartonkova et al. found that the essential oil in nutmeg induced CYP3A4 in human intestinal cancer cells, human hepatocytes, and human progenitor cells by the activation of PXR. Along with controlling drug metabolism, PXR was involved in the pathogenesis of cancer, inflammatory bowel disease, regulation of lipid, and carbohydrate metabolism. Moreover, blockage of PXR did not induce the expression of CYP3A4.[6]

2.5.6   PARP-1 and NF-κB Inhibitory Effects

Inhibition of Poly(adenosine 5'-diphosphate (ADP)-ribose) polymerase 1(PARP-1) and transcription factor nuclear factor kappa-light chain-enhancer of activated B cells (NF-kB) by neolignans and acyclic bisphenyl-propanoid in nutmeg produced in vitro antiproliferative effects. Inhibition of Poly(adenosine 5'-diphosphate (ADP)-ribose) polymerase 1(PARP-1) protected DNA damage and sensitized cancer cells to cytotoxic agents. Apoptosis of cancer cells and modulation in the inflammatory pathway was resulted from NF-κB inhibition.[1]

2.5.7   Antidiarrheal Activity

Extract of *M. fragrans* inhibited the propagation of simian (SA-11) and human (HCR3) rotaviruses (causative agents of diarrhea) in African Rhesus monkey kidney cells (MA-104). Antiviral assay suggested the toxicity against the rotaviruses due to the presence of flavonoids in the extract prevented viral invasion of the cells.[13] Ether extract and hexane fraction of alcohol extract of flowers and seeds of *M. fragrans* had the antidiarrheal effect in the ileum of rabbit and guinea pig against the enterotoxins of *E. coli*. Both the extracts inhibited fluid accumulation and secretory response. According to Gupta et al.,[14] nonpolar compounds present in the extracts may be responsible for the antidiarrheal effect.

2.5.8   Inhibition of Hepatic Lipogenesis

Nectandrin-B (a lignan from *M. fragrans*) inhibited hepatic lipogenesis stimulated by liver X receptor-α (LXR-α) and sterol regulatory element-binding protein (SREBP)-1c in HepG2 cells. Inhibition was a direct consequence of LXR-α, (SREBP)-1c, and m-RNA expression of LXR-α genes. Nectandrin-B also activated AMP-activated protein kinase (AMPK), which inhibits LXR-α and (SREBP)-1c activities. Nectandrin-B inhibited the lipid accumulation in the liver; hence has an application in nonalcoholic fatty liver disease.[9]

2.5.9   Modulation of Colon Cancer

Toxic uremic derivatives produced by the gut flora in mice bearing adenomatous polyposis coli (APC: gene mutation-induced colon cancer) led to intestinal tumorigenesis, inflammatory responses (increased Interleukin-6). Modulation of colon cancer was due to the improved lipid metabolism, antimicrobial (inhibition of gut flora producing toxic uremic products), anti-inflammatory (decreased IL-6, proinflammatory cytokine), and antioxidant activities of nutmeg.[21]

2.5.10   Protection against Colitis

M. fragrans extract (MFE) exhibited dose-dependent protective effects against dextran sulfate sodium (DSS)-induced colitis in a mouse model by reducing the mucosal inflammatory cytokines (IFN-c, TNF-a, IL-1b, and IL-6) in the colon mucosa, severity of inflammation, epithelial damage, ulceration, and colon shortening.[19]

2.5.11   Anti-Inflammatory Effect of Nutmeg

Myristicin exerts anti-inflammatory action against the edema induced by carrageenan and increased vascular permeability induced by acetic acid in mice. Inhibition of edema and vascular permeability proved the anti-inflammatory effect of myristicin.[2,3,26] Traditional marketed formulations of nutmeg are indicated below:

- Babbularishta: Ayurvedic
- Dashamularishta: Ayurvedic
- Khadirarishta: Ayurvedic
- Kumaryasava: Ayurvedic
- Madhusnuhirasayana: Ayurvedic
- Jatiphaladichurna: Ayurvedic
- Jawarish Pudina Wilayti: Unani
- Jawarish-E-Bisbasa: Unani

2.6 SUMMARY

Varous parts of *M. fragrans* Houtt (such as: mace, mace oil, kernel, and kernel oil) are reported to have significant medicinal value to provide traditional treatments of: insomnia, depression, helminth, and oligospermia, etc. Anticancer benefits of nutmeg extract is attributed to the antimicrobial activity in GI flora. Methanol extract of nutmeg is effective in *H. pylori*-induced gastritis and DSS-induced colitis.

KEYWORDS

- **colitis**
- **gastritis**
- **hepatoprotective**
- **myrcene**
- **myristagenol**
- **myristic acid**
- ***Myristica fragrans***
- **trimyristin**
- **TRPM ion channel**

REFERENCES

1. Acuña, U. M.; Carcache, P. J. B.; Matthew, S.; de Blanco, E. J. C. New Acyclic Bisphenylpropanoid and Neolignans, From *Myristica fragrans* Houtt., Exhibiting PARP-1 and NF-κB Inhibitory Effects. *Food Chem.* **2016,** *202,* 269–275.
2. Anonymous. *The Ayurvedic Pharmacopoeia of India (formulations): Volume 2.* 1st ed.; Government of India, Ministry of Health and Family Welfare, Department of Ayurveda, Yoga & Naturopathy, Unani: Siddha and Homoeopathy: New Delhi, 2016; pp 23, 32, 48, 52, 107, 120.
3. Anonymous. *The Unani Pharmacopoeia of India, Volume III (Formulations)*; 1st edition; Government of India—Ministry of AYUSH; Pharmacopoeia Commission For Indian Medicine & Homoeopathy, Ghaziabad: New Delhi: 2016; pp 57, 61.
4. Asgarpanah, J.; Kazemivash, N. Phytochemistry and Pharmacologic Properties of *Myristica Fragrans* Hoyutt—A Review. *Afr. J. Biotechnol.* **2012,** *11* (65), 12787–12793.
5. Bafna, P.; Bodhankar, S. Gastrointestinal Effects of Mebarid®, an Ayurvedic Formulation, in Experimental Animals. *J. Ethnopharmacol.* **2003,** *86* (2–3), 173–176.
6. Bartonkova, I.; Dvorak, Z. Essential Oils of Culinary Herbs and Spices Activate PXR and Induce CYP3A4 in Human Intestinal and Hepatic In Vitro Models. *Toxicol. Lett.* **2018,** *296,* 1–9.
7. Beckerman, B.; Persaud, H. Nutmeg Overdose: Spice Not So Nice. *Complem. Therap. Med.* **2019,** *46,* 44–46.
8. Carstairs, S. D.; Cantrell, F. L. The Spice of Life: An Analysis Of Nutmeg Exposures in California. *Clin. Toxicol.* **2011,** *49* (3), 177–180.
9. Choi, D. G.; Kim, E. K.; Yang, J. W.; Song, J. S.; Kim, Y. M. Nectandrin B: Lignan Isolated From Nutmeg, Inhibits Liver X Receptor-a-Induced Hepatic Lipogenesis Through AMP-Activated Protein Kinase Activation. *Die Pharmazie-An Int. J. Pharm. Sci.* **2015,** *70* (11), 733–739.
10. Chung, J. Y.; Choo, J. H.; Lee, M. H.; Hwang, J. K. Anticariogenic Activity of Macelignan Isolated from *Myristica fragrans* (nutmeg) Against Streptococcus Mutans. *Phytomedicine* **2006,** *13* (4), 261–266.
11. Duarte, R. C.; Fanaro, G. B.; Koike, A. C.; Villavicencio, A. L. C. Irradiation Effect on Antifungal Potential *Myristica fragrans* (nutmeg) Essential Oil. *2011 Int. Nucl. Atlantic Conf.*; Belo Horizonte – Brazil: Brazil Association of Nuclear Energy (ABEN); 24–28 October of **2011**; Online; p 108.
12. Farzaei, M. H.; Shams-Ardekani. M. R; Abbasabadi. Z.; Rahimi, R. Scientific Evaluation of Edible Fruits and Spices Used for the Treatment of Peptic Ulcer in Traditional Iranian Medicine. *ISRN Gastroenterol.* **2013,** *2013,* 1–12.
13. Gonçalves, J. L. S.; Lopes, R. C. In Vitro Anti-rotavirus Activity of Some Medicinal Plants used in Brazil against Diarrhea. *J. Ethnopharmacol.* **2005,** *99* (3), 403–407.
14. Gupta, S.; Yadava, J. N. S.; Mehrotra, R.; Tandon, J. S. Anti-diarrhoeal Profile of an Extract and Some Fractions from *Myristica fragrans* (Nut-meg) on Escherichia coli Enterotoxin-induced Secretory Response. *Int. J. Pharmacognosy* **1992,** *30* (3), 179–183.
15. https://www.flowersofindia.net/catalog/slides/Nutmeg.html; accessed on 6th January, 2020.

16. https://www.indianspices.com/sites/default/files/Major%20Item%20wise%20 Export%202019.pdf; accessed on 6th January, 2020.

17. Jaiswal, P.; Kumar, P.; Singh, V. K.; Singh, D. K. Biological Effects of *Myristica fragrans*. *Ann. Rev. Biomed. Sci.* **2009**, *11*, 21–29.

18. Jose, H.; Arya, K. R.; Sindhu, T. J.; Syamjith, P.; Vinod, K. R.; Sandhya, S. A Descriptive Review on *Myristica fragrans* Houtt. *Hygeua: Journal For Drugs and Medicines*, **2016**, *8 (1)*, 35-43.

19. Kim, H.; Bu, Y.; Lee, B. J.; Bae, J. *Myristica fragrans* Seed Extract Protects against Dextran Sulfate Sodium–Induced Colitis in Mice. *J. Med. Food*, **2013**, *16* (10), 953–956.

20. Kimura, Y.; Ito, H.; Hatano, T. Effects of Mace and Nutmeg on Human Cytochrome P450 3A4 and 2C9 activity. *Biol. Pharm. Bull.*, **2010**, *33* (12), 1977–1982.

21. Li, F.; Yang, X. W.; Krausz, K. W. Modulation of Colon Cancer by Nutmeg. *J. Proteome Res.* **2015**, *14* (4), 1937–1946.

22. Mahady, G. B.; Pendland, S. L. In Vitro Susceptibility of *Helicobacter pylori* to Botanical Extracts Used Traditionally for the Treatment of Gastrointestinal Disorders. *Phytotherap. Res.* **2005**, *19* (11), 988–991.

23. Mbadugha, C. C.; Edem, G. D.; Emmanuel, U.; Udoudo, I. E. Haematologic and Gastric Histological Changes Associated with Administration of Ground Nutmeg Seed on Adult Male Albino Wistar Rats. *J. Adv. Med. Pharm. Sci.* **2018**, *2018*, 1–10.

24. Morita, T.; Jinno, K.; Kawagishi, H. Hepatoprotective Effect of Myristicin from Nutmeg (*Myristica fragrans*) on Lipopolysaccharide/d-galactosamine-Induced Liver Injury. *J. Agric. Food Chem.* **2003**, *51* (6), 1560–1565.

25. Omoruyi, I. M.; Emefo, O. T. In Vitro Evaluation of the Antibiogramic Activities of the Seeds of *Myristica fragrans* on Food borne Pathogens. *Malaysian J. Microbiol.* **2012**, *8* (4), 253–258.

26. Ozaki, Y.; Soedigdo, S.; Wattimena, Y. R.; Suganda, A. G. Antiinflammatory Effect of Mace, Aril of *Myristica fragrans* Houtt., and Its Active Principles. *Japanese J. Pharmacol.* **1989**, *49* (2), 155–163.

27. Shafiei, Z.; Shuhairi, N. N. Antibacterial Activity of Nutmeg Against Oral Pathogens. *Evidence-Based Complem. Altern. Med.* **2012**, *2012*, 1–7.

28. Shirai, T.; Kumihashi, K.; Sakasai, M.; Kusuoku, H.; Shibuya, Y.; Ohuchi, A. Identification of A Novel TRPM8 Agonist From Nutmeg: A Promising Cooling Compound. *ACS Med. Chem. Lett.* **2017**, *8* (7), 715–719.

29. Stein, U.; Greyer, H.; Hentschel, H. Nutmeg (myristicin) Poisoning—Report on a Fatal Case and A Series of Cases Recorded by A Poison Information Centre. *Foren. Sci. Int.* **2001**, *118* (1), 87–90.

30. Van Gils, C.; Cox, P. A. Ethnobotany of Nutmeg in the Spice Islands. *J. Ethnopharmacol.* **1994**, *42* (2), 117–124.

31. Yadav, A.; Kujur, A.; Kumar, A.; Singh, P. P.; Prakash, B.; Dubey, N. K. Assessing the Preservative Efficacy of Nano Encapsulated Mace Essential Oil Against Food Borne Molds, Aflatoxin B1 Contamination, and Free Radical Generation. *LWT* **2019**, *108*, 429–436.

32. Yang, A. H.; He, X.; Chen, J. X. Identification and Characterization of Reactive Metabolites in Myristicin-mediated Mechanism-based Inhibition of CYP1A2. *Chem. Biol. Inter.*, **2015**, *237*, 133–140.

33. Yang, X. N.; Liu, X. M.; Fang, J. H.; Zhu, X.; Yang, X. W.; Xiao, X. R.; Li, F. The PPARα Mediates the Hepatoprotective Effects of Nutmeg. *J. Proteome Res.* **2018,** *17* (5), 1887–1897.

34. Yimam, M.; Jiao, P.; Hong, M.; Jia, Q. Hepatoprotective Activity of an Herbal Composition, MAP, a Standardized Blend Comprising *Myristica fragrans*, *Astragalus membranaceus*, and Poriacocos. *J. Med. Food* **2016,** *19* (10), 952–960.

Plant-Based Phytochemicals in the Prevention of Colorectal Cancer

YANA PUCKETT and KYLE DRINNON

ABSTRACT

Research has shown that natural secondary metabolites have some anticancer properties and can play a role in the prevention and treatment of colon cancer. These metabolites are found in various berries and vegetables and work via different mechanisms, such as by suppressing inflammation, suppressing angiogenesis and proliferation, and suppressing oxidative stress. The effectiveness and/or harm of these plant-based metabolites on the prevention and treatment of colon cancer are controversial and largely unproven. This chapter presents a review on how plant-based metabolites work and their efficacy in the prevention of colon cancer.

3.1 INTRODUCTION

Colorectal cancer affects the population worldwide. Approximately 52,000 patients die annually due to colorectal cancer in the United States. It is a major leading cause of deaths among men and women, ranking third most common in women and second in men (Fig. 3.1).

Colorectal cancer is screened for in the United States via an annual fecal occult blood test, fecal immunochemical test (FIT), and FIT-DNA (multitarget stool DNA test); with colonoscopy starting at the age of 45 and repeated every 5 years if no positive findings occur; or with flexible sigmoidoscopy every 5 years. If colorectal cancer is found through symptoms, typically the tumor is in a more advanced stage. The staging of colorectal cancer provides the physician with a framework for a treatment plan.

Currently, the typical treatment plan consists of surgical resection, neoadjuvant chemotherapy or radiation, or adjuvant chemotherapy and radiation depending on the stage of a tumor. Metastatic disease, which is present in approximately 20% of newly diagnosed colorectal cancer, is also treated typically with resection of metastases and systemic chemotherapy. The overall 5-year survival based on SEER (seasonal energy efficiency rating) data is about 80%; however, survival depends largely on the stage of cancer at presentation.[9,15] Multiple data are available to clinicians regarding the prevention and treatment of colorectal cancer with plant-based phytochemicals.

The research data from many articles show that the plant-based metabolites have a positive effect on colon cancer by suppressing inflammation, suppressing angiogenesis and proliferation, and suppressing oxidative stress, among other things. In addition, plant-based metabolites may have a potentiating effect on chemotherapeutic drugs, such as, in the case of gallic acid and cisplatin in lung cancer. The effects of polyethylene-coated, iron magnetite nanoparticles loaded with gallic acid showed better results than free gallic acid, which allowed for a decreased number of viable colon cancer cells. *Rosa canina* was found to exhibit selective cytotoxic effects by neutralizing free radicals allowing healthy cells to not be affected while causing apoptosis in cancerous cells.

Berries have anticancer activities due to the presence of metabolites, such as, flavonoids, anthocyanins, phenolic acids, and stilbenes, which can neutralize free radicals and fight the proliferation of cancer cells. By preventing crucial features of cancer, berries have been shown to reduce metastatic activity. Lastly, salicylic acid (a phenolic compound found in plants), has been shown in a large epidemiologic study to prevent colorectal cancer when taken as a low dose aspirin starting at the age of 50. What is limited is the unknown side effects of such compounds in cancer patients taking them, especially in conjunction with chemotherapeutic drugs.

This chapter explores the potential benefits of plant-based metabolites, such as, *R. canina*, gallic acid, berries, and salicylic acid in the prevention and adjunct treatment of colorectal cancer.

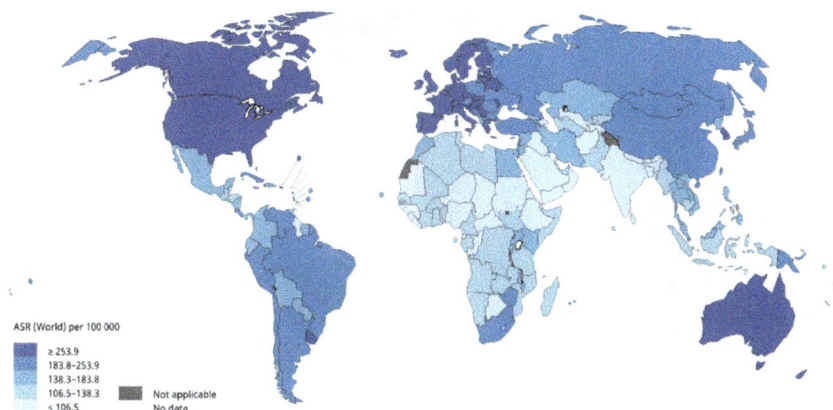

FIGURE 3.1   Cancer rates in each country for all ages and both genders for 2018 according to World Health Organization.

3.2   ROSA CANINA

The plant, *R. canina* (Fig. 3.2, known commonly as Rosehip or Dog-Rose), is shown to have cytotoxic characteristics and has been used in specific treatments in medicine. This plant was experimentally tested against colon cancer and non-cancerous colon cells to see its cytotoxic activity. The results showed that there was a reduction of cell viability and an increase in the number of cells in early apoptosis when compared to the untreated cell lines while showing some selective cytotoxic activity.[36] The active compounds in *R. canina* with antioxidative properties are Vitamin C and flavonoids and with cytotoxic characteristic is polyphenols.[16,35,36] The results of this experiment showed that *R. canina* can arrest the colon cancer cells in the S-phase of cell division and also showed that *R. canina* increased the death rate of cancer cell via mitochondrial-dependent apoptosis. It can affect telomerase in cancer cells to reduce its expression, which can lead to an increase in cell death and antiproliferation.[16,35,36]

The flower of *R. canina* is not edible in its natural state; but the rosehips are often dried and have a high dose of antioxidants and Vitamin C and are prepared as a traditional herbal tea. Rosehips can also be prepared in many ways, such as, jams or other food items. The phenolic content of this fruit is responsible for fighting free radicals responsible for human diseases, such as cancer, aging, and atherosclerosis.[16,35,36]

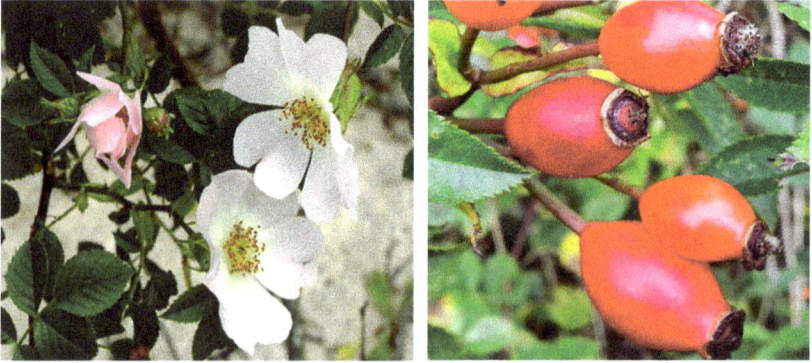

FIGURE 3.2   Rosehip of the *Rosa canina* (also known as Dog-Rose): flowers can appear in white or pink.

3.3   GALLIC ACID

Gallic acid is commonly found in white tea, gallnuts, sumac, tealeaves, oak bark, and witch hazel as well as other foods and plants. It is known to have antioxidant, anti-inflammatory, and anticancer properties, and protective properties for healthy cells. In a research study, the polyethylene-coated, iron magnetite nanoparticles loaded with gallic acid were designed with a specific anticancer nanocomposite formulation to determine the effects on lung and colon cancers. The results did show a decrease in colon cancer HT-29 viability with increasing dose of this combination.[11]

Gallic acid has been observed to induce apoptosis in SMMC-7721 human hepatocellular carcinoma selectively.[5,6,11] Through the PTEN/AKT/HIF-1a/VEGF signaling pathway, gallic acid has been observed in studies to reduce angiogenesis in ovarian cancer cells.[13,14,19] By upregulating miR-518b in SW1353 human chondrosarcoma cells, gallic acid inhibited cell migration and induced apoptosis. It has also been shown to enhance cisplatin's anticancer effects via the ROS-dependent mitochondrial apoptotic pathway in human H446 cell line of lung cancer.[5,6,11,13,14,17,20,21,23,24,28,29]

3.4   EDIBLE BERRIES

Selected studies have shown that fruits and berries (Fig.s 3.3 and 3.4) can be beneficial in the prevention and treatment of some cancers, due to their antioxidant properties and the presence of phytochemicals.[10,18,31,33] The pathways used for this action can be the ERK/MAPK, PI3K/AKT/ PKB/mTOR, Wnt/β-catenin, and NF-κB pathways. The studies[10,18,32] have indicated molecular activities of berries with benefits in patients with colon cancer. The metabolites differed for each type of berries which had different effects on colon cancer. The effects varied from inhibiting invasion, inhibiting proliferation, reducing inflammation, suppressing Wnt pathway, inducing apoptosis, cell-cycle arrest, to preventing oxidative damage, and so on. Other research on human studies for chemopreventive effects has focused on black raspberries and bilberries.

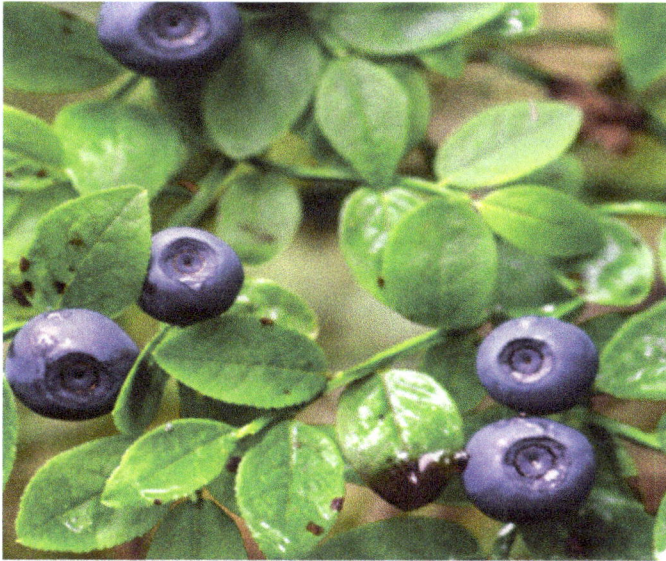

FIGURE 3.3   Blueberries growing on bush.

3.5   SALICYLIC ACID

The use of aspirin on a regular basis has been shown to decrease the incidence and mortality of colon cancer. No clear explanation is available on the mechanism of chemopreventive effects. Some possible mechanisms include the downregulation of c-Myc protein levels in the human colon. Northern blot analysis showed that the drug caused decreased levels of c-Myc mRNA. Salicylic acid, a plant-based phenolic compound found in aspirin, has been shown to potentially prevent colon cancer in persons on this therapy. A study looked at the mechanism of colon cancer prevention in a rat model. It was found that salicylic acid might prevent cancerous colon cells from proliferating by decreasing inflammation and oxidative stress. Cytoskeletal regulation, energy metabolism, redox, transport, and protein folding were assisted with actions of salicylic proteins.[3,4,8,34]

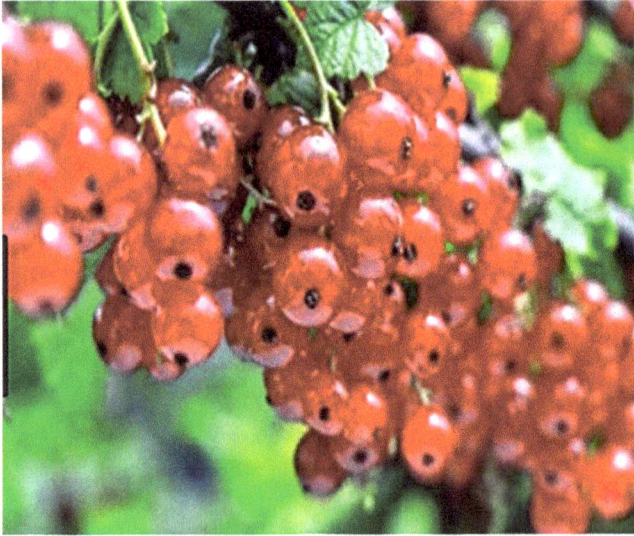

FIGURE 3.4   Edible wild berries: Partridge berries.

Inhibition of COX-1 is a known and verified mechanism of salicylic acid (Fig. 3.5). COX-1 inhibition in platelets may cause a decrease in COX-2 in nearby cells, specifically, the intestinal mucosa, which will lead to neoplasia inhibition in intestinal polyps. In addition, activation of platelets at the site of mucosal injury in the intestines may decrease inflammation by reducing apoptosis and enhancing angiogenesis.[2,7,12,22,25]

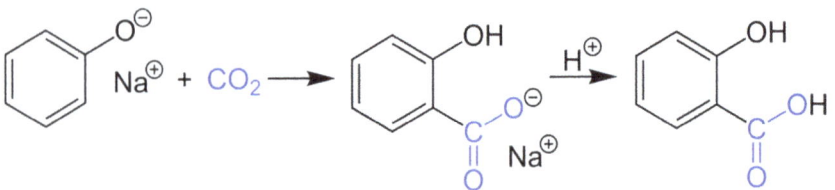

FIGURE 3.5   The acidification of sodium salicylate can result in salicylic acid.

Salicylic acid is found naturally in high amounts in fruits, such as apricots, apples, cranberries, currants, dates and figs, grapes, and pineapples. Dried fruits are good source of salicylic acid.

3.6 SUMMARY

Different phytochemicals from different sources (such as, berries and *R. canina*) can provide anticancer effects. *R. canina* can cause the arrest of cancer cells and prevent proliferation. Polyethylene coated, iron magnetite nanoparticles loaded with gallic acid have been shown to reduce cancer cell viability. Many fruits and berries have expressed the ability to protect cells from oxidative damage. The use of plant-based metabolites has the potential to provide aid in the treatment and prevention of colon cancer, due to neutralizing properties of natural phenolic compounds.

KEYWORDS

- **berries**
- **chemoprevention**
- **colon cancer**
- **gallic acid**
- ***Rosa canina***
- **salicylic acid**

REFERENCES

1. Afrin, S.; Giampieri, F.; Gasparrini, M. Chemopreventive and Therapeutic Effects of Edible Berries: A Focus on Colon Cancer Prevention and Treatment. *Molecules* **2016**, *21* (2), 169–174.
2. Ai, G.; Dachineni, R.; Muley, P.; Tummala, H.; Bhat, G.J. Aspirin and Salicylic Acid Decrease c-Myc Expression in Cancer Cells: A Potential Role in Chemoprevention. *Tumour Biol.* **2016**, *37* (2), 1727–1738.

3. Arvind, P.; Qiao, L.; Papavassiliou, E.; Goldin, E.; Koutsos, M.; Rigas, B. Aspirin and Aspirin-Like Drugs Induce HLA-DR Expression in HT29 Colon Cancer Cells. *Int. J. Oncol.* **1996,** *8* (6), 1207–1211.

4. Baron, J. A.; Greenberg, E. R. Could Aspirin Really Prevent Colon Cancer? *New Engl. J. Med.* **1991,** *325* (23), 1644–1646.

5. Chen, H.; Wu, Y.; Chia, Y.; Chang, F.; Hsu, H. Gallic Acid, A Major Component Of *Toona sinensis* Leaf Extracts, Contains A ROS-Mediated Anti-Cancer Activity In Human Prostate Cancer Cells. *Cancer Lett.* **2009,** *286* (2), 161–171.

6. Choi, K.; Lee, Y.; Jung, M. G.; Kwon, S. H. Gallic Acid Suppresses Lipopolysaccha-ride-Induced Nuclear Factor-B Signaling By Preventing RelA Acetylation in A549 Lung Cancer Cells. *Mol. Cancer Res.* **2009,** *7* (12), 2011–2021.

7. Coyle, B.; McCann, M.; Kavanagh, K. Synthesis, X-ray Crystal Structure, Anti-Fungal and Anti-Cancer Activity Of [Ag2(NH3)2(salH)2] (salH2=salicylic acid). *J. Inorg. Biochem.* **2004,** *98* (8), 1361–1366.

8. Doubilet, P.; Donowitz, M.; Pauker, S. G. Evaluation for Colon Cancer in Patients With Occult Fecal Blood Loss While Taking Aspirin. *Med. Decision Making* **1982,** *2* (2), 147–160.

9. Engstrom, P. F.; Arnoletti, J. P.; Benson, A. B. NCCN Clinical Practice Guidelines in Oncology: Colon Cancer. *J. Natl. Compreh. Cancer Netw. (JNCCN)* **2009,** *7* (8), 778–831.

10. Flis, S.; Jastrzebski, Z.; Namiesnik, J.; Arancibia-Avila, P. Evaluation of Inhibition of Cancer Cell Proliferation in Vitro With Different Berries and Correlation With Their Antioxidant Levels By Advanced Analytical Methods. *J. Pharm. Biomed. Anal.* **2012,** *62,* 68–78.

11. García-Rivera, D.; Delgado, R.; Bougarne, N. Gallic Acid Indanone and Mangiferin Xanthone are Strong Determinants of Immunosuppressive Anti-Tumor Effects of *Mangifera indica* L. Bark In MDA-MB231 Breast Cancer Cells. *Cancer Lett.* **2011,** *305* (1), 21–31.

12. Gunther, J.; Frambach, M.; Deinert, I. Effects of Acetylic Salicylic Acid and Pent-oxifylline on the Efficacy of Intravesicalbcg Therapy in Orthotopic Murine Bladder Cancer (Mb49). *J. Urol.* **1999,** *161* (5), 1702–1706.

13. Ho, H.; Chang, C.; Ho, W.; Liao, S.; Wu, C.; Wang, C. Anti-Metastasis Effects of Gallic Acid on Gastric Cancer Cells Involves Inhibition of NF-κb Activity and Downregulation of PI3K/AKT/small GTPase Signals. *Food Chem. Toxicol.* **2010,** *48* (8–9), 2508–2516.

14. Hsu, J.; Kao, S.; Ou, T.; Chen, Y.; Li, Y.; Wang, C. Gallic Acid Induces G2/M Phase Arrest of Breast Cancer Cell MCF-7 Through Stabilization of p27Kip1 Attributed to Disruption of p27Kip1/Skp2 Complex. *J. Agric. Food Chem.* **2011,** *59* (5), 1996–2003.

15. Yusuf, M. A.; Kapoor, V. K.; Kamel, R. R. Modification and Implementation of NCCN Guidelines™ on Hepatobiliary Cancers in the Middle East and North Africa Region. *J. Natl. Compreh. Cancer Netw.* **2010,** *8* (Suppl. 3), S36–S40.

16. Jiménez, S.; Gascón, S.; Luquin, A. *Rosa Canina* Extracts Have Antiproliferative and Antioxidant Effects On Caco-2 Human Colon Cancer. *Plos One* **2016,** *11* (7), e0159136.

17. Kawada, M.; Ohno, Y.; Ri, Y.; Ikoma, T. Anti-Tumor Effect of Gallic Acid on LL-2 Lung Cancer Cells Transplanted in Mice. *Anti-Cancer Drugs* **2001,** *12* (10), 847–852.

18. Kedzierska, M.; Olas, B.; Wachowicz, B. An Extract From Berries of *Aronia Melanocarpa* Modulates The Generation of Superoxide Anion Radicals in Blood Platelets from Breast Cancer Patients. *Planta Medica* **2009,** *75* (13), 1405–1409.

19. Liu, K.; Ho, H.; Huang, A.; Ji, B. Gallic Acid Provokes DNA Damage and Suppresses DNA Repair Gene Expression in Human Prostate Cancer PC-3 Cells. *Environ. Toxicol.* **2011,** *28* (10), 579–587.

20. Liu, K.: Huang, A.: Wu, P.; Lin, H. Gallic Acid Suppresses Migration and Invasion of PC-3 Human Prostate Cancer Cells via Inhibition of Matrix Metalloproteinase-2 and Metalloproteinase-9 Signaling Pathways. *Oncol. Rep.* **2011,** *26* (1), 177–184.

21. Liu, Z.; Li, D.; Yu, L.; Niu, F. Gallic Acid as a Cancer-Selective Agent Induces Apoptosis in Pancreatic Cancer Cells. *Chemotherapy* **2012,** *58* (3), 185–194.

22. O'Connor, M.; Kellett, A.; McCann, M. Copper (II) Complexes of Salicylic Acid Combining Superoxide Dismutase Mimetic Properties With DNA Binding and Cleaving Capabilities Display Promising Chemotherapeutic Potential with Fast Acting in vitro Cytotoxicity Against Cisplatin Sensitive and Resistant Cancer Cell Lines. *J. Med. Chem.* **2012,** *55* (5), 1957–1968.

23. Ohno, Y.; Fukuda, K.; Takemura, G. Induction of Apoptosis By Gallic Acid in Lung Cancer Cells. *Anti-Cancer Drugs* **1999,** *10* (9), 845–852.

24. Parihar, S.; Gupta, A.; Chaturvedi, A. K. Gallic Acid Based Steroidal Phenstatin Analogues for Selective Targeting of Breast Cancer Cells Through Inhibiting Tubulin Polymerization. *Steroids* **2012,** *77* (8–9), 878–886.

25. Paterson, J. Salicylic Acid: A Link between Aspirin, Diet and the Prevention of Colorectal Cancer. *QJM* **2001,** *94* (8), 445–448.

26. Reddivari, L.; Vanamala, J.; Safe, S. H. The Bioactive Compounds α-Chaconine and Gallic Acid in Potato Extracts Decrease Survival and Induce Apoptosis in LNCaP and PC3 Prostate Cancer Cells. *Nutr. Cancer* **2010,** *62* (5), 601–610.

27. Rosman, R.; Saifullah, B.; Maniam, S. Improved Anticancer Effect of Magnetite Nanocomposite Formulation of GALLIC Acid (Fe3O4-PEG-GA) Against Lung, Breast and Colon Cancer Cells. *Nanomaterials* **2018,** *8* (2), 83–90.

28. Russell, L.H.; Mazzio, E.A.; Badisa, R.B. Differential Cytotoxicity of Triphala and Its Phenolic Constituent Gallic Acid on Human Prostate Cancer LNCap And Normal Cells. *Anticancer Res.* **2011,** *31* (11), 3739–3745.

29. Russell, L.H.; Mazzio, E.A.; Badisa, R.B. Autoxidation of Gallic Acid Induces ROS-dependent Death in Human Prostate Cancer LNCaP cells. *Anticancer Res.* **2012,** *32* (5), 1595–1602.

30. Siegel, R.L., Miller, K.D.; Jemal, A. Cancer Statistics, 2019. *CA: Cancer J. Clin.* **2019,** *69* (1), 7–34.

31. Stoner, G. D.; Chen, T.; Kresty, L. A.; Aziz, R. M.; Reinemann, T.; Nines, R. Protection Against Esophageal Cancer in Rodents With Lyophilized Berries: Potential Mechanisms. *Nutr. Cancer* **2006,** *54* (1), 33–46.

32. Stoner, G. D.; Wang, L.; Casto, B. C. Laboratory and Clinical Studies of Cancer Chemoprevention By Antioxidants in Berries. *Carcinogenesis* **2008,** *29* (9), 1665–1674.

33. Stoner, G.D.; Wang, L.; Zikri, N.N. Cancer Prevention with Freeze-Dried Berries and Berry Components. *Semin. Cancer Biol.* **2007,** *17* (5), 403–410.

34. Thun, M. J.; Namboodiri, M. M.; Heath, C. W. Aspirin Use and Reduced Risk of Fatal Colon Cancer. *New Engl. J. Med.* **1991,** *325* (23), 1593–1596.

35. Tumbas, V. T.; Čanadanović-Brunet, J. M. Effect of Rosehip (*Rosa canina* L.) Phytochemicals on Stable Free Radicals and Human Cancer Cells. *J. Sci. Food Agric.* **2011,** *92* (6), 1273–1281.

36. Turan, I.; Demir, S.; Kilinc, K.; Yaman, S. O. Cytotoxic Effect of *Rosa Canina* Extract on Human Colon Cancer Cells through Repression of Telomerase Expression. *J. Pharm. Anal.* **2018,** *8* (6), 394–399.

CHAPTER 4

Role of Medicinal Plants in the Treatment of Hemorrhoids

YAW DUAH BOAKYE, DANIEL OBENG MENSAH,
EUGENE KUSI AGYEI, RICHARD AGYEN, and CHRISTIAN AGYARE

ABSTRACT

Many individuals of varicose range and nonspecific gender have reported signs and symptoms that include inflammation, pain, bleeding, anal itching, and pain during defecation. Most drugs therapies in ancient Persian and Turkish medicines have proved to be beneficial against hemorrhoids. In this chapter, 20 medicinal plants have been discussed with anti-hemorrhoidal activities.

4.1 INTRODUCTION

Hemorrhoids are vascular cushions with a thick submucosa comprising of blood vessels, connective tissues, and Treitz muscle around the anus.[48] Any enlargement, bleeding, and protrusion of these cushions will lead to pathologic hemorrhoids (Fig. 4.1). The bright red color of hemorrhoidal bleeding, coupled with the blood having same pH as arterial pH, has led to the identification of hemorrhoidal bleeding being arterial and not venous.[46] Hemorrhoids are categorized as either internal or external hemorrhoids based on their position with respect to the dentate line and their anatomic origin within the anal canal.[37]

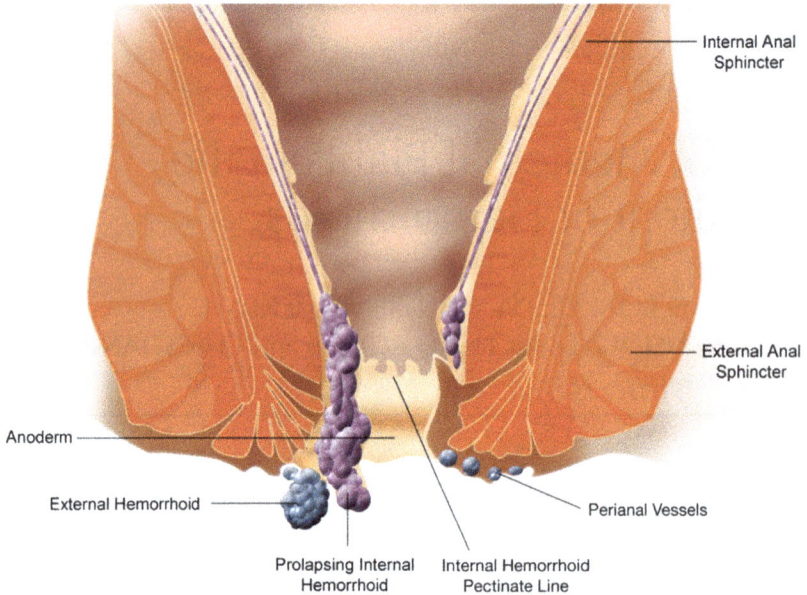

FIGURE 4.1 Anatomy of hemorrhoids.

Source: WikipedianProlific. https://creativecommons.org/licenses/by-sa/3.0/deed.en

4.1.1   Etiology and Pathophysiology of Hemorrhoids

Hemorrhoids are present in every individual; and its pathological condition occurs when these vascular cushions become inflamed, enlarged, prolapsed, or obstructed by a blood clot.[37,46] Swelling of the anal cushions causes distension and engorgement of the arteriovenous plexuses. This leads to a stretch in the suspensory muscles and eventual prolapse of rectal tissue through the anal canal. The engorged anal mucosa is easily traumatized, leading to rectal bleeding that is typically bright red due to high blood oxygen content within the arteriovenous anastomoses. Prolapse leads to soiling and mucus discharge (triggering pruritus) and predisposes to incarceration and strangulation.[22]

Constipation and its related vigorous straining and prolonged sitting have been the common causes of hemorrhoids. These causative links have very limited evidence to support them. However, some of these likely etiologies are discussed below:

- Small caliber stools due to low fiber diets lead to straining during defecation, which in turn results in increased pressure causing engorgement of the hemorrhoids. The engorgement of the hemorrhoids then interferes or reduces venous return. It has also been observed that the canal resting tone of patients with hemorrhoids is higher than normal.[27,46,55]

- Another common contributing factor cited is prolonged sitting (while working, reading, or on the toilet). There is a tourniquet effect (reduced venous return in the perianal area) in these positions, hence resulting in the hemorrhoids getting enlarged.[27,46,55]

- Also, aging leads to the loss of strength of the support structures, which facilitates prolapse. This loss of strength of the support systems may occur as early as the third decade of life.[27,37,46]

- Due to direct pressure and hormonal changes, pregnant women are predisposed to symptoms from hemorrhoids. As the gravid uterus expands, it presses on the inferior vena cava, causing decreased venous return and distal engorgement. Notably, most pregnant women return to their previously asymptomatic state after delivery. [25,27,37,46]

4.1.2 Epidemiology

The United States has about 33.33% prevalence of pathologic hemorrhoids among 10 million people with hemorrhoids seeking medical treatment, accounting for 1.5 million hemorrhoid-related prescriptions per annum.[46] White people from rural areas and higher socioeconomic status mostly present with hemorrhoidal disease. There is no specific sex preference, although men are more likely to seek treatment. External hemorrhoids occur more commonly in young and middle-aged adults than in older adults. The prevalence of hemorrhoids increases with age, with a peak among persons aged 45–65 years.[46]

4.1.3 Prognosis

Most hemorrhoids resolve spontaneously or with conservative medical therapy alone. Complications such as secondary infection, abscess, thrombosis, incontinence, and ulceration may occur. The rate of recurrence in nonsurgical management techniques is 10–50% over a 5-year period, whereas that of surgical hemorrhoidectomy is less than 5%.[46]

In most traditional and folk medicines of different countries, many plants have shown to be used successfully in the treatment of hemorrhoids, with lower incidence of side effects. These plants have been shown to improve the symptoms of hemorrhoids (such as bleeding, rectal prolapse, pain, heaviness and tenesmus, number of hemorrhoidal cushions, itching, and recurrence), and increase the rate of wound healing.[28]

Their mechanisms of action include anti-inflammatory, venotonic, antinociceptive, and venoprotective activities. Mostly tripterpenes, flavonoids, terpenoids, and tannins have been suggested to be responsible for the anti-hemorrhoidal activity of most of these medicinal plants.[28]

This chapter discusses anti-hemorrhoidal activity of medicinal plants and their active metabolites.

4.2   MEDICINAL PLANTS FOR THE TREATMENT OF HEMORRHOIDS

4.2.1   *Aesculus hippocastanum (Sapindaceae)*

Extracts of *Aesculus hippocastanum* L. contain flavonoids and aescin as its main active biocomponents, with antioxidant activity, venotonic properties, anti-inflammatory activity, and vascular protective effects.[25,32] The seed extract of *A. hippocastanum* could decrease capillary permeability, edema, and antagonize enzymes involved in the degradation of proteoglycan.[47] In a clinical study, the gel from the 20% glycerolic extract of *A. hippocastanum* seeds induced a statistically significant reduction of hind paw edema. In other clinical trials, it was observed that acute symptomatic hemorrhoids were improved after 6 days of administration to patients.[48]

4.2.2   *Vitis vinifera (Vitaceae)*

Several pharmacological studies conducted on extracts of *Vitis vinifera* showed antioxidant, antipyretic, antinociceptive, hepatoprotection, and cardioprotection properties.[37] Also, the use of *V. vinifera* extracts for their anti-hemorrhoidal property in traditional medicine has been reported. *V. vinifera* extracts are rich in polyphenols, such as stilbenes, catechins, and flavonoids.[40] Caffeic acid, kaempferol glycosides, resveratrol, and quercetin have been identified as the main compounds responsible for the antinociceptive and anti-inflammatory activities.[6,25]

4.2.3   Allium iranicum (Amaryllidaceae)

Allium iranicum (leek) is a common edible vegetable in Persian people's diet. Steroidal saponin (such as furostane-type saponin and spirostane-type saponin) with anti-inflammatory and anti-ulcerogenic effects has been extracted from leek.[9,10] This plant has been used in the treatment of hemorrhoids in the traditional Persian medicines, either topically or orally. In a double-blinded randomized controlled clinical study trial, a cream containing 1.38 g of leek extract was used against placebo in hemorrhoid patients. This study showed a general reduction in anal pain, anal itching, bleeding severity, and defecation discomfort among all patients, with very significant reduction in bleeding severity.[35]

4.2.4   Commiphora mukul (Burseraceae)

Commiphora mukul is one of the best herbal monotherapies for hemorrhoids, which can be used orally or topically. The resin of *C. mukul* is a delicate mixture of different classes of phytochemical compounds, such as, diterpenoids, lipids and lignans, and steroids. One clinical trial demonstrated a significant reduction in symptoms of hemorrhoids (such as, concomitant GI symptoms including GE-reflux, colonoscopic stage, and flatulence). Also, there was a significant improvement in most of hemorrhoidal symptoms after 4 weeks of follow-up.[58]

4.2.5   Boswellia species (Burseraceae)

In Iran, gum resins of *Boswellia serrata* Roxb. ex Colebr. and *B. carterii* Bird. have been used for the management of hemorrhoids for all age groups.[7] The gum resins from *Boswellia* species mainly contain boswellic acid; a mixture of tetracyclic triterpenes and pentacyclic triterpenes are reported to be responsible for its anti-inflammatory effect.[18] In a study done on boswellic acid, it was observed that these acids are specific, non-redox inhibitors of leukotriene synthesis either by interacting immediately with 5-lipoxygenase (5-LOX) or restricting its translocation and thus acting as anti-inflammatory agent.[49] Al-Harrasi et al.[2] used formalin-induced pain and acetic acid-induced writhing to investigate the analgesic activity *of B. sacra* in mice. They observed that polar subfraction of *B. sacra* had the highest analgesic activity, almost double of aspirin (control treatment). The study proposed that *Boswellia* seems to produce an antinociceptive effect by both peripheral and central mechanism.[2]

4.2.6   *Adiantum capillus-veneris (Pteridaceae)*

Adiantum capillus-veneris has been used by medieval Persian practitioners in the treatment of various inflammatory conditions, such as hemorrhoids. In a study to ascertain the maidenhair fern's pharmacological activity, the ethanol extract of *A. capillus-veneris* aerial parts (200 mg) was evaluated for anti-inflammatory activities by evaluating the spleen index and the protein expression related to tumor necrosis factor (TNF) in lipopolysaccharide-induced mice. The extract of *A. capillus-veneris* was able to normalize the lipopolysaccharide-induced elevation of the spleen index and TNF and thus could be introduced as a natural anti-inflammatory resource.[59] Both ethyl acetate fraction and ethanolic extract of *A. capillus-veneris* demonstrated antinociceptive effects (300 mg/kg orally) in a tail-flick method and writhing test.[19]

4.2.7   *Myrtus communis L. (Myrtaceae)*

Iranian traditional medicine *Myrtus communis* is a popular medicinal plant to reduce the swelling and pain in patients with hemorrhoids. *M. communis* leaves have been used to cause the cessation of bleeding. The poultice from *M. communis* leaves is also used for the treatment of hemorrhoids. Sitting in a decoction of *M. communis* leaves was recommended for anal protrusion.[30] *M. communis* leaves contain gallo-tannin-sacylphloroglucinols (myrtucommulone-A and -B), volatile oils (0.1–0.5%), and condensed tannins.[57] *M. communis* is mainly used in the treatment of hemorrhoids due to its antinociceptive and anti-inflammatory properties. The major compound of *M. communis* essential oil, 1,8-Cineole, reduced inflammatory cytokines mediators, TNF-α, and interleukin-6 (IL-6) and inhibited the movement of white blood cells in areas with inflammation.[52] The hemostatic and analgesic effects of *M. communis* essential oil are attributed to the anti-inflammatory effects.[30]

4.2.8   Acacia ferruginea D.C. (Fabaceae)

Acacia ferruginea is a drought-resistant tree found in western region of India. The bitter bark of *A. ferruginea* has been used traditionally as an astringent cure for itching and ulcers. Phytochemical constituents of *A. ferruginea* include phenols, alkaloids, anthraquinones, terpenoids, tannins, and flavonoids. In a study using the hydroalcoholic extract of the bark of *A. ferruginea* (400 mg/kg body weight orally) for treatment of hemorrhoids in wistar albino rats, there was significant reduction of rectoanal damage and restoration to the near-normal structure of the rectoanal region. There was a significant reduction in inflammatory cytokines (IL-6, PGE2, and TNF-α), which showed that the anti-inflammatory effect of *A. ferruginea* mediates its anti-hemorrhoidal activity.[16]

4.2.9   Terminalia chebula Retz. (Combretaceae)

Terminalia chebula Retz. is a major medicinal plant for treatment of hemorrhoids in Persian medicine. This herb could shrink the hemorrhoid mass size and stop the bleeding in other traditional systems of medicines, such as Ayurveda.[15] Possibly, the efficacy of *T. chebula* against pain could be attributed to its central analgesic effects and triterpenoids saponin, which blocks the cholecystokinin (CCK) receptors.[54] This, in turn, may be due to anti-inflammatory and analgesic characters of tannins (chebulinic acid, ellagic acid, corilagin, and gallic acid) via reducing the serum levels of pro-inflammatory cytokines (TNF-α, IL-6, and IL-1β) or inhibiting enzyme cyclooxygenase (COX) and prostaglandin synthesis.[13,33,55] Gallic acid and its metabolites can also control the pain by acting as a glucocorticoid receptor agonist.[38] Chebulagic acid relieves the pain due to inhibition of COX and 5-LOX[11] along with flavonoids (quercetin and kaempferol).[44,17] The efficacy of *T. chebula* against hemorrhoid mass size can be due to its venotonic characteristic (chebulinic acid and terflavin

B)[4,13] and venoprotective (via cytoprotective characteristics with inhibiting oxidative stress) features.[4,39]

4.2.10   *Cissus quadrangularis (Vitaceae)*

The major phytochemicals in *Cissus quadrangularis* are flavonoids. Bioflavonoids have been shown to exhibit phelotonic, vasculoprotective, and anti-inflammatory activities. Luteolin and β-sitosterol from the crude extract of *C. quadrangularis* have been shown to produce its anti-inflammatorry effect. The venotonic effect of *C. quadrangularis* has been postulated to be due to the flavonoids present in its crude extract, which act in the same way as that of diosmin and hesperidin (found in Daflon).[53]

Several other medicinal plants have been studied with regard to the treatment of hemorrhoids, and are presented in Table 4.1.

4.3   SUMMARY

As the search for effective drug treatment options for hemorrhoids with lower incidence of side effects continues, this review has reinforced the fact that medicinal plants could serve as priceless repository of these drugs. The medicinal plants evaluated in this review in different stages of experimental studies showed significant anti-hemorrhoid activity by varying mechanisms of action.

KEYWORDS

- anti-hemorrhoidal
- anti-inflammatory
- antinociceptive
- hemorrhoids
- traditional medicine
- venotonic

TABLE 4.1 Some Medicinal Plants Studied for Treatment of Hemorrhoids.

Scientific name (family)	Common name	Part used	Chemical constituents	Activity	Dose used	Reference
Acacia ferruginea (Fabaceae)	Arimedah	Bark	Phenolics Flavonoids Saponins	Anti-inflammatory	400 mg/kg BW of hydroalcoholic extract	[16]
Adiantum capillus-veneris (Pteridaceae)	Maidenhair fern	Aerial part	Triterpinoids (capillirone 1 and 2)	Anti-inflammatory Antinociceptive	200–300 mg/kg	[19, 59]
Aesculus hippocastanum (Sapindaceae)	Horse chestnut	Glycerol extract of seeds	Aescin Flavonoids	Anti-inflammatory Venotonic Antioxidant	0.50 g of 20% glycerol extract	[26, 29, 32, 33]
Allium iranicum (Amaryllidaceae)	Leek (wendelbo)	Leaves	Steroidal Saponins Flavonoids	Anti-inflammatory Anti-ulcerogenic Anti-oxidant	2 mL of the leek cream (contains 1.38 g of leek extract)	[9, 10, 35]
Boswellia serrata (Burseraceae)	Salai guggal	Gum resins	Boswellic acid	Anti-inflammatory Antinociceptive	100 mg/kg orally	[2, 3, 18, 47, 49]
Cissus quadrangularis (Vitaceae)	Bone setter		Flavonoids Luteolin β-sitosterol	Anti-inflammatory Venotonic		[53]
Commiphora mukul (Burseraceae)	Indian bdellium	Gum resins	Steroids Guggulusteroids Terpenoidss	Anti-hemorrhoidal	3 g orally in three divided doses	[58]
Ficus carica (Moraceae)	Common fig	leaves	Phenolics Volatile compounds	Anti-inflammatory	600 mg/kg	[45]

TABLE 4.1 *(Continued)*

Scientific name (family)	Common name	Part used	Chemical constituents	Activity	Dose used	Reference
Myrtus communis (Myrtaceae)	Myrtle	Leaves	Volatile oils Gallotannins Condensed tannins AcylphloroGlucinols	Anti-inflammatory Antinociceptive		[30, 52, 57]
Pistacia terebinthus (Anacardiaceae)	Turpentine tree	Seed	Tannins Trierpenes Oleanonic acid	Anti-inflammatory	18 g orally	[27, 50]
Plantago major (Plantaginaceae)	Ribwort	Leaves	Flavonoids Steroids Terpenes	Anti-inflammatory Antinociceptive	1 g/kg per oral of aqueous leave extract	[43]
Sesamum indicum (Pedaliaceae)	Sesame	Seed	Oleic acid Linoleic acid	Anti-inflammatory Analgesia	400 mg/kg of seed oil	[34]
Smilax china (Smilacaceae)	China root	Root	Kaempferol 7-O-glycoside Sieboldogenin	Anti-inflammatory Antinociceptive	1000 mg/kg aqueous extract	[24]
Tamarindus indica (Fabaceae)	Tamarind	Leaves	Polyphenols Flavonoids	Anti-inflammatory Antinociceptive	1000 mg/kg hydroethanolic extract	[8]
Terminalia bellirica (Combretaceae)	Bibhitaki	Fruit	Saponins Triterpenoids Tannins	Anti-inflammatory Antinociceptive	800 mg/kg of ethanolic extract	[23, 41]
Terminalia chebula (Combretaceae)	Chebulic myrobalan	Fruit	Triterpenoid Saponins Tannins Flavonoids	Anti-inflammatory Antinociceptive Venoprotective	30 g per oral	[41]

TABLE 4.1 *(Continued)*

Scientific name (family)	Common name	Part used	Chemical constituents	Activity	Dose used	Reference
Trigonella foenum-graecum (Fabaceae)	Fenugreek	Seeds	Alkaloids Flavonoids	Anti-inflammatory Antinociceptive	100 mg/kg methanolic extracts	[31]
Verbascum pterocalycinum (Scrophulariaceae)	Mullein	Flowers	Saponin Iridoid glycosides	Anti-inflammatory Antinociceptive	100–200 mg/kg	[1]
Vitis vinifera (Vitaceae)	Grape vine	Ethanolic extract of leaves	Caffeic acid quercetin Kaempferol glycosides resveratrol	Analgesia Anti-inflammatory	0.20 mL/10 g BW ethanolic extract	[6, 25, 33, 40]

REFERENCES

1. Akkol, E. K.; Tatli I. I.; Akdemir Z. S. Antinociceptive and Anti-Inflammatory Effects of Saponin and Iridoid Glucosides from *Verbascum Pterocalycinum*. *Zeitschrift für Naturforschung (J. Nat. Res.)* **2007,** *62* (11–12), 813–820.
2. Al-Harrasi, A.; Ali, L.; Hussain, J.; Rehman, N. U.; Ahmed, M.; Al-Rawahi, A. Analgesic Effects of Crude Extracts and Fractions of Omani Frankincense Obtained From Traditional Medicinal Plant *Boswellia Sacra* on Animal Models. *Asian Pacific J. Trop. Med.* **2014,** *7,* S485–S490.
3. Al-Harrasi, A.; Ali, L.; Rehman, N. U.; Hussain, H.; Hussain, J.; Al-Rawahi, A. Nine Triterpenes from *Boswellia Sacra* Fluckiger and Their Chemotaxonomic Importance. *Biochem. Syst. Ecol.* **2013,** *51,* 113–116.
4. Anwesa, B.; Bhattacharyya, S. K.; Chattopadhyay, R. R. Development of *Terminalia Chebula* Retz. in Clinical Research. *Asian Pacific J. Trop. Biomed.* **2013,** *3* (3), 244–252.
5. Anwesa, B.; Kumar, B. S.; Kumar, P. N.; Ranjan, C. R. Antiinflammatory, Anti-Lipid Peroxidative, Antioxidant and Membrane Stabilizing Activities of Hydroalcoholic Extract of *Terminalia Chebula* Fruits. *Pharm. Biol.* **2013,** *51,* 1515–1520.
6. Aouey B.; Samet, A. M.; Fetoui, H.; Simmonds, M. S. J.; Bouaziz, M. Anti-Oxidant, Anti-Inflammatory, Analgesic and Antipyretic Activities of Grapevine Leaf Extract (*Vitis Vinifera*) in Mice and Identification of its Active Constituents by LC–MS/MS Analyses. *Biomed. Pharmacotherap.* **2016,** *84,* 1088–1098.
7. Arzani M. A.; Tebb-e A. *Institute of Medical History, Islamic and Complementary Medicine.* Iran University of Medical Sciences: Tehran; **2005**; pp 33–40.
8. Bhadoriya, S. S.; Mishra, V.; Raut, S. Anti-Inflammatory and Antinociceptive Activities of a Hydroethanolic Extract of *Tamarindus Indica* Leaves. *Scientia Pharmaceutica* **2012,** *80,* 685–700.
9. Camila, R. A.; da Silva, B. P.; Inoco, L. W., Parente, J. P. Haemolytic Activity and Immunological Adjuvant Effect of a New Steroidal Saponin from *Allium Ampeloprasum* Var. Porrum. *Chemistry and Biodiversity* **2012,** *9,* 58–67.
10. Camila, R. A.; da Silva, B. P.; Parente, J. P. Steroidal Saponin with Anti-Inflammatory and Antiulcerogenic Properties from the Bulbs of *Allium Ampeloprasum*. *Fitoterapia* **2011,** *82,*1175–1180.
11. Christine, T. P.; Denniston, K.; Chopra, D. Therapeutic Uses of Triphala in Ayurvedic Medicine. *J. Altern. Complem. Med.* **2017,** *23,* 607–614.
12. Cloinical Practice Committee, American Gastroenterological Association (AGA). Medical Position Statement: Diagnosis and Treatment of Hemorrhoids. *Gastroenterology* **2004,** *126,* 1461–1462.
13. Cock, I. E. The Medicinal Properties and Phytochemistry of Plants of the Genus *Terminalia*. *Inflammopharmacol.* **2015,** *23,* 203–229.
14. Dehdari, S.; Hajimehdipoor, H.; Esmaeili, S.; Choopani, R.; Mortazavi, S. A. Traditional and Modern Aspects of Hemorrhoid Treatment in Iran: A Review. *Journal of Integrative Medicine* **2018,** *16,* 90–98.
15. Dodke, P.; Pansare, T. Ayurvedic and Modern Aspect of *Terminalia chebula* Retz. Haritaki: An Overview. *Int. J. Ayurverdic Herbal Med.* **2017,** *7,* 2508–2517.

16. Faujdar, S.; Bhawana, S.; Swapnil, S.; Pathak, A. K.; Paliwal, S. K. Phytochemical Evaluation and Anti-Hemorrhoidal Activity of Bark of *Acacia Ferruginea*. *J. Traditional Complem. Med.* **2019**, *9*, 85–89.
17. García-Mediavilla, V.; Crespo, I.; Collado, P.S. The Anti-Inflammatory Flavones Quercetin and Kaempferol Cause Inhibition of Inducible Nitric Oxide Synthase, Cyclooxygenase-2 and Reactive C-Protein, and Down-Regulation of the Nuclear Factor Kappa B Pathway in Chang Liver Cells. *Eur. J. Pharmacol.* **2007**, *557*, 221–229.
18. Gerbeth, K.; Meins, J.; Kirste, S.; Momm, F. Determination of major boswellic acids in plasma by high-pressure liquid chromatography/mass spectrometry. *J. Pharm. Biomed. Anal.* **2011**, 56, 998–1005.
19. Haider, S.; Nazreen, S.; Alam, M. M.; Gupta, A.; Hamid, H.; Alam, M. S. Anti-Inflammatory and Anti-Nociceptive Activities of Ethanolic Extract and Its Various Fractions from *Adiantum capillus veneris* Linn. *J. Ethnopharmacol.* **2011**, *138*, 741–747.
20. Iqbal, P.; Ahmed, D.; Asghar, M. N. A Comparative *In Vitro* Antioxidant Potential Profile of Extracts from Different Parts of *Fagonia Cretica*. *Asian Pacific J. Tropical Med.* **2014**, *7* (Suppl. 1), S473–S480.
21. Johanson, J. F.; Sonnenberg, A. The Prevalence of Hemorrhoids and Chronic Constipation: An Epidemiologic Study. *Gastroenterology* **1990**, *98*, 380–386.
22. Kaidar-Person, O.; Person, B.; Wexner, S. D. Hemorrhoidal Disease: A Comprehensive Review. *J. Am. Coll. Surg.* **2007**, *204* (1), 102–117.
23. Kaur S.; Jaggi R. K. Antinociceptive Activity of Chronic Administration of Different Extracts of *Terminalia bellerica* and *Terminalia chebula* Fruits. *Ind. J. Exp. Biol.* **2010**, *48*, 925–930.
24. Khan, I.; Nisar, M.; Ebad, F.; Nadeem, S. Anti-Inflammatory Activities of Sieboldogenin from *Smilax China* Linn.: Experimental and Computational Studies. *J. Ethnopharmacol.* **2009**, *121*, 175–177.
25. Kosar, M.; Küpeli, E.; Malyer, H.; Uylaser, V.; Türkben, C.; Baser, K. H. C. Effect of Brining on Biological Activity of Leaves of *Vitis vinifera* L. (Cv. Sultani Çekirdeksiz) from Turkey. *J. Agric. Food Chem.* **2007**, *55*, 4596–4603.
26. Küçükkurt, I.; Ince, S.; Kele, S. H.; Küpeli, A. E. Beneficial Effects of *Aesculus hippocastanum* L. Seed Extract on the Body's Own Antioxidant Defense System on Subacute Administration. *J. Ethnopharmacol.* **2010**, *129*, 18–22.
27. Lohsiriwat, V. Hemorrhoids: from Basic Pathophysiology to Clinical Management. *World J. Gastroenterol.* **2012**, *18* (17), 9–17.
28. Lorenzo-Rivero, S. Hemorrhoids: Diagnosis and Current Management. *American Journal of Surgery* **2009**, *75*, 635–642.
29. MacKay, D. Hemorrhoids and Varicose Veins: A Review of Treatment Options. *Altern. Med. Rev.* **2001**, *6*, 126–140.
30. Mahboubi, M. Effectiveness of *Myrtus Communis* in the Treatment of Hemorrhoids. *J. Integr. Med.* **2017**, *15* (5), 351–358.
31. Mandegary, A.; Pournamdari, M.; Sharififar, F. Alkaloid and Flavonoid Rich Fractions of Fenugreek Seeds (*Trigonella foenum-graecum* L.) with Antinociceptive and Anti-Inflammatory Effects. *Food Chem. Toxicol.* **2012**, *50*, 2503–2507.
32. Margina, D.; Olaru, O.T.; Ilie, M. Assessment of The Potential Health Benefits of Certain Total Extracts from *Vitis Vinifera, Aesculus Hyppocastanum* and *Curcuma Longa*. *Exp. Therap. Med.* **2015**, *10*, 1681–1688.

33. Mihai, D. P.; Seremet, O. C.; Nitulescu, G. Evaluation of Natural Extracts in Animal Models of Pain and Inflammation for a Potential Therapy of Hemorrhoidal Disease. *Scientia Pharm.* **2019,** *87,* 14–18.

34. Monteiro, É. M. H.; Chibli, L. A. Antinociceptive and Anti-Inflammatory Activities of the Sesame Oil and Sesamin. *Nutrients* **2014,** *6,* 1931–1944.

35. Mosavat, S. H.; Ghahramani, L.; Sobhani, Z. The Effect of Leek (*Allium iranicum*) Leaves Extract Cream on Hemorrhoid Patients: A Double Blind Randomized Controlled Clinical Trial. *Eur. J. Integr. Med.* **2015,** 7, 669–673.

36. Mosavat, S. H.; Ghahramani, L.; Sobhani, Z.; Haghighi, E. R., Heydar M. Topical *Allium ampeloprasum* (Leek) Extract Cream in Patients with Symptomatic Hemorrhoids: A Pilot Randomized and Controlled Clinical Trial. *J. Evidence Based Complem. Altern. Med.* **2015,** *20,* 132–136.

37. Mott, T.; Latimer, K.; Edwards, C. Hemorrhoids: Diagnosis and Treatment Options. *Am. Fam. Phys.* **2018,** *97* (3), 172–179.

38. Muhammed S.; Khan B. A.; Akhtar N. The Morphology, Extractions, Chemical Constituents and Uses of *Terminalia Chebula*: A Review. *J. Med. Plants Res.* **2012,** *6,* 4772–4775.

39. Na, M.; Bae, K.; Sik Kang, S.; Sun M. B. Cytoprotective Effect on Oxidative Stress and Inhibitory Effect on Cellular Aging of *Terminalia Chebula* Fruits. *Phytotherap. Res.* **2004,** *18,* 737–741.

40. Nadia, Z.; Aicha, M.; Sihem, H.; Abdelmalik, B. *In Vivo* Analgesic Activities and Safety Assessment of *Vitis Vinifera* L. and *Punica Granatum* L. Fruit Extracts. *Tropical Journal Pharmaceutical Research* **2017,** *16,* 553–561.

41. Nair V.; Ingh S.; Gupta Y. K. Anti-Arthritic and Disease Modifying Activity of *Terminalia Chebula*: Experimental Model. *J. Pharm. Pharmacol.* **2010,** *62,* 1801–1806.

42. Nassiri-Asl, M.; Hosseinzadeh, H. Review of the Pharmacological Effects of *Vitis vinifera* (Grape) and its Bioactive Compounds. *Phytotherap. Res.* **2009,** *23,* 1197–1204.

43. Nunez-Guille, M. E.; da Silva Emim, J. A.; Souccar, C.; Lapa, A. J. Analgesic and Anti-Inflammatory Activities of Aqueous Extract of *Plantago Major* L. *Pharm. Biol.* **1997,** *35,* 99–104.

44. Pablo, A.; Zhou, Q.; Martinez-Zapata, M. J.; Mills, E. Meta-analysis of Flavonoids For The Treatment of Haemorrhoids. *Br. J. Surg.* **2006,** *93,* 909–920.

45. Patil, V. V.; Patil V. R. Evaluation of Anti-Inflammatory Activity of *Ficus Carica* Linn. Leaves. *Ind. J. Nat. Prod. Res.* **2011,** *2,* 151–155.

46. Perry, R. K. *Personal data.* **2019**; https://emedicine.medscape.com/article/775407-overview#a5; Accessed on December 23, 2020.

47. Pilkhwal, N.; Dhaneshwar, S. An Update on Pharmacological Profile of *Boswella serrta. Asian J. Pharm. Clin. Res.* **2019,** *12* (5), 49–56.

48. Pirard, J.; Gillet P.; Guffens, J. M.; Defrance, P. Double Blind Study of Reparil in Proctology. *Revue Medicale de Liege* **1976,** *31* (10), 343–345.

49. Poeckel D.; Werz O. Boswellic Acids: Biological Actions and Molecular Targets. *Curr. Med. Chem.* **2006,** *13,* 59–69.

50. Reese, G. E.; von Roon, A. C.; Tekkis, P. P. Haemorrhoids. *Clinical Evidence (Online)* **2009,** article ID: 0415; pages 8.

51. Roja, R.; Mohammad, A. Evidence-based Review of Medicinal Plants Used for the Treatment of Hemorrhoids. *Int. J. Pharmacol.* **2013,** *9,* 1–11.

52. Santos, F. A.; Silva, R. M.; Campos, A. R. 1,8-Cineole (eucalyptol): A Monoterpene Oxide Attenuates the Colonic Damage in Rats on Acute TNBS-Colitis. *Food Chem. Toxicol.* **2004,** *42* (4), 579–584.

53. Siddiqua, A.; Mittapally, S. Review on *Cissus Quadrangularis*. *Pharma Innov. J.* **2017,** *6* (7), 329–334.

54. Sukwinder, K.; Jaggi, R. K. Antinociceptive Activity of Chronic Administration of Different Extracts of *Terminalia bellerica* and *Terminalia chebula* Fruits. *Ind. J. Exp. Biol.* **2010,** *48* (9), 925–930.

55. Sukwinder, K.; Surveswaran, Y.Z.; Cai, C. H.; Sun, M. Systematic Evaluation of Natural Phenolic Antioxidants from 133 Indian Medicinal Plants. *Food Chem.* **2007,** *102,* 938–953.

56. Sun, Z.; Migaly, J. Review Of Hemorrhoid Disease: Presentation and Management. *Clin. Colon Rectal Surg.* **2016,** *29* (1), 22–29.

57. Tuberoso, C. I.; Barra, A.; Angioni, A.; Sarritzu, E.; Pirisi, F.M. Chemical Composition of Volatiles in Sardinian Myrtle (*Myrtus communis* L.) Alcoholic Extracts and Essential Oils. *J. Agric. Food Chem.* **2006,** *54* (4), 1420–1426.

58. Yousefi, M.; Mahdavi, M. R. V.; Hosseini, S.M. Clinical Evaluation of *Commiphora Mukul,* a Botanical resin, in the Management of Hemorrhoids: A Randomized Controlled trial. *Pharmacognosy Magaz.* **2013,** *9* (36), 350–356.

59. Yuan Q.; Zhang X.; Liu Z. Liu, Z.; Song, S.; Xue, P.; Wang, J.; Ruan, J. Ethanol Extract of *Adiantum capillus-veneris* L. Suppresses the Production of Inflammatory Mediators by Inhibiting NF-kappaB Activation. *J. Ethnopharmacol.* **2013,** *147,* 603–611.

PART II

Role of Spices and Herbs in the Management of Gastrointestinal Disorders

CHAPTER 5

Health Benefits of Garlic (*Allium sativum*) in Gastrointestinal Disorders

YAW DUAH BOAKYE, DANIEL OBENG MENSAH,
EUGENE KUSI AGYEI, RICHARD AGYEN,
DOREEN KWANKYEWAA ADJEI, and CHRISTIAN AGYARE

ABSTRACT

The medicinal plant, garlic, is used traditionally as a spice and flavoring agent and for therapeutic purposes for the management of an array of disease conditions. The literature provided scientific evidence on promising potential of garlic to treat gastrointestinal neoplasms, gastrointestinal infections and ulcers, inflammatory bowel disease, gastritis, and diarrhea of varied etiologies. This chapter identifies both experimental and epidemiological studies carried out on garlic and its bioactive compounds that justifies its use in the management of gastrointestinal disorders.

5.1 INTRODUCTION

Traditional Medicine/Complementary and Alternative Medicine (TCAM) has enjoyed patronage in advanced and as well in developing countries due to ease of access, relatively low cost and low toxicity in comparison to allopathic medicine.[25] In the era where antibiotics and other pharmaceutical products had not been developed, garlic has constituted a pharmacy industry due to wide range of health benefits. This includes its use in the management of different gastrointestinal (GI) disorders.

This review chapter seeks to comb through literature to identify studies carried out on the garlic and use of bioactive compounds to treat GI disorders.

5.2 GARLIC

5.2.1 *Botanical Description*

Garlic (Allium sativum) belongs to the family Liliaceae, along with chives, shallots, and onions.[13] It is a bulbous perennial plant characterized by its pungent taste and peculiar aroma. The plant can grow up to a height of about 1.2 m. The part of the plant that is most important for use medicinally is the compound bulb. About 4–20 cloves constitute each bulb with each clove weighing about 1 g. The dried bulbs, fresh bulbs, and oil extracted from the garlic bulbs are often the forms that are used traditionally for medicinal purposes.[34] Based on the geographical area, garlic is cultivated under other names, such as, clove garlic, stinking rose, nectar of the gods, poor man's treacle, camphor of the poor man, etc. Vernacular names of garlic (*Allium sativum*) are listed below:

- Arabic: ThumThawm, Thoum, Toum, Toom, Saum
- Armenian: Sekhdor
- Bengali: Rasun
- Burmese: Chyet, phew, thon
- Croatian : Češnjak
- Danish: Hvidløg
- Dutch: Knoflook
- Finnish: Valkosipuli
- German: Echter, Knoblauch, Knoblauch, Gewöhnlicher & Gemeiner Knoblauch
- Greek: Skordo, Skorda, Skordon, Skortho
- Hebrew: Shoum, Shum
- Hindi: Larsan, Lahsan, Lahasun, Lasun
- Italian: Aglio, Agliocomune
- Japanese: Gaarikku, Ninniku
- Kannada: Lashuna, Bellulli
- Khmer: Khtümsââ
- Korean: MaNul
- Laotian: Kath'ièm
- Madurese: Bhabangpoté
- Malay: Bawangputeh, Bawangputih
- Malayalam: Vallaipundu
- Marathi: Lasuun

- Nepalese: Lasun
- Norwegian: Hvitløk
- Persian: Seer, Sir
- Polish: Czosnek, Czosnek, pospolity
- Portuguese: Alho
- Punjabi: Lasun, Lasan
- Russian: Lukchesnok, Chesnok, Lukposevnoi
- Sanskrit: Lashunaa
- Serbian: Beliluk
- Sinhalese: Sudulunu
- Slovenian: Česen
- Spanish: Ajo, Ajocomun, Ajo vulgar
- Sudanese: Bawangbodas
- Swahili: Kitunguusaumu
- Swedish: Vitloek, Vitlök, Hvitlök
- Tamil: Vellaippuuntu, Vellaypoondoo, Wullaypoondoo
- Telugu: Vellulli
- Thai: Krathiam, Homtiam
- Turkish: Sarmesak, Sarımsak, Sarmusak
- Urdu: Leshun
- Vietnamese: Toi

Consumption of garlic ranks second to onion among the bulbs. Garlic is distributed in both temperate and tropical regions. It exists in various subspecies or types, the predominant ones being hard-neck and the soft-neck garlic. Evidence of the domestication of garlic can be found in ancient Greek, Egyptian, Chinese, and Indian writings. Production of garlic worldwide is reported to be nearly 10 million tons with China, Turkey, Egypt, India, USA, Spain, and Korea being the largest producers in the world.[28]

5.3 PHYTOCHEMICAL COMPOSITION OF GARLIC

Fresh garlic is composed of water, carbohydrates (such as fructose), lipids, vitamins (predominantly A and C), minerals (magnesium, potassium, iron, sodium, calcium, and phosphorus), phenolic compounds, phytosterols, and different organic compounds of sulfur. Based on the solubility of the compound, the chemical components in garlic can be categorized into two main groups: (1) Lipid-soluble allyl sulfur compounds (Fig. 5.1), such as, DADS (diallyl disulfide), DATS (diallyl trisulfide) and DAS (diallyl sulfur). (2) Water-soluble allyl sulfur compounds (Fig. 5.2), such as, S-allyl-cysteine and G-glutamyl-S-allyl-cysteine.

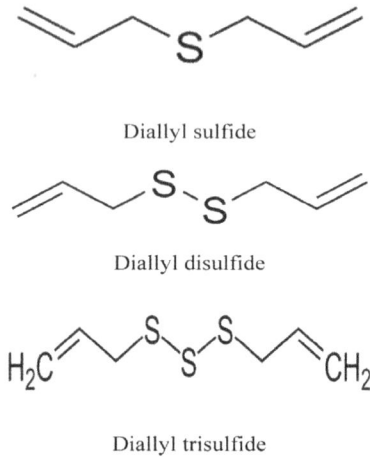

Diallyl sulfide

Diallyl disulfide

Diallyl trisulfide

FIGURE 5.1   Examples of compounds that are lipid-soluble.

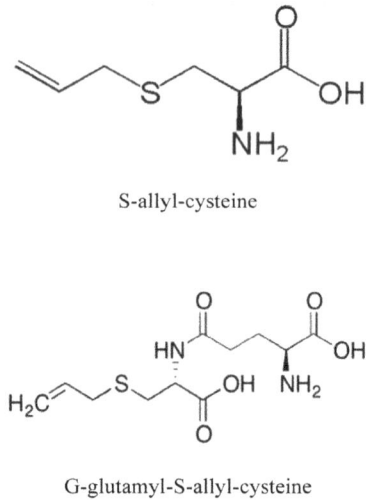

S-allyl-cysteine

G-glutamyl-S-allyl-cysteine

FIGURE 5.2   Examples of compounds that are water-soluble.

The principal bioactive compound in the aqueous extract of garlic is allicin (diallylthiosulfinate or allyl-2-propenethiosulfinate). Chopping or crushing garlic causes allinase, an enzyme found in garlic to be activated. The activation of allinase causes allicin to be produced from allin (S-allyl cysteine sulfoxide), which is found in intact garlic. Other biocompounds (Fig. 5.3) in garlic homogenate are y-L-glutamyl-S-alkyl-L-cysteine, (E, Z)-4,5,9-trithiadodeca-1,6,11-triene-9-oxide (ajoene), 1-propenyl-allyl-thiosulfonate, allyl-methyl-thiosulfonate.[5]

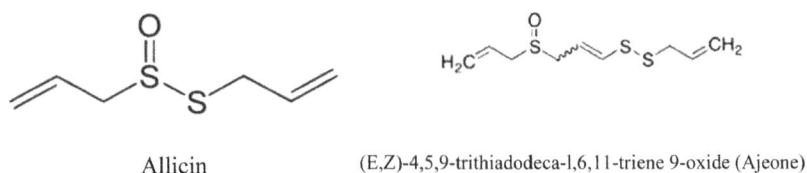

Allicin   (E,Z)-4,5,9-trithiadodeca-1,6,11-triene 9-oxide (Ajeone)

FIGURE 5.3 Major compounds in garlic.

Garlic oil, which is obtained from a steam distillation process, consists of the lipid-soluble allyl-sulfur compounds, which includes diallyl, allyl-methyl, and dimethyl mono to hexa sufides. Aged garlic extract (AGE) (obtained by storing sliced raw garlic in ethanol at a concentration of 15%–20% for more than a year) is another garlic preparation that has been widely used. The long period of storage causes significant breakdown of allicin and increases the activity of newly generated compounds, such as, N-0-(Ideoxy-D-fructose-1-yl)-L-arginine, allixin, S-allylcysteine, and sallylmercaptocysteine, which are relatively stable and possess significant antioxidant properties.[24]

5.4 TRADITIONAL USES OF GARLIC

5.4.1 *Culinary Uses*

Garlic is one the most important bulb vegetables, and is widely used as a spice and flavoring agent for foods because of its peculiar pungent flavor. Organosulfur compounds (such as allicin and DAS) account for the spicy aroma and lachrymatory effects of garlic. It is usually dehydrated into different forms, such as, slices, flakes, and powder.[35]

5.4.2 Therapeutic Uses

Therapeutic uses of *Allium sativum* goes back to 4000 years. The Egyptian papyrus of the Ebers Codex mentions 22 formulations of garlic as efficient remedies for cephalea, snake bites, and cardiac problems. In Greece, garlic was employed in the management of intestinal and pulmonary disorders. The garlic was used an antiseptic agent in the treatment of wounds and ulcers during the Second World War. Pliny the Elder, Galen, Dioscorides, and Hippocrates mentioned the use of garlic for parasitic infections, low vitality, and digestive and respiratory diseases. Garlic's notoriety in the practice of medicine in the west came to be known in 1858 as a result of Louis Pasteur's affirmation of its antibacterial effects.

Garlic has also been known to Traditional Chinese Medicine since A.D. 510 and it is still utilized in the management of scalp ringworm, amoebic and bacterial dysentery, vaginal trichomoniasis, and tuberculosis. Other Folkloric medicine cultures have customarily utilized garlic for the management of colds and influenza, fever, hacks, cerebral pain, asthma, arteriosclerosis, hemorrhoids, low-circulatory strain, both hyperglycemia and hypoglycemia and other malignancies.[33]

5.5 POTENTIAL USE OF GARLIC IN GASTROINTESTINAL DISORDERS

5.5.1 Gastrointestinal Neoplasms

Epidemiological studies bolster the claim that the intake of vegetables from the *Allium* genus (such as garlic) diminishes the risks of colorectal and stomach tumors.[9] Additionally, garlic has been proven to offer huge protection against gastric cancers in the Chinese populace caused by *Helicobacter pylori* disease.[38] Research has demonstrated the antibacterial and anticarcinogenic properties of garlic due to the presence of organosulfur compounds, such as DATS, DADS, and DAS, out of which DATS has demonstrated the most superior effect.[31,39]

In a study by Wang et al.,[37] sulferedoxin, malondialdehyde, and reactive oxygen species levels, which show a positive correlation with gastric cancer and tumor malignancy, were able to markedly inhibit the gastric cancer cell line BGC823 with DATS treatment. The conclusion of this study points to antioxidation as the possible mechanism of action of DATS.[37]

In another study to elucidate the molecular basis of the anticancer properties of garlic by utilizing HCT-15 and DLD-1 (which are human colon cancer cell lines), Chihara et al.[7] indicated that DATS disrupted microtubule network formation of cells. Possible involvement of the mitogen-activated protein kinase (MAPKS) pathways in the apoptosis induced by DATS has also been reported by Jiang et al.[16] based on the activation of c-Jun N-terminal Kinase (JNK), extracellular signal-regulated (ERK), and p38 phosphorylation in SGC-7901 cancer cells treated with DATS. They indicate that there may be several mechanisms of actions in the antineoplastic effect of garlic mediated by DATS.

Epidemiological data on the usage of garlic for primary prevention of gastric and colorectal neoplasms have not been correlated significantly with experimental studies. Garlic intake was protective for gastric cancer based on a study of Cangshan County of Shandong Province, which ranks lowest in terms of gastric cancer rates in China.[38]

Garlic intake has also been found to have an inverse association with gastric cancer from several case-control studies. A recently conducted meta-analysis incorporating 12 case-control studies yielded a relative risk of 0.60 with 95% confidence interval of 0.47–0.76 for the highest versus lowest category based on the intake of garlic. The Shandong Intervention Trial conducted in 2011 also confirmed the earlier studies. Antibiotic treatment for a duration of 2 weeks in *H. pylori* infection reduced the prevalence of precancerous gastric lesions. Garlic extract and oil (garlic treatment), selenium (vitamin treatment), vitamin E, and vitamin C failed to reduce the prevalence of *H. pylori*.

However, in a large prospective cohort study, Kim and Kwon[21] failed to provide the support for the assertion that high garlic intake reduces the risk of gastric cancer. This is supported by another study carried out by Hu et al.[12] on garlic intake or garlic supplement use in colorectal carcinogenesis.

5.5.2 Inflammatory Bowel Disease

Inflammatory bowel disease (IBD) refers to ulcerative colitis and Chron's disease that involves inflammation of chronic nature of the GI tract. The development of targeted, monoclonal antibody-based therapies has greatly improved the treatment of IBD. Key interventions have been the use of tumor necrosis factor antagonists, but its utilization has been associated with side effects and their efficacy has been shown to decrease with time.

The resort to nonconventional remedies, which includes nutraceuticals, has increased in recent times among the patients with IBD.[27]

Garlic is marketed in several countries as a dietary supplement for the management of inflammatory conditions including inflammatory bowel disease. Experimental studies to assess its effectiveness has therefore been carried out recently. Raw garlic has been shown to be beneficial in acetic acid-induced colitis in an in vivo study using rat models. Oral pretreatments of the rats with garlic @ 0.25 mg/kg body weight for four consecutive weeks to a large extent quelled the increase in colon weight induced by acetic acid and also helped to forestall changes in oxidant and antioxidant parameters.[10]

Based on the involvement of cytokines in inflammatory bowel disease, garlic has also been studied for its modulatory effects on cytokine production and leukocyte cell proliferation. The pro-inflammatory cytokines IL-8, I-1 alpha, IL-6, IL-2, IL-12, and tumor necrosis factor-alpha were significantly reduced. while IL-10 (anti-inflammatory cytokine) was upregulated in the presence of garlic extract from the in vitro analysis of whole blood and peripheral blood mononuclear cells.[11] In vivo studies on garlic oil and its effects on colitis-induced by endotoxin in Wistar rats showed that doses of 10 and 50 mg/kg bodyweight of garlic oil extract was successful in inhibiting neutrophil infiltration and in reducing serum levels for other inflammatory cytokines.[23] The immunomodulatory effects of garlic provide evidence of its possible role in the management of IBD.

5.5.3 Gastrointestinal Infections

Garlic in all its available forms (such as alcoholic and aqueous extracts, fresh garlic juice, steam-distilled oil, and other commercial preparations) has been found to have antibacterial effects.[32] Its broad-spectrum antibacterial actions have coverage against Gram-negative and Gram-positive organisms, such as *Staphylococcus*, *Streptococcus Micrococcus*, *Aerobacter*, *Citrobacter*, *Enterobacter*, *Aeromonas*, *Pseudomonas*, *Lactobacillus*, *Bacillus*, *Citrella*, *Clostridium*, *Escherichia*, *Salmonella*, *Shigella*, *Klebsiella*, *Leuconostoc*, *Mycobacterium*, *Proteus* and *Providencia*.[6,19,22]

In a study to assess the effects of garlic on *Salmonella typhi* infection and other gastrointestinal flora, it was found that the crude garlic extract inhibited the growth of *Salmonella typhi* with an inhibition zone diameter of about 24 mm from the agar diffusion assay. Conventional antibiotics (streptomycin, gentamycin, chloramphenicol, ofloxacin, erythromycin, penicillin, ampicillin, cloxacillin, and streptomycin) except streptomycin gave inferior inhibitions compared with crude garlic extract. Streptomycin rather gave a growth inhibitory value of 24 mm.

An in vivo study of the antibacterial activity of garlic in rats demonstrated that the consumption of crude garlic extracts resulted in a substantial (p<0.05) reduction in *Salmonella typhi* in the feces. The duration of infection was also a significant drop from 5 to 3 days. Feeding the rats with garlic @ 1 mL of the extract daily for 7 weeks resulted in a decrease in the number of microbial species to one from an initial six. Microbial flora load was also reduced significantly from 1.64×10^{12} to 1.3×10^7 cfu/mL.[2]

Several studies have also attested to the antibacterial properties of garlic against *H. pylori*, which has been thought to be the reason why stomach cancer incidence is low in populations in both developed and developing countries, where allium vegetable intake including garlic is high.[32] The various forms of garlic (such as garlic oil, garlic powder, etc.) and their diallyl compounds have been evaluated for their antibacterial activity against *H. pylori*. Results from these studies have shown significant anti-*H. pylori* activity against all the strains of the organism. O'Gara et al.[26] showed that the MIC (minimum inhibitory concentrations) and MBC (minimum bactericidal concentrations) of undiluted garlic oil were about 8–32 mcg/mL and 16–32 mcg/mL, respectively. However, this was lower as compared with garlic powder, which recorded both MIC and MBC of 250–500 mcg/mL.

Of the bioactive compounds, allicin demonstrated a high potency showing the MIC and MBC of 6 mcg/mL as compared with 100–200 mcg/mL of its corresponding sulfide, diallyl disulfide compounds. However, allicin's antibacterial activity was comparable to diallyl-tetrasulfide which has both MIC and MBC in the range of 3–6 mcg/mL. This reveals that the number of atoms of sulfur has an influence on the antimicrobial activity of diallyl sulfides with activity increasing with an increase in the number of atoms of sulfur.[26] Jonkers et al.[17] has also reported that the synergistic effect of garlic (raw garlic extract, commercially available garlic tablet) has with omeprazole based on studies on the killing curves of clinical isolates of *H. pylori*.

5.5.4   Gastrointestinal Ulcers

Akinbo et al.[3] reported the antiulcer effect of garlic on indomethacin-induced gastrointestinal injury among albino Wistar rats. In the study, 100–300 mg/kg of the aqueous garlic extract was sufficient to prevent macroscopic signs of ulceration or perforation.[3] In a similar study with AGE, pretreatment of male Wistar rats with the extract generated similar results with those obtained in the control group pretreated with omeprazole; and the preventive index in the AGE group was 83.4% as compared with 94.5% in the group pretreated with omeprazole

The gastroprotective properties of garlic oil against ulcers induced by ethanol and its involvement in holding back the oxidation process generated in gastric tissue was evaluated. Pretreatment doses of 0.25 and 0.5 mg/kg of garlic administered 30 min before ethanol administration caused lipid peroxidation and ulcer index to decrease and it forestalled the dwindling of antioxidant enzyme levels induced by ethanol thereby providing evidence that it can help to prevent ethanol-induced gastric injury.[20]

The DAS and DADS isolated from garlic serve as a source of hydrogen sulfide, which helps to maintain gastrointestinal mucosal defense and repair by acting as a gaseous mediator. In addition, DAS and DADS exhibited antioxidant action, which is important based on the observation that inflammation in gastrointestinal ulcers is driven by free radicals.[36]

5.5.5   Diarrhea

Research studies have shown the potential of garlic in the management of diarrhea of different etiologies. Joshi et al.[10] evaluated the effects of commercial garlic oil on gastrointestinal transit of castor oil and charcoal meal-induced diarrhea in an in vivo study in rats. They found that garlic oil at a concentration of 0.25% w/w demonstrated an approximate reduction of 75% in charcoal meal propulsion within the gastrointestinal tract ($p < 0.001$) at a dose of 0.1 mL/10 g. Garlic oil at the same dose was also successful in preventing the onset of diarrhea with only 17.6% of animals treated with garlic oil exhibiting a positive diarrheal response as against the 90% of the control group.[18] Although the exact mechanism of its antidiarrheal effect has not been elucidated, yet it has been thought to be due to its ability to relax the gastrointestinal smooth muscle. This is based on a study by Abdo et al.,[1] where it demonstrated the ability to cause relaxation of the smooth muscle of the uterus of guinea pigs thus showing its potential as an important remedy in patients suffering from hypermotility disorders in the gastrointestinal tract.

Aged garlic extract has also been studied as a possible remedy for the gastrointestinal intestinal side effects of the anticancer agent methotrexate. AGE has also been proven anti-inflammatory. The onset of diarrheas was reported for 40% of animals treated with Methotrexate + AGE as against Methotrexate-treated group. The study also provides evidence of the extract's ability to reduce gastrointestinal damage associated with methotrexate, which has been attributed to its antioxidant effects due to the presence of tetrahydro-βcarboline derivatives (THβCs) and S-Allyl cysteine (SAC).[13]

Eja et al.[8] highlighted the antimicrobial action of raw garlic extract against diarrheagenic organisms, such as, *Salmonella* sp, *Shigella* sp, *Proteus mirabilis* and *Escherichia coli*, which was comparable to ciprofloxacin. This has been attributed to the similarity in garlic's mechanism of action and that of ciprofloxacin. Allicin, the principal bioactive compound in garlic, has been shown to act by inhibiting DNA and protein synthesis and also halting RNA synthesis. Ciprofloxacin similarly interferes with DNA transcription and other activities involving DNA by inhibiting bacteria DNA gyrase.[30]

5.5.6   Gastritis

Gastritis describes the condition, where the stomach lining becomes inflamed, often resulting in discomfort. Prolongation of the inflammation causes atrophic gastritis (when the glands of the lining of the stomach) or ulcers to develop. Excess secretion of acid, autoimmune processes, *H. pylori* infection and damage induced by alcohol, nonsteroidal anti-inflammatory drugs and corticosteroids are underlying causes of gastritis. *H. pylori* are however thought to account for a majority of cases of gastritis. The antibacterial effects of garlic against *H. pylori* have been well established and confirmed in *in vitro* studies.

Iimuro et al.[15] evaluated the ability of garlic oil to suppress gastritis induced by *H. pylori* in Mongolian gerbils; and they concluded that garlic extract could be an important treatment agent. The garlic extract caused a dose-dependent decrement in *H. pylori* gastritis with most significant effect at a concentration of 4% of the extract. There was a reduction in hemorrhagic spot numbers in the glandular stomach from 19.2+/−15.6 to 8.1+/−11.2. The microscopic score for gastritis was also substantially reduced from 5.9+/−0.8 in the control gerbils to 4.2+/−1.5 in the garlic extract treated group.[15]

Karinat is a dietary supplement, which contains 5 mg of alpha-tocopherol, 30 mg of ascorbic acid, 150 mg of garlic powder, 2.5 mg of beta-carotene. It was taken through a randomized placebo-controlled and double-blind trial by patients suffering from chronic multifocal atrophic gastritis; and the study has been shown to improve digestion, the fibro-gastroscopic pattern of mucosa, to inhibit *H. pylori* infection, to stimulate stomach activity, to mitigate intestinal metaplasia and to interfere with the epithelial proliferation of gastric mucosa. This lends more credence to the possible role of garlic in the treatment of gastritis.[5]

5.6 SUMMARY

The literature supports the traditional use of *Allium sativum* (garlic) in the management of the gastrointestinal disorders. The bioactive compounds isolated from *Allium sativum* have demonstrated their efficacy through varied mechanisms of actions and these provide the basis for conducting further research to optimize their use.

KEYWORDS

- diarrhea
- garlic
- gastritis
- gastrointestinal neoplasms
- gastrointestinal ulcers
- *H. pylori*
- inflammatory bowel disease

REFERENCES

1. Abdo, M.S.; Al-Kafawi, A. A. Biological Activities of *Allium sativum*. *Japanese J. Pharmacol.* **1969**, *19* (1), 1–4.
2. Adebolu T.T.; Adeoye, O.O.; Oyetayo, V.O. Effect Of Garlic (*Allium sativum*) On *Salmonella typhi* Infection, Gastrointestinal Flora and Hematological Parameters of Albino Rats. *Afr. J. Biotechnol.* **2011**, *10* (35), 6804–6808.
3. Akinbo, F.; Eze, G. Combined Effects of Medicinal Plants on Induced Upper Gastrointestinal Tract Injury in Wistar Rats. *Ethiopian J. Health Sci.* **2016**, *26* (6), 573–580.
4. Bayan, L.; Koulivand, P.H.; Gorji, A. Garlic: A Review of Potential Therapeutic Effects. *Avicenna J. Phytomed.* **2014**, *4* (1), 1–14.
5. Berspalov, V.G.; Shcherbakov, A. Study of Antioxidant Drug "Karinat" in Patients with Chronic Atrophic Gastritis. *Voprosyonkologii* (Oncology issues) **2004**, *50* (1), 81–85.
6. Caldwell, D. R.; Danzer, C. J. Effects of Allyl Sulfides on Growth of Predominant Gut Anaerobes. *Curr. Microbiol.* **1988**, *16* (5), 237–241.
7. Chihara, T.; Shimpo, K.; Kaneko, T. Inhibition of 1,2-Dimethylhydrazine- Induced Mucin - Depleted Foci and O-6 -Methylguanine DNA Adducts in Rat Colorectum By Boiled Garlic Powder. *Asian Pacific J. Cancer Prev.: APJCP* **2010**, *11* (5), 1301–1304.
8. Eja, M.E.; Asikong, B.E.; Abriba, C.; Arikpo, G.E. Comparative Assessment of the Antimicrobial Effects of Garlic (*Allium sativum*) and Antibiotics on Diarrheagenic Organisms. *Southeast Asian J. Trop. Med. Public Health* **2007**, *38* (2), 343–348.
9. Fleischauer, A. T.; Poole, C.; Arab, L. Garlic Consumption and Cancer Prevention: Meta-Analyses of Colorectal and Stomach Cancers. *Am. J. Clin. Nutr.* **2000**, *72* (4), 1047–1052.
10. Harisa, G. E.; Abo-Salem, O. M.; El-Sayed, S. M.; Taha, E. I. L-arginine Augments the Antioxidant Effect of Garlic Against Acetic Acid-Induced Ulcerative Colitis in Rats. *Pak. J. Pharm. Sci.* **2009**, *22* (4), 373–380.
11. Hodge, G.; Hodge, S.; Han, P. *Allium sativum* Suppresses Leukocyte Inflammatory Cytokine Production *In Vitro*: Potential Therapeutic Use in the Treatment of Inflammatory Bowel Disease. *Cytometry* **2002**, *48* (4), 209–215.
12. Hu, J.; Hu, Y.; Zhou, J.; Zhang, M.; Li, D.; Zheng, S. Consumption of Garlic and Risk of Colorectal Cancer: An Updated Meta-Analysis of Prospective Studies. *World J. Gastroenterol.* **2014**, *20* (41), 15413–15422.
13. Iciek, M.; Kwiecień, I.; Włodek, L. Biological Properties of Garlic and Garlic-Derived Organosulfur Compounds. *Environ. Mol. Mutagenesis* **2009**, *50* (3), 247–265.
14. Ide, N.; Ichikawa, M.; Ryu, K.; Ogasawara, K. Antioxidants in Processed Garlic, Part II: Tetrahydro-B-Carboline Derivatives Identified in Aged Garlic Extract. *Int. Congress Ser.* **2002**, *1245*, 449–450.
15. Iimuro, M.; Shibata, H.; Kawamori, T. Suppressive Effects of Garlic Extract on Helicobacter Pylori-Induced Gastritis in Mongolian Gerbils. *Cancer Lett.* **2002**, *187* (1–2), 61–68.
16. Jiang, X.; Zhu, X.; Huang, W.; Xu, H.; Zhao, Z. Garlic-Derived Organosulfur Compound Exerts Antitumor Efficacy via Activation of MAPK Pathway and Modulation of Cytokines In SGC-7901 Tumor-Bearing Mice. *Int. Immunopharmacol.* **2017**, *48*, 135–145.

17. Jonkers, D.; Vanden-Broek, E.; VanDooren, I. Antibacterial Effect of Garlic and Omeprazole on Helicobacter Pylori. *J. Antimicrob. Chemotherap.* **1999,** *43* (6), 837–839.

18. Joshi, D. J.; Dikshit, R. K.; Mansuri, S. M. Gastrointestinal Actions of Garlic Oil. *Phytotherap. Res.* **1987,** *1* (3), 140–145.

19. Kabelik, J.; Hejtmankova-Uhrova, N. The Antifungal and Antibacterial Effects of Certain Drugs and Other Substances. *Veterinary Med. (Pragu)* **1968,** *13,* 295–303.

20. Khosla, P.; Karan, R. S.; Bhargava, V. K. Effect of Garlic Oil on Ethanol Induced Gastric Ulcers in Rats. *Phytotherap. Res.* **2004,** *18* (1), 87–91.

21. Kim J.Y.; Kwon, O. Garlic Intake and Cancer Risk: An Analysis Using the Food and Drug Administration's Evidence-Based Review System for the Scientific Evaluation of Health Claims. *Am. J. Clin. Nutr.* **2009,** 89 (1), 257–264,

22. Kumar, A.; Sharma, V.D. Inhibitory Effect of Garlic (*Allium Sativum* Linn.) on Entero toxigenic *Escherichia coli. Ind. J. Med. Res.* **1982,** *76* (Supp. l), 66–70.

23. Kuo, C.H.; Lee, S.H.; Chen, K.M.; Lii, C.K. Effect of Garlic Oil on Neutrophil Infiltration in the Small Intestine of Endotoxin-Injected Rats and its Association with Levels of Soluble and Cellular Adhesion Molecules. *J. Agric. Food Chem,* **2011,** *59* (14), 7717–7725

24. Lawson, L.D.; Bauer, R. Garlic: Review of Its Medicinal Effects and Indicated Active Compounds. In *Phytomedicines of Europe. Chemistry and Biological Activity, Series 69–1*; Washington, DC: American Chemical Society, 1998; pp 176–209.

25. Morales-González, J. A. Garlic (*Allium Sativum* L.): A Brief Review of its Antigenotoxic Effects. *Foods* **2019,** *8* (8), 343–347.

26. O'Gara, E. A.; Hill, D. J.; Maslin, D. J. Activities of Garlic Oil, Garlic Powder and their Diallyl Constituents against *Helicobacter Pylori. Appl. Environ. Microbiol.* **2000,** *66* (5), 2269–2273.

27. Opheim, R.; Hoivik, M.L.; Solberg, I.C.; Moum, B. Complementary and Alternative Medicine in Patients with Inflammatory Bowel Disease: The Results of a Population-Based Inception Cohort Study (IBSEN). *J. Crohn's Colitis* **2012,** *6* (3), 345–353.

28. Petrovska, B.; Cekovska, S. Extracts from the History and Medical Properties of Garlic. *Pharmacognosy Rev.* **2010,** *4* (7), 6–10.

29. Philippine medicinal Plants—Garlic. http://www.stuartxchange.com/Bawang.html; (accessed on Dec 18, 2019)

30. Prescott L.M.; Harley J.P.; Klein D.A. *Microbiology*, 6th ed.; Boston: McGraw-Hill, 2005; p 992.

31. Seki, T.; Hosono, T.; Hosono-Fukao, T. Anticancer Effects of Diallyl Trisulfide Derived from Garlic. *Asia Pacific J. Clin. Nutr.* **2008,** *17* (1), 249–252.

32. Sivam, G. P. Protection against *Helicobacter Pylori* and Other Bacterial Infections by Garlic. *J. Nutr.* **2001,** *131* (3), 1106S–1108S.

33. Tattelman, E. Health Effects of Garlic. *Am. Fam. Phys.* **2005,** *72* (1), 103.

34. UMM. Garlic Effects on GI; University of Maryland Medical Center, 2004; p 8.

35. Velíšek, J.; Kubec, R.; Davídek, J. Chemical Composition and Classification of Culinary and Pharmaceutical Garlic-Based Products. *Zeitschrift for Lebensmitteluntersuchung und -Forschung A (J. Food Inspec. Res. A)* **1997,** *204* (2), 161–164.

36. Wallace, J. L. Physiological and Pathophysiological Roles of Hydrogen Sulfide in Gastrointestinal Tract. *Antioxidants Redox Signal.* **2010,** *12* (9), 1125–1133.

37. Wang, J.; Si, L.; Wang, G.; Bai, Z.; Li, W. Increased Sulfiredoxin Expression in Gastric Cancer Cells May be a Molecular Target of the Anticancer Component Diallyl Trisulfide. *BioMed Res. Int.* **2019,** *2019,* 1–8.

38. You, W. *Helicobacter Pylori* Infection, Garlic Intake and Precancerous Lesions in a Chinese Population at Low Risk of Gastric Cancer. *Int. J. Epidemiol.* **1998,** *27* (6), 941–944.

39. Zhou, Y.; Zhuang, W.; Hu, W.; Liu, G.; Wu, T.; Wu, X. Consumption of Large Amounts of *Allium* Reduces Risk for Gastric Cancer in a Meta-Analysis. *Gastroenterology* **2011,** *141* (1), 80–89.

CHAPTER 6

Role of Onion (*Allium cepa*) in Gastrointestinal Disorders

YAW DUAH BOAKYE, RICHARD AGYEN, EUGENE KUSI AGYEI, DANIEL OBENG MENSAH, DOREEN KWANKYEWAA ADJEI, and CHRISTIAN AGYARE

ABSTRACT

Onion is widely used as ethnomedicine with several health benefits, such as antiviral, antidiabetic, antihyperlipidemic, antithrombotic, antioxidant, and anti-inflammatory activity. This review chapter identifies studies on *Allium cepa* for its activity against gastrointestinal disorders, such as gastrointestinal neoplasms, gastrointestinal ulcers, diarrhea, and helminthic, etc.

6.1 HISTORICAL ASPECTS OF ONION

Onion (*Allium cepa* L.) is consumed and grown worldwide and is the most cultivated vegetable after tomato.[14] The word onion originated from the Latin word "*unus*," which means one. It was later introduced in the United Kingdom by Romans, and from there probably got to Americas.[6] Onion was suggested as a laxative, emmenagogue, and a diuretic by Hippocrates, and was also used for healing wounds and treatment of pneumonia.[19]

A. cepa belongs to the family Liliaceae, which is composed of >252 genera and 3600 species. They possess rhizomes, bulbs, and tubers, which enable them to grow or survive under very harsh conditions. Naturally, plants that contain tannins as their main components are often used for the treatment of dysentery and diarrhea.[3] Corea et al. listed 30 disorders for which onion could be used to treat.[8] There is an inverse association between the risk of human diseases and onion consumption based on several epidemiological studies.

This chapter focuses on healing benefits of onion (*A. cepa*) in the management of gastrointestinal disorders.

6.2   ONION DESCRIPTION AND PROFILING

Onion is one of the largest perennial flowering herbaceous plants in its genera.[33] *A. sativum* (garlic), *A. Chinense* (scallion), *A. hookeri* (hooker chive), *A. ascalonicum* (shallot), *A. schoenoprasum L.* (chives), *A. cepa, L.* (onion), and *A. ampeloprasum* (leek) are examples of the many species of *Allium*[4] that have been utilized over the years as ornaments, vegetables, and spices and in ethnomedicine. Members of this genus contain sulfur compounds and enriched substantive oil,[5] which confers unique taste and healing properties to different species.[24]

The onion plant consists of tubular leaves, a bulb, and fibrous adventitious roots.[30] In the second cycle of the plant's life, the stem grows up to about 50–100 cm. Onion contains an umbel-like inflorescence, which contains from 200 to 600 small singly flowers.[35] Onion has 16 chromosomes in its diploid state. Vernacular names of *A. cepa* are mentioned below:

- Albanians: Qepe
- Arabic: Basal
- Armenian: Soch
- Azerbaijan: Sogan
- Bosnian: Crni, Luk, Sogan, Crveni, Zvibel
- Bulgarian: Ognon
- Chinese: Chhang, Cong Tou
- Dutch: Ajuin, Ui
- Estonian: Sibul
- French: Oignon
- German: Bolle, Gartenzwiebel, Zwiebel, Sommerzwiebel
- Hebrew: Bazal, Besalim
- Hungarian: Hagyma
- Indian: Piyaj, Palandu, Kando, Pyaaz, Nirulli, Erra
- Italian: Cipolla
- Japanese: Tamanegi, Tama Negi, Tamane
- Korean: Dungulpha, Yangp'a

- Malaysian: Bawang, Bawang Besar, Bawang Merah
- Persian: Piyaaz
- Philippines: Sibuyas, Si-Bolyas
- Polish: Cebula, Cebula-Jadalna, Cebula-Zwyczajna
- Russian: Louk Zepchatnyi, Louk Repka

6.3 DISTRIBUTION OF ONION PLANT

Onion is substantially cultivated as a biennial bulb crop largely in China and India. Countries including Brazil, Turkey, Iran, USA, Pakistan, the Russian Federation, Republic of Korea and Egypt also cultivate onion.[14] The Republic of Korea has the highest onion productivity, followed by USA, Spain, and the Netherlands. The mean productivity of onion in the world is about 19.8 tons/ha. The Netherlands exports greatest amount of onion worldwide with Argentina exporting the least (Table 6.1).[14]

TABLE 6.1 Top 10 Onion Producing Countries in the World.

Country	Onion Production (tons)
Republic of Korea	1,411,650
Russia	1,536,300
Brazil	1,556,000
Pakistan	1,701,100
Turkey	1,900,000
Iran	1,922,970
Egypt	2,208,080
USA	3,320,870
India	13,372,100
China	20,507,759

6.4 NUTRITIONAL VALUE OF ONION

Onion leaves can be used for dietary purpose. The leaves are used for preparing food, while the flowers are used in preparing salads.[7] Onion is highly rich in various important nutrients, vitamins and minerals, all amino acids except glutamine and asparagine,[37] and high levels of vitamin A and vitamin K (which are cofactors (coenzymes)), hence may improve cell functions when consumed (Table 6.2).[12,34]

TABLE 6.2　Nutritional Composition and Proximate Values of Onion Bulbs (per 100 g).

Component	Mean value (unit)
Proximate	
Energy	40 (kcal)
Sugar total	4.24(g)
Carbohydrates	0.34 (g)
Fiber	1.7 (g)
Lipids	0.1 (g)
Protein	1.1 (g)
Water	89.11 (g)
Vitamins	
Folate	19 (µg)
Thiamine	0.046 (mg)
Vitamin A	2 (IU)
Vitamin C	7.4 (mg)
Vitamin E	0.02 (mg)
Vitamin K	0.4 (µg)
Minerals	
Calcium	23 (mg)
Iron	0.21 (mg)
Phosphorus	29 (mg)
Potassium	146 (mg)
Sodium	4 (mg)
Zinc	0.17 (mg)
Lipids	
Palmitic acid	0.034 (g)
Phytosterols	15 (mg)
Stearic acid	0.004 (g)
Total monounsaturated acids	0.013 (g)
Total polyunsaturated acids	0.017 (g)
Total saturated acids	0.42

6.5　TRADITIONAL USES OF ONION

6.5.1　Culinary Use

Onions are usually chopped and utilized as ingredients in several dishes, but sometimes used as main ingredient, for example, in onion rings, creamed onions, and onion chutney. Onion is usually eaten boiled, baked, raw in salads, and roasted. Sometimes, they are eaten as snacks by pickling in vinegar, and as side servings in pubs throughout the United Kingdom.

6.5.2 Nonculinary Use

The large cells of onions help in educational settings, especially in laboratories to view them under the microscope during experiment and also for breeding purpose.[40,44]

6.5.3 Medicinal Use

Onions contain important phytochemicals that are potent against many medical conditions including cancers, diarrhea, and ulcers. According to Dini et al.[11] while determining the constituents of red onion, it was revealed that onions possess strong antioxidant properties.

6.6 PHYTOCHEMICAL CONSTITUENTS OF ONION

Onion is known to contain quercetin, flavonoid, trace minerals, and chromium,[27,29] but saponins, quercetin, and anthocyanin are the primary phytochemicals. They contain sulfur compounds, such as allyl-propyl-disulfide that gives the pungent smell.[22,37] S-propenylcysteine sulfoxide (major component), S-methylcysteine sulfoxide, S-propylcysteine sulfoxide, and dipropyl disulfide are organosulfur compounds, which are found in onion.[13,43]

6.7 PHARMACOLOGICAL ACTIVITIES

Based on attestations from several investigations, onions have biological and medical functions primarily because of their high concentration of organosulfur compounds[41] with health benefits, such as

- anti-inflammatory activity,[38]
- antibacterial,[24]
- antidiabetic,[25]
- antifungal,[28]

- antihyperlipidemic,[17]
- antihypertensive,[2]
- antioxidant,[9,10] and
- antiviral.[32]

Based on several research studies and clinical trials, onion can be used to treat many disorders, such as, hypercholesterolemia,[20] asthma,[15] diabetes,[15,16,37] viral diseases,[30,32] cancer,[9] and osteoporosis.[1,3]

6.7.1   Gastrointestinal (GI) Neoplasm

The flavonoids in *A. cepa* inhibit proliferation or growth of colorectal cancer at very high doses and aid in treating hyperlipidemic colorectal cancer also at high doses.[17] Hence, onion can reduce blood fat and protect heart and blood vessels based on their deductions.[23,31] The flavonoids from onion can help in regulating the level of low-density lipoprotein (LDL).

Onion consumption has been seen to have an inverse association with stomach cancer risk in Shanghai and Qingdao, China.[36] As onion consumption was increased, there was a decrease in distal stomach cancer risk.

6.7.2   Gastrointestinal Ulcer

Onion consumption can prevent ethanol-induced gastric ulcers.[36] When onion is consumed, glutathione S-transferase activity is increased in all tissues due to the incorporation of the organosulfur compounds (S-propenylcysteine sulfoxide (major component), S- methylcysteine sulfoxide, S-propylcysteine sulfoxide, and dipropyl disulfide).[16,36,39,43] Thus, the gastric mucosa was protected by combining the usage of garlic and onion due to increase in glutathione S-tranferase levels, which in turn could increase prostaglandin synthesis leading to cytoprotection.

6.7.3   Diarrhea

The onion has shown an effective antidiarrheal activity in rats.[21] The aqueous extract of onion tested at 150 and 300 mg/kg gave an effect similar to that of standard drug, loperamide, which inhibited the rate of defecation droppings compared with the untreated rats. It was postulated that onion contains significant amounts of tannins and tannic acid, which can denature proteins thus forming protein tannate. This was able to increase the resistance of the intestinal mucosa and to reduce secretion.[42]

Quercetin and taxifolin were also identified by Corea et al.[8] to affect the gastrointestinal tract due to antispasmodic, antiulcer, and antidiarrheal propeties.[9,10]

6.7.4   Helminth Infection

A research study indicated that the coconut powder together with onion was efficient against both nematodes and cestodes in sheep.[16] This synergistic effect was also effective in the hatching stages of eggs and the adult stages of the parasites.

6.8   SUMMARY

This chapter has shown evidence to justify the traditional use of onion in the management of gastrointestinal disorders, such as gastrointestinal ulcers, gastrointestinal neoplasms, diarrhea, and helminthic infections. Literature has provided the scientific basis for its continuous use and the avenue for further research toward the discovery of potential drug candidates.

KEYWORDS

- *Allium cepa*
- flavonoids
- onion
- quercetin
- sulfur

REFERENCES

1. Aiyegoro, O. A.; Akinpelu, D. A.; Afolayan, A. J.; Okoh, A.I. Antibacterial Activities of Crude Stem Bark Extracts of *Distemonanthus benthamianus* Baill. *J. Biol. Sci.* **2008,** *8* (2), 356–361.

2. Amalia, L.; Sukandar, E.; Roesli, R.; Sigit, J. The Effect of Ethanol Extract of Kucai (*Allium schoenoprasum* L.) Bulbs on Serum Nitric Oxide Level in Male Wistar Rats. *Int. J. Pharmacol.* **2008,** *4* (6), 487–491.

3. American Chemical Society. Onion Compound May Help Fight Osteoporosis. *Sci. Daily.* (**2005,** April 11); www.sciencedaily.com/releases/2005/04/050411112150.htm; accessed on April 30, 2020.

4. Amir, N.; Dhaheri, A.A.; Jaberi, N.A.; Marzouqi, F.A.; Bastaki, S.M. Comparative Effect of Garlic (*Allium sativum*), Onion (*Allium cepa*), and Black Seed (*Nigella sativa*) on Gastric Acid Secretion and Gastric Ulcer. *Res. Rep. Med. Chem.* **2011,** *1*, 3–9.

5. Barazani, O.; Dudai, N.; Khadka, U.R.; Golan-Goldhirsh, A. Cadmium Accumulation in *Allium schoenoprasum* Grown in an Aqueous Medium. *Chemosphere* **2004,** *57*, 1213–1218.

6. Burnie, G.; Forrester, S.; Greig, D. *Botanica: The Illustrated A-Z of over 10,000 Garden Plants*, 3rd ed.; Random House: New South Wales, 1999; p 74.

7. Charles, D.J. *Antioxidant Properties of Spices, Herbs and Other Sources*; New York, NY: Springer- Verlag, 2013; pp 225–230.

8. Corea, G.; Fattorusso, E.; Lanzotti, V.; Capasso, R.; Izzo, A. A. Antispasmodic Saponins from Bulbs of Red Onion (*Allium cepa* L.) var. Tropea. *J. Agric. Food Chem.* **2005,** *53* (4), 935–940.

9. Craig, W. J. Health-Promoting Properties of Common Herbs. *Am. J. Clin. Nutr.* **1999,** *70* (3), 491–499.

10. Di Carlo, G.; Mascolo, N.; Izzo, A. A.; Capasso, F. Flavonoids: Old and New Aspects of Class of Natural Therapeutic Drugs. *Life Sci.* **1999,** *65* (4), 337–353.

11. Dini, I.; Tenore, G. C.; Dini, A. Chemical Composition, Nutritional Value and Antioxidant Properties of *Allium cepae* L. Var. Tropeana (Red Onion) Seeds. *Food Chem.* **2008,** *107* (2), 613–621.

12. DiNicolantonio, J.J.; Bhutani J.; O'Keefe, J.H. The Health Benefits of Vitamin K. *Open Heart* **2015,** 2, article ID: e000300.

13. Dorsch, W.; Schneider, E.; Bayer, T.; Breu, W.; Wagner, H. Anti-Inflammatory Effects of Onions: Inhibition of Chemotaxis of Human Polymorphonuclear Leukocytes by Thiosulfinates and Cepaenes. *Int. Arch. Allerg. Immunol.* **1990,** *92* (1), 39–42.

14. Edwards, S. J.; Musker, D. The Analysis of s-alk(en)yl-L-Cysteine Sulphoxides (Flavor Precursors) from Species Ofallium by High Performance Liquid Chromatography. *Phytochem. Analy.* **1994,** *5* (1), 4–9.

15. Egert, M.; Tevini, M. Influence of Drought on Some Physiological Parameters Symptomatic for Oxidative Stress in Leaves of Chives (*Allium schoenoprasum*). *Environ. Exp. Bot.* **2002,** *48* (1), 43–49.

16. FAO. World Onion Production. Rome: Food and Agriculture Organization (FAO) of the United Nations, 2012; http://faostat.fao.org; accessed on April 30, 2020.

17. He, Y.; Jin, H.; Zhang, C.; Gong, W.; Zhou, A. Effect of Onion Flavonoids on Colorectal Cancer with Hyperlipidemia: An In Vivo Study. *OncoTargets Therap.* **2014**, *7*, 101–110.
18. Kadan, S.; Saad, B.; Sasson, Y.; Zaid, H. In Vitro Evaluations of Cytotoxicity of Eight Antidiabetic Medicinal Plants and Their Effect on GLUT4 Translocation. *Evidence-Based Complem. Altern. Med.* **2013**, *2013*, 1–9.
19. Klimpel, S.; Abdel-Ghaffar, F.A. The Effects of Different Plant Extracts on Nematodes. *Parasitol. Res.* **2010**, *108*, 1047–1054.
20. Koch, H.P.; Lawson, L.D. *Garlic: The Science and Therapeutic Application of Allium sativum L. and Related Species*, 2nd ed.; Williams & Wilkins: Baltimore, MD, 1996; pp 19–24.
21. Kumar, K. R.; Shaik, A.; Gopal, J. V.; Raveesha, P. Evaluation of Antidiarrhoeal Activity of Aqueous Bulb Extract of *Allium cepa* Against Castor Oil-Induced Diarrhoea. *Int. J. Herb. Med.* **2013**, *1* (3), 64–67.
22. Kumari, K.; Augusti, K.T. Lipid Lowering Effect of S-Methyl Cysteine Sulfoxide from *Allium cepa* Linn in High Cholesterol Diet-fed Rats. *J. Ethnopharmacol.* **2007**, *109* (3), 367–371.
23. Liliana, G.; Rodica. D.; Camelia.N.; Loredana. D. Sulphur Compound Identification and Quantification from Allium Spp. Fresh Leaves. *J. Food Drug Analy.* **2014**, *22* (4), 425–430.
24. Majewska-Wierzbicka, M.; Czeczot, H. Flavonoids in the Prevention and Treatment of Cardiovascular Diseases. *Pol Merkur Lekarski* **2012**, *32* (187), 50–54.
25. Mehlhorn, H.; Al-Quraishy, S. Addition of A Combination of Onion (*Allium cepa*) and Coconut (*Cocos nucifera*) to Food of Sheep Stops Gastrointestinal Helminthic Infections. *Parasitol. Res.* **2010**, *108* (4), 1041–1046.
26. Mnayer, D.; Fabiano-Tixier, A.S. Chemical Composition, Antibacterial and Antioxidant Activities of Six Essentials Oils from the Alliaceae Family. *Molecules* **2014**, *19*, 20034–20053.
27. Pareek, S.; Sagar, N.A.; Sharma, S.; Kumar, V. Onion (*Allium Cepa* L.). In *Fruit and Vegetable Phytochemicals: Chemistry and Human Health*; Yahia, E.M., Eds., Vol. 2, 2nd ed.; John Wiley & Sons Ltd.: New York, USA, 2018; pp 1145–1161.
28. Pârvu, A.E.; Pârvu, M.; Vlase, L. Anti-inflammatory Effects of *Allium schoenoprasum* L. Leaves. *J. Physiol. Pharmacol.* **2014**, *65* (2), 309–315.
29. Platt, E.S. *Garlic, Onion and Other Alliums*; Mechanicsburg, PA: Stackpole Books, 2003; p 71.
30. Ranjitkar, H.D. (Ed.). *Handbook of Practical Botany*; Arun Kumar Ranjitkar: Kathmandu, 2003; p 319.
31. Rao, J. J.; Jin, H.; Pang, J.X. The Lipid-Lower Effect of Onion's Extraction on Hyperlipidemia Mice. *J. Branch Camp. First Military Med.* **2004**, *27* (2), 103–104.
32. Rastogi, R.P.; Dhawan, B.N. Anticancer and Antiviral Activities in Indian Medicinal Plants: A Review. *Drug Dev. Res.* **1990**, *19* (1), 1–12.
33. Rattanachaikunsopon, P.; Phumkhachorn, P. Diallyl Sulfide Content and Antimicrobial Activity Against Food-Borne Pathogenic Bacteria of Chives (*Allium schoenoprasum*). *Biosci. Biotechnol. Biochem.* **2008**, *72* (11), 2987–2991.
34. Ross, A. C.; Gardner, E. M. The Function of Vitamin A in Cellular Growth and Differentiation and its Roles During Pregnancy and Lactation. *Adv. Exp. Med. Biol.* **1994**, *352*, 187–200.

35. Ross, I.A. *Medicinal Plants of the World: Chemical Constituents, Traditional and Modern Medicinal Uses*, Vol. 2; Humana: Totowa, NJ, 2001; pp 3–9.

36. Setiawan, V.W.; Yu, G.; Lu, Q. Allium Vegetables and Stomach Cancer Risk in China. *Asian Pacific Journal of Cancer Prevention* **2005**, *6* (3), 387–395.

37. Sharma, K.K.; Gupta, R.K.; Gupta, S.; Samuel, K.C. Antihyperglycemic Effect of Onion: Effect on Fasting Blood Sugar and Induced Hyperglycemia in Men. *Indian Journal of Medical Research* **1977**, *65* (3), 422–429.

38. Sima, N.; Mahdieh, A.; Narges, K. Evaluation of Analgesic and Anti-Inflammatory Effects of Fresh Onion Juice in Experimental Animals. *Afr. J. Pharm. Pharmacol.* **2012**, *6* (23), 1679–1684.

39. Sparnins, V.L.; Barany, G.; Wattenberg, I.W. Effects of Organosulfur Compounds From Garlic and Onions of Benzopyrone-Induced Neoplasia and Glutathione S-Transferase Activity in Mouse. *Carcinogenesis.* **1988**, *9*, 131–134.

40. Suslov, D.; Verbelen, J.P.; Vissenberg, K. Onion Epidermis as New Model to Study the Control of Growth Anisotropy in Higher Plants. *J. Exp. Bot.* **2009**, *60* (14), 4175–4187.

41. Tocmo, R.; Liang, D.; Lin, Y.; Huang, D. Chemical and Biochemical Mechanisms Underlying the Cardioprotective Role of Dietary Organopolysulfides. *Front. Nutr.* **2015**, *2*, 1–6.

42. Tripathi, K.D., Ed. *Essentials of Medical Pharmacology*; Jaypee Brothers Medical Publishers: New Delhi, 1994; p 775.

43. Virtanen, A. I.; Matikkala, E. J.; Laland, S. Isolation of S-Methylcysteine - Sulphoxide and S-N-Propylcysteine-Sulfoxide from Onion (*Allium cepa*) and the Antibiotic Activity of Crushed Onion. *Acta Chem. Scand.* **1959**, *13*, 1898–1900.

44. Xu, K.; Huang, X.; Wu, M. Efficient and Economical Method of Agrobacterium— Mediated in Planta Transient Transformation in Onion Epidermis. *Plos One* **2014**, *9* (1), article ID: e83556.

CHAPTER 7

Role of Lectins in Gastrointestinal Disorders

HUGH JAMES FREEMAN

ABSTRACT

The intestinal tract is particularly useful for the topographic evaluation of normal epithelial cells that undergo increasing differentiation and maturation. Topographic mapping of the intestinal tract has been done as stem cells in the base of intestinal crypts divide and migrate toward the lumen. The aim of this chapter is to review the role of lectins in nature, their binding to receptors in normal, premalignant and malignant intestinal cells along with other intestinal diseases, and finally, it addresses some of the potential directions for future research.

7.1 INTRODUCTION

Lectins are proteins derived largely from plants and some animals, that they bind to specific sugar residues in tissues including the intestinal tract. Using lectin histochemical methods, the gastrointestinal tract has been explored to define the location of carbohydrate-containing structures. In addition, there are alterations in disease states, including the poorly differentiated, but nonmalignant, epithelial cells in celiac disease, and malignant intestinal epithelial cell disorders in cancer.

Reported changes in the normal upper gastrointestinal (GI) tract are reviewed including changes with different diseases, particularly malignancy. In addition, some future directions in evolving technical methods are mentioned to permit future evaluation in conjunction with lectin histochemical methods.

This chapter will review some of the lectin histochemical work focused on premalignant and malignant diseases of the gastrointestinal tract.

7.2   LECTINS IN NATURE

Lectins are proteins or glycoproteins that are largely derived from plants, although some have been detected in animals, including some invertebrates. An important family of mammalian lectins are the selectins that are critical in lymphocyte migration and homing during immune surveillance. Most important for humans, lectins are often found in foods and food products, such as peas, beans, potatoes, soybeans, tomatoes, and wheat germ. Although their role in nature has not been precisely defined for each lectin, yet some appear to have potent biological properties.

Some proteins play a role in biological recognition, attachment and binding to specific targets. This binding is very specific for sugar residues and appears to be largely dependent on their ability to attach to surface sugar-containing structures along the length of the mammalian, and particularly, human intestinal tract. Subsequent to binding to their intended targets, lectins may (1) cause agglutination of fetal or neoplastic cells, (2) stimulate lymphocyte proliferation, and (3) inhibit tumor growth both in vivo and in vitro.[52] Given this information, it is difficult to ignore the possible positive role of lectins.

In nature, lectins may provide some protection against harmful agents (e.g., fungal invasion). Other lectins may act in a negative fashion as potent toxins, such as ricin (an agent used by terrorists). Previously, their sugar specificity has been used in the laboratory analysis of blood types and in genetic engineering of crops to aid in the promotion of resistance to pests and diseases. In animals and humans, evidence indicates that lectins bind to the surface of normal and diseased tissues. Evaluation of the binding patterns in these tissues has been of particular interest during the past 2–3 decades especially with discovery and application of lectin histochemical methods to determine if binding patterns may be altered in disease, particularly in disorders of the intestinal tract.

Often, a lectin specificity may focus on a simple sugar residue, occasionally a series of sugars, as in a disaccharide or trisaccharide, and this may be reflected in the sugars that inhibit binding. However, lectins may actually recognize a larger or more complicated sugar-containing three-dimensional structure. As a result, lectins may have the same sugar specificity but may yield different or distinctive binding profiles.[47] In a breast cancer study, for example, application of 26 different lectins, specific for the N-acetyl-D-galactosamine sugar, produced different binding patterns.[29]

7.3   TOPOGRAPHIC BINDING IN THE NORMAL INTESTINAL TRACT

Lectins may be linked to markers, such as fluorescein, peroxidase, rhodamine and electron dense markers, and are used to evaluate the topographic distribution of binding along the length of the gastrointestinal tract. Simply, the intestinal tract epithelium lines the lumen from the mouth through the stomach and small/large intestine. Multiple cell types are present, particularly in different areas of the GI tract. In addition, developmental structures that emerged from the intestinal tract during fetal life, such as the pancreas and biliary tract are also lined with epithelial cells. Many of these cells have been subjected to intense anatomical study and contain different intracellular structures, including a luminal membrane lipid bilayer. Inserted into this membrane are proteins and lipids with attached sugar residues, so-called membrane or structural glycoproteins. Some of these function in the GI tract as recognition molecules, others as enzymes involved in nutrient digestion and transport uptake into epithelial cells, and eventually into the circulation.

Some epithelial cells are highly specialized, including goblet cells that produce mucous, consisting of mucin-type glycoproteins, eventually being secreted from these cells into the lumen. These membrane and mucin components of the GI tract may be mapped by labeling with lectins to define the topographic localization of different lectins (and their specific sugar residues) along the length of the GI tract. To some extent, these can be viewed as a form of evaluation or mapping of carbohydrate structures, potentially providing an increased dimension of specificity compared with traditional methods, such as staining with periodic acid Schiff or Alcan blue. Some of these individual lectins and their distribution in the GI tract have been explored and will be discussed later in this chapter.

Some of these proteins associated with the epithelial cell membrane may not be an integral part of the membrane or cell structure, but may also represent complex products resulting from the luminal digestive process or sloughed cellular products associated with the continuous epithelial cell renewal process. These ultimately find their way into the intestinal lumen itself and then may be adsorbed to the luminal cell surface. Very little quantitative or qualitative information is available on the source and derivation of much of the intestinal luminal content. Further studies in future are needed to elucidate this important component of intestinal epithelial cell biology along with their implications in human health.

The intestinal epithelial cells are very heterogenous and this inherently hinders the analysis of lectin-binding evaluation. In part, this reflects their site along the length of the intestinal tract. In some sites, the epithelium consists of stratified squamous in type, while in others, most mucus-producing cells are columnar cell-type. In addition to the topographic differentiation in epithelial cells based on their site along the length of the intestinal tract, the GI tract is in a state of constant (and relatively rapid) renewal as individual cells from the crypt region migrate to the villus region, and eventually to the lumen. During this process, increasing differentiation of individual epithelial cells and maturation occur.

Closely related, individual glycoproteins also change with individual sugar residues added sequentially to individual glycoprotein molecules, eventually producing a completed glycoprotein structure. Structural changes are accompanied by functional changes so that more mature villus cells appear to perform most of the digestive and transport functions in the GI tract, while these activities are limited quantitatively and qualitatively in individual crypt cells. It may be anticipated that these structural and functional changes along the crypt–villus column may be mirrored by topographic differences in the distribution of lectin-binding sites, not only along the length of the intestinal tract but also with the degree of enterocyte differentiation in the crypt–villus column.

7.4   GASTROINTESTINAL TRACT TRANSIT AND EFFECTS ON NUTRIENT AND DRUG ASSIMILATION

Lectins detected in food products have led to further exploration of their transit and disposition within the human intestine. During digestion, lectins may be released from food and remain intact for variable distances within the intestinal tract. The lectin from wheat germ may be detected in effluent from the small bowel (in ileostomies) and large bowel (fecal material) after feeding and transit through the intestine.[11] Potentially, it is likely that lectins of various types have some differential biological effects on biochemical and physiologic processes within the intestine, including the assimilation of specific micro- and macronutrients.

Carbohydrate assimilation from the lumen of the small intestine may be altered by the presence of different foods, in particular, vegetable protein, fat, fiber, and antinutrients. The latter include phytates and lectins.[27,58] The potential antinutritive and toxic effects of some plant lectins may be based largely on their binding effect to carbohydrate associated with membrane glycoconjugates (i.e., glycoproteins and glycolipids). As noted earlier, these are integral to the luminal epithelial cell membrane surface, and critical to survival in the digestive environment of the small intestine.

Turnover of epithelial cells, as they migrate toward the lumen, may be impaired causing altered digestion and assimilation, alterations in the luminal microbiome and the local intestinal immune system. As a result, particularly with large amounts of ingested lectins, normal growth and health of different animal species may be affected. Lectins also appear to mediate cellular adhesion and invasion of some therapeutic agents, particularly orally administered drugs. In the future, further studies may lead to improvements in drug absorption and the bioavailability of drugs, peptides and proteins that are normally poorly transported from the lumen.[23]

7.5   LECTIN BINDING IN THE NORMAL INTESTINE

Earlier studies with different fluorescein-labeled lectins showed regional differences in the labeling patterns of both small bowel and colonic mucosa from the mammalian intestine.[21,22] In small intestinal studies, frozen cryostat sections were initially used to explore the pattern with lectins derived from *Riccinus communis* and *Triticum vulgare* (wheat germ). These two lectins bind to end-terminal nonreducing *beta*-D-galactosyl and *beta*-N-acetyl-D-glucosaminyl residues, respectively. Labeling differences for normal proximal and distal small intestine were seen. In addition, differences in the intensity of labeling from the crypt to villus region were observed. Later, colonic biopsy sections from proximal and distal colonic mucosa, which were fixed with Bouin's solution (picric acid and formalin-based fixation) and embedded in paraffin, were used to explore the goblet cell mucin differences.

An array of nine different fluorescein-labeled lectins (see Table 7.1 and Figure 7.1 for sugar specificities) showing binding were used to compare these two different sites.[21,22] Different patterns of binding to mucins in goblet cells and the colonic crypt epithelial cell surface were noted including unique differential labeling patterns with increasing differentiation of colonic epithelial cells in the crypt regions. Based on these studies, significant differences in biologic characteristics of the mammalian colonic mucosa from these two different sites was suggested, in part reflecting both their location or site within the colon and the degree of cellular differentiation within crypt as the epithelial cells migrate from the crypt bases to the lumen. This application of labeled lectins to formalin-fixed sections opened the door for future pathological studies in different tissues. Similar changes in lectin binding of the intestinal tract were confirmed later by other investigators in different mammalian species.

TABLE 7.1   Sugar Specificities for Some Lectins.

Lectin	Plant origin	Major sugar specificities*	Binding inhibitor*#
Wheat germ (WGA)	*Triticum vulgare*	GlcNAc)n; NeuNAc	GlcNAc
Castor bean (RCA1)	*Riccinus communis*	Gal	Gal
Gorse (UEA1)	*Ulex europeus*	L-Fuc	L-Fuc
Horse gram (DBA)	*Dolichos biflorus*	GalNAc	GalNAc
Jack bean (ConA)	*Canavalia ensiformis*	Man; Glc	MM
Peanut (PNA)	*Arachis hypogaea*	Gal-GalNAc > Gal	Gal

L-Fuc, alpha-L-fucose; MM, alpha-methyl-mannoside; GalNAc, N-acetylgalactosamine; Glc, Glucose; GlcNAc, N-acetylglucosamine; Man, mannose; NeuNAc, N-acetylneuraminic acid (sialic acid). Note: All sugars are beta-D-configuration unless otherwise stated.
To inhibit lectin binding, sugars used at 0.2 M except for PNA binding, which required 0.3 M.[21,22]

Differentiation-based changes in the goblet cells in the distal colonic epithelium of a specific strain of mice (i.e., the CF-1)[7] and differences in lectin binding for the proximal and distal colon of Sprague-Dawley rats[36] were later reported. In the latter study,[36] rhodamine and fluorescein-conjugated lectins were used. Similar regional lectin labeling differences were subsequently reported from human fetal and normal adult colon[12] and normal-appearing colonic mucosa of patients with irritable bowel syndrome.[51] Subsequent studies showed that rat colon lectin binding may be altered by starvation and re-feeding under controlled conditions, another important consideration in research studies even in genetically closely related species.[2]

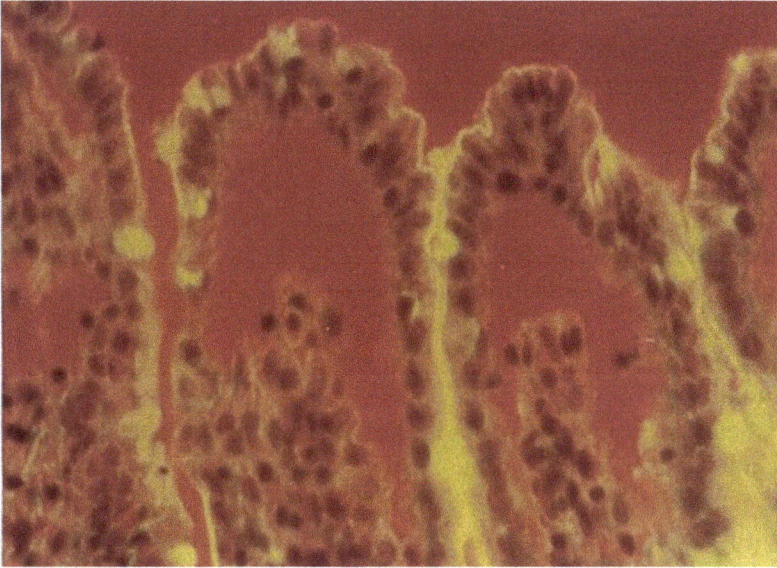

FIGURE 7.1 Fluoroscein-labeled lectin (wheat germ agglutinin, WGA) labeling the small intestinal epithelial cell surface including goblet cells. A red filter was added for enhancement.

Later, preliminary lectin labeling studies of other gastrointestinal tissues including normal human stratified squamous epithelium in the esophagus were noted, along with lectin labeling binding patterns for columnar epithelium in the stomach and duodenum confirming that the glycoconjugate structures in the mucosa of these different anatomical sites may also be examined with lectin histochemical methods.[52] Interestingly, several lectin studies by other investigators were also reported on normal tissues embryologically derived from the upper gastrointestinal tract, specifically, the biliary tract and pancreas.[5,15,32,33,48,49,57]

7.6 LECTIN BINDING IN PREMALIGNANT AND MALIGNANT INTESTINE

Early studies demonstrated significant alterations in the metabolism of glycoproteins in human colon cancer.[30] Specifically, the carbohydrate content and the enzymatic activities of some glycosyltransferases involved in the synthesis of mucosal glycoproteins were reduced in neoplastic colonic tissues compared with the normal human colonic mucosa. Carcinogen-induced animal models of human colon cancer were developed using chemicals, such as 1,2-dimethylhydrazine. This agent caused colonic cancers similar to the pathological appearance and distal colonic distribution in human colon cancer.

In male Wistar rats, reduced labeling of goblet cell mucin was noted with lectins derived from *Triticum vulgare* lectin, *Riccinus communis* lectin, and *Limulus polyphemus* lectin, while binding with *Arachis hypogaea*, a lectin that ordinarily failed to bind the mucin of normal colon, was present.[17] Similar changes were noted in the normal mucosa near the neoplastic lesions, the so-called "transitional" zone mucosa. These findings indicated for the first time in a well-controlled laboratory setting that significant histochemical alterations in glycoconjugate metabolism occur in colon cancer along with the nearby normal-appearing mucosa in this animal model of human colon cancer. These initial observations were later confirmed in a chemically treated (i.e., CF-1) mouse strain model with the detection of this cancer-associated mucin in cancer and in normal-appearing, but potentially premalignant colonic epithelium.[7]

Similar observations were described in human colon cancer specimens with an alteration in colon mucin and in transitional mucosa suggesting a potential marker for early malignant transformation.[10] In addition, more recent studies noted some similarities and differences between peanut lectin binding, the lectin of *Amarantus caudatus*, and a cancer-associated antigen (i.e., Thomsen-Friedenreich antigen) in polyps and cancer[50,63] and these have implicated specific sugar binding properties of lectins during malignant progression in human colon cancer.[25]

Patients with long-standing inflammatory bowel disease (IBD) are thought to be at increased risk for later development of colon cancer. Abnormal goblet cell glycoconjugates, reflected in alterations in lectin staining patterns, were reported in patients with ulcerative colitis.[9] Similar findings were reported in New World monkeys with spontaneously developing colitis, although the precise significance was uncertain.[8] Though other investigators have found peanut lectin-binding sites in the colon of patients with ulcerative colitis,[16] yet changes appeared to be similar to controls and reversible with the development of quiescence of colonic mucosal inflammation. In a subsequent study of colonic biopsies from patients with ulcerative colitis or Crohn's disease, changes, particularly in peanut agglutinin positivity, could not be confirmed.[46]

Eight of 21 ulcerative colitis rectal biopsies and 10 of 17 Crohn's disease rectal biopsies were reported to be positive for peanut agglutinin, particularly in the supranuclear region of surface epithelial cells. And yet, no correlation was found with the duration of disease or inflammation and none of these 38 biopsies showed dysplasia. It was concluded that the changes observed in this setting may reflect a fundamental abnormality in glycoprotein synthesis with inflammatory bowel disease. In a later study in Japanese patients with ulcerative colitis and Crohn's disease, changes in lectin binding were detected; but appeared to only reflect the underlying inflammatory process rather than specificity for development of later neoplasia.[62]

In a separate study of South Asians from Birmingham, altered lectin binding was noted in ulcerative colitis after application of 10 biotinylated lectins compared with matched European cases with ulcerative colitis.[37] In summary, these studies in patients with inflammatory bowel disease have provided evidence for altered lectin-labeling patterns consistent with an ongoing inflammatory process, but not as a specific premalignant marker.

7.7   ROLE OF LECTIN BINDING IN OTHER DISEASES OF THE GASTROINTESTINAL TRACT

Studies in the upper GI tract have explored changes in lectin-binding patterns in normal, metaplastic, and neoplastic biopsies from the esophagus, stomach, and duodenum. Barrett's epithelium refers to the replacement of normal stratified squamous epithelium in the esophagus with columnar epithelial cells, possibly due to chronic reflux of contents in the stomach to the esophagus. It is believed to be a preneoplastic disorder with the eventual development in some, but not all, patients with esophageal adenocarcinoma. In high-grade dysplasia and carcinoma associated with Barrett's esophagus, deletion of glycoconjugate expression was reported.[53]

A subsequent study in biopsies from Barrett's epithelium with fluorescein-linked peanut agglutinin showed variable labeling, suggesting that Barrett's epithelium represents a much more heterogeneous preneoplastic mucosal change than had previously been appreciated using routine histochemical methods.[18]

Chronological long-term lectin studies might be conducted during surveillance to determine the natural history of these alterations in these mucosal cells, since prior cell biological studies have already documented the complex nature of these cell types in this mucosa.[14] Others have reported a binding pattern with *Ulex europeus* lectin that is distinct in Barrett's mucosa and not detected in reflux disease.[38] Studies in gastroesophageal reflux disease, including both squamous and columnar epithelium, were also reported with prominent binding in deep glandular elements of the columnar epithelium.[39]

Recently, the possible use of fluorescent lectins (i.e., wheat germ lectin) for molecular imaging during endoscopic surveillance was reported to be particularly sensitive for the detection of high-grade dysplastic lesions that were not detectable with conventional endoscopic studies.[6]

Research studies have also explored the gastric mucosa in different diseases. In peptic ulcer disease, a significant difference in peanut lectin binding was observed between *Helicobacter pylori*—positive and *Helicobacter pylori*—negative patients,[45] suggesting that exposure of sialic acid residues was present in gastric epithelium colonized with this specific organism. Similar studies were reported with different lectins in *Helicobacter*—associated gastritis in humans[3,34] as well as a guinea pig animal model of this disease.[34]

Lectin-binding patterns have also been examined in *Helicobacter pylori*-infected gastric mucosa as a tool to explore the presence of dysplastic changes in the gastric mucosa with the hope of new insights into gastric carcinogenesis and the treatment of precancerous lesions.[59] Others have focused on the *Helicobacter pylori* organism and its binding to epithelial cells, particularly gastric mucins that may prohibit the organisms from reaching the epithelium and later promoting infection and inflammation.[44]

Extensive lectin-binding studies have also been completed in celiac disease. During the recent couple of decades, this has become an increasingly recognized immune-mediated small intestinal mucosal disorder that results in malabsorption of different nutrients, diarrhea, and weight loss. Pathologic changes in small intestinal biopsies may be reversed with a gluten-free diet. Studies with different lectins showed different lectin-binding patterns in celiac biopsies compared with control; also changes within the crypt and villi were thought to be reflective of increasing differentiation of epithelial cells with migration from the crypt regions to the lumen. Interestingly, in untreated adult celiac disease, lectin-binding studies also showed increasing differentiation within the small intestinal crypt regions per se even in the presence of villous atrophy.[19]

Lectin studies have also been reported in children with celiac disease and others with post-enteritis syndrome.[4,43] These findings have also suggested a possible relationship between the pathogenesis of this disorder, the so-called and controversial "lectin hypothesis."[60] Here, specific binding to the small intestinal epithelial cell surface by gluten (or a gluten component) in a genetically predisposed individual may cause toxicity followed by an immunological cellular cascade damaging the mucosa. Interestingly, lectin activity has been previously identified as wheat germ agglutinin[31]; and serum antibodies to wheat germ agglutinin and gluten have been identified in patients with celiac disease[54] and dermatitis herpetiformis,[55] a skin disorder closely linked to celiac disease. A change in the luminal microbiome might also have similar effects.

Further topographic mapping studies of the luminal surface in celiac disease may require additional: (1) studies after normalization of the small intestinal mucosa to a gluten-free diet, (2) studies on the specificity of mucosal changes since other diseases may mimic celiac disease (i.e., sprue-like enteropathy), and (3) effects of adsorbed luminal sugar residues on the small intestine.[20]

7.8 FUTURE RESEARCH DIRECTIONS

A major problem of histochemical approach in this chapter is the recognition that the underlying molecular structures are only now becoming increasingly appreciated. Although employed for decades as a method of mapping glycosylated structures, yet the binding patterns for some lectins may not be fully characterized and their functions poorly understood.[13] In addition, a widening range of investigative tools has emerged.[1,26]

Recombinant forms of lectins[24] have been developed that may permit the use of better characterized and more homogeneous tools for exploring the ability of a specific lectin to identify a precancer or cancer marker, compared with the current use of natural lectins (e.g., seed products) that may be less uniform.[13] High throughput screening technologies are being developed to permit increased speed of lectin carbohydrate microarrays for the evaluation of mammalian and bacterial glycome.[26,41,42,56]

Recently, specific glycoproteins that bind to *Helico pomatia*, a lectin used to explore the development of colorectal cancer, were employed.[40] Lectin histochemistry combined with lectin affinity chromatography was used to isolate the critically increased proteins. Then further analysis with western blotting, two-dimensional electrophoresis and matrix-assisted laser desorption ionization mass spectroscopy methods were done. By combining these methods with lectin histochemistry, potential glycosylation sites on proteins were evaluated using silicon bioinformatics and correlations were done with clinical and pathological features in the patients with cancer-related genes (specifically, P53 gene, using a defined immunohistochemical method, and KRAS gene (using the polymerase chain reaction method). Others have employed wide array of evolving methodologies for further exploration.[28,61,64]

7.9   SUMMARY

Lectins are potentially powerful tools to explore binding receptors on the intestinal cell surface of normal, premalignant and malignant cells, and in other intestinal diseases. In the past, lectin binding has largely been explored using immunological and immunohistochemical methods, but novel technologies have recently been employed that may permit further critical research efforts and likely critical discoveries for improved understanding and treatment of intestinal diseases.

KEYWORDS

- **agglutinins**
- **celiac disease**
- **Crohn's disease**
- *Helicobacter pylori*
- **gastritis**
- **lectins**
- **ulcerative colitis**

REFERENCES

1. Adamczyk, B.; Tharmalingham, T.; Rudd, P.M. Glycans as Cancer Biomarkers. *Biochim. Biophys. Acta* **2012,** *1820* (9), 1347–1353.

2. Atillasoy, E. O.; Kapetenakis, A; Itzkowitz, S. H.; Holt, P.R. Amaranthin Lectin Binding in the Rat Colon: Response to Dietary Manipulation. *Mt. Sinai J. Med.—New York* **1998**, *65* (2), 46–53.

3. Baczako, K.; Kuhl, P.; Malfertheiner, P. Lectin-binding Properties of the Antral and Body Surface Mucosa in the Human Stomach are Differences relevant for *Helicobacter pylori* Affinity? *J. Pathol.* **1995**, *176* (1), 77–86.

4. Barresi, G.; Tuccari, G.; Tedeschi, A.; Magazzu, G. Lectin Binding Site in Duodeno-jejunal Mucosa from Celiac Children. *Histochemistry* **1988**, *88*, 105–112.

5. Barresi, G.; Vitarelli, E.; Grosso, M.; Tuccari, G. Peanut Lectin Binding Sites in Human Fetal and Neonatal Pancreas. *Eur. J. Histochem.: EJH* **1993**, *27*, 329–334.

6. Bird-Lieberman, E. L.; Neves, A. A. Molecular Imaging using Fluorescent Lectins Permits Rapid Endoscopic Identification of Dysplasia in Barrett's Esophagus. *Nat. Med.* **2012**, *18*, 315–321.

7. Boland, C.R.; Ahnen, D.J. Binding of Lectins to Goblet Cell Mucin in Malignant and Premalignant Colonic Epithelium in the CF-1 Mouse. *Gastroenterology*, **1985**, *89* (1), 127–137.

8. Boland, C.R.; Clapp, N.K. Glycoconjugates in the Colon of Monkeys with Spontaneous Colitis: Association between inflammation and neoplasia. *Gastroenterology* **1987**, *92* (3), 625–634.

9. Boland, C.R.; Lance, P.; Levin, B.; Riddell, R.H.; Kim, Y.S. Abnormal Goblet Cell Glycoconjugates in Rectal Biopsies associated with Increased Risk of Neoplasia in Patients with Ulcerative Colitis: Early Results of a Prospective Study. *Gut* **1984**, *25* (12), 1364–1371.

10. Boland, C.R.; Montgomery, C.K.; Kim, Y.S. Alterations in Human Colonic Mucin occurring with Cellular Differentiation and Malignant Transformation. *Proc. Natl Acad. Sci. USA* **1982**, *79* (6), 2051–2055.

11. Brady, P.G.; Vannier, A.M.; Banwell, J.G. Identification of Dietary Lectin: Wheat Germ Agglutinin in Human Intestinal Contents. *Gastroenterology* **1978**, *75* (2), 236–239.

12. Bresalier, R.S.; Boland, C.R.; Kim, Y.S. Regional Differences in Normal and Cancer-associated Glycoconjugates of the Human Colon. *J. Natl. Cancer Inst.* **1985**, *75* (2), 249–260.

13. Brooks, S.A. Lectin Histochemistry: Historical Perspectives, State of the Art, and the Future. *Methods Mol. Biol.* **2017**, *1560*, 93–107.

14. Buchan, A.M.; Grant, S.; Freeman, H.J. Regulatory Peptides in Barrett's Esophagus. *J. Pathol.* **1985**, *146* (3), 227–234.

15. Ching, C.K.; Black, R.; Helliwell, T.; Savage, A.; Barr, H.; Rhodes, J.M. Use of Lectin Histochemistry in Pancreatic Cancer. *J. Clin. Pathol.* **1988**, *41* (3), 324–328.

16. Cooper, H.S.; Farano, P.; Chapman, R.A. Peanut Lectin Binding Sites in Colons of Patients with Ulcerative Colitis. *Arch. Pathol. Lab. Med.* **1987**, *111* (3), 270–275.

17. Freeman, H.J. Lectin Histochemistry of 1,2-Dimethylhydrazine-induced Rat Colon Neoplasia. *J. Histochem. Cytochem.: Off. J. Histochem. Soc.* **1983**, *31*, 1241–1245.

18. Freeman, H. J. Peanut Lectin Histochemistry of Barrett's Esophagus. *Can. J. Gastroenterol.* **1989**, *3* (5), 185–188.

19. Freeman, H.J. Topography of Lectin Binding Sites in Celiac Sprue. *Can. J. Gastroenterol.* **1992**, *6* (5), 271–276.

20. Freeman, H.J. Topographic Lectin Mapping of the Epithelial Cell Surface in Normal Intestine and Celiac Disease. *Int. J. Celiac Dis.* **2019,** 7 (3), 69–73.
21. Freeman, H.J.; Etzler, M.E.; Garrido, A.B.; Kim, Y.S. Alterations in Cell Surface Membrane Components of Adapting Rat Small Intestinal Epithelium. *Gastroenterology* **1978,** 75 (6), 405–412.
22. Freeman, H.J.; Lotan, R.; Kim, Y.S. Application of Lectins for Detection of Goblet Cell Glycoconjugate Differences in Proximal and Distal Colon of the Rat. *Lab. Invest. J. Tech. Methods Pathol.* **1980,** *42* (4), 405–412.
23. Gabor, F.; Bogner, E.; Weissenboeck, A.; Wirth, M. The Lectin-cell Interaction and Its Implications of Intestinal-lectin Mediated Drug Delivery. *Adv. Drug Deliv. Rev.* **2004,** 56 (4), 459–480.
24. Habermann, F. A.; Andre, S.; Kaltner, H. Galectins as Tools for Glycol Mapping in Histology: Comparison of Their Binding Profiles to Bovine Zone Pellucid by Confocal Scanning Electron Microscopy. *Histochem. Cell Biol.* **2011,** *135* (6), 539–552.
25. Hagerbaumer, P.; Veith, M.; Anders, M.; Schumacher, U. Lectin Histochemistry shows WGA, PHA-L and HPA Binding Increases During Progression of Human Colorectal Cancer. *Anticancer Res.* **2015,** *35* (10), 5333–5339.
26. Hu, D.; Tateno, H.; Hirabayashi, J. Lectin Engineering, a Molecularly Evolutionary Approach to Expanding Lectin Utilities. *Molecules* **2015,** *20*, 7637–7656.
27. Jenkins, D. J.; Josse, R. G.; Jenkins, A.L.; Wolever, T.M.; Vuksan, V. Implications of Altering the Rate of Carbohydrate Adsorption from the Gastrointestinal Tract. *Clin. Invest. Med.* **1995,** *18* (4), 296–302.
28. Johnson, Q.R.; Lindsay, R.J.; Petridis, L. Investigation of Carbohydrate Recognition via Computer Simulation. *Molecules* **2015,** *20*, 7700–7718.
29. Khan, S.; Brooks, S.A.; Leathem, A.J. GalNAc-type Glycoproteins in Breast Cancer: 126 Lectin Study. *J. Pathol.* **1994,** *172* (suppl.), 134A.
30. Kim, Y.S.; Isaacs, R. Glycoprotein Metabolism in Inflammatory and Neoplastic Disease of the Human Colon. *Cancer Res.* **1975,** *35* (8), 2092–2097.
31. Kolberg, J.; Sollid, L. Lectin Reactivity of Gluten Identified as Wheat Germ Agglutinin. *Biochem. Biophys. Res. Commun.* **1985,** *130* (2), 867–872.
32. Lee, K.T.; Sheen, P.C. Lectin Histochemical Study of Cholangiocarcinoma Arising from Stone-bearing Intrahepatic Bile Duct. *J. Surg. Oncol.* **1995,** *59* (2), 1331–1335.
33. Lee, K.T.; Sheen, P.C. A Lectin Histochemical Study of Intrahepatic Bile Ducts in Patients with Hepatolithiasis. *Digest. Dis. Sci.* **1995,** *40*, 757–762.
34. Lueth, M.; Sturegard, E.; Sjunnesson, H.; Wadstrom, T.; Schumacher, U. Lectin Histochemistry of the Gastric Mucosa in Normal and *Helicobacter pylori* Infected Guinea Pigs. *J. Mol. Histol.* **2004,** *36*, 51–58.
35. Lynch, C. V.; Pedersen, O. The Human Intestinal Microbiome in Health and Disease. *New Engl. J. Med.* **2016,** *375* (24), 2369–2379.
36. McGarrity, T. J.; Pfeiffer, L.P.; Colony, P.C. Alterations in Lectin Binding in the Proximal and Distal Colon of Sprague-Dawley Rats with 1,2-Dimethyl-hydazine Administration. *Exp. Pathol.* **1991,** *41* (4), 175–183.
37. McMahon, R.F.; Warren, B.F.; Jones, C.J. South Asians with Ulcerative Colitis Exhibit Altered Lectin Binding Compared with Matched European Cases. *Histochem. J.* **1997,** *29*, 469–477.

38. Neumann, H.; Wex, T.; Monkemuller, K.; Vietch, M.; Fry, L.C.; Malfertheiner, P. Lectin UEA-1 Binding Proteins are Specifically Increased in Squamous Epithelium of Patients with Barrett's Esophagus. *Digestion* **2008**, *78*, 201–207.

39. Neumann, H.; Wex, T.; Vietch, M. Gastroesophageal Reflux Disease Leads to Major Alterations in Lectin-binding in the Columnar Epithelium of the Gastroesophageal Junction. *Scand. J. Gastroenterol.* **2007**, *42* (7), 791–798.

40. Peiris, D.; Ossondo, M.; Fry, S. Identification of O-linked Glycoproteins Binding to the Lectin *Helix pomatia* Agglutinin as Markers of Metastatic Colorectal Cancer. *PloS One* **2015**, *10* (10), article ID: e0138345.

41. Pilobello, K.; Mahal, L.K. Lectin Microarrays for Glycoprotein Analysis. *Methods Mol. Biol.* **2007**, 193–203.

42. Pilobello, K.; Slawek, D.E.; Mahal, L.K. Radiometric Lectin Micro Assay Approach to Analysis of the Dynamic Mammalian Glycol. *Proc. Natl. Acad. Sci. USA* **2007**, *104* (28), 11534–11539.

43. Pittschieler, K.; Ladinser, B.; Petell, J.K. Reactivity of Gliadin and Lectins with Celiac Intestinal Mucosa. *Pediatr. Res.* **1994**, *36* (5), 635–641.

44. Radziejewska, I.; Borzym-Kluczyk, M.; Leszczynska, K. *Lotus tetragonolobus, Ulex europeus, Maackia amurensis* and *Arachis hypogaea* (peanut) Lectins Influence the Binding of *Helicobacter pylori* to Gastric Carbohydrates. *Adv. Clin. Exp. Med.: Off. Org. Wroclaw Med. Univ.* **2018**, *27* (6), 807–811.

45. Rameshkumar, K.; Cooper, R.; Jalihal, A.; Nirmala, V. Peanut Agglutinin Binding by Gastric Mucosal Epithelial Cells in *Helicobacter pylori* Associated Gastritis. *Ind. J. Med. Res.* **1994**, *100*, 26–30.

46. Rhodes, J.M.; Black, R.R.; Savage, A. Altered Lectin Binding by Colonic Epithelial Glycoconjugates in Ulcerative Colitis and Crohn's Disease. *Digest. Dis. Sci.* **2005**, *33*, 1359–1363.

47. Roth, J. Lectins for Histochemical Demonstration of Glycans. *Histochem. Cell Biol.* **2011**, *136*, 117–130.

48. Saito, K.; Nakanuma, Y. Lectin Binding of Intrahepatic Bile Ducts and Peribilary Glands in Normal Livers and Hepatoliasis. *Tohoku J. Exp. Med.* **1990**, *160* (1), 81–92.

49. Sanzen, T.; Yoshida, K.; Sasaki, M.; Tereda, T.; Nakanuma, Y. Expression of Glyco-conjugates During Intrahepatic Bile Duct Development in the Rat: An Immunohisto-chemical and Lectin-histochemical Study. *Hepatology* **1995**, *22* (3), 944–951.

50. Sata, T.; Roth, J.; Zuber, C.; Stamm, B. Studies on the Thomsen-Friedenreich Antigen in Human Colon with the Lectin Amaranthin. Normal and Neoplastic Epithelium Express Only Cryptic T-Antigen. *Lab. Invest. J. Tech. Methods Pathol.* **1992**, *66* (2), 175–186.

51. Shah, M.; Shrikhande, S.S.; Swaroop, V.S. Lectin Binding in Colorectal Mucosa. *Ind. J/ Gastroenterol. Off. J. Ind. Soc. Gastroenterol.* **1989**, *8* (1), 31–33.

52. Sharon, N.; Lis, H. History of Lectins: from Hemagglutinin to Biological Recognition Molecules. *Glycobiology* **2004**, *14* (11), 53R-63R.

53. Shimamoto, C.; Weinstein, W.M.; Boland, C.R. Glycoconjugate Expression in Normal, Metaplastic, and Neoplastic Human Upper Gastrointestinal Mucosa. *J. Clin. Invest.* **1987**, *80* (6), 1670–1678.

54. Sollid, L. M.; Kolberg, J.; Scott, H.; Ek, J.; Fausa, O.; Brandtzaeg, P. Antibodies to Wheat Germ in Celiac Disease. *Clin. Exp. Immunol.* **1986**, *63* (1), 95–100.

55. Sollid, L.M.; Scott, H.; Kolberg, J.; Brandtzaeg, P. Serum Antibodies to Wheat Germ Agglutinin and Gluten in Patients with *Dermatitis herpetiformis*. *Arch. Dermatol. Res.* **1986,** *278*, 433–436.

56. Tateno, H.; Utchiyama, N.; Kuno, A. A Novel Strategy for Mammalian Cell Surface Glycol Profiling using Lectin Microarray. *Glycobiology* **2007,** *17* (10), 1138–1146.

57. Tereda, T.; Nakanuma, Y. Profiles of Expression of Carbohydrate Chain Structures During Human Intrahepatic Bile Duct Development and Maturation: A Lectin-Histochemical and Immuno-histochemical Study. *Hepatology* **1994,** *20* (2), 388–397.

58. Vasconceios, I.M.; Oliveira, J.T. Antinutritional Properties of Plant Lectins. *Toxicon* **2004,** *44* (4), 385–403.

59. Vernygorodskyi, S.; Shkolnikov, V.; Suhan, D. Lectin Binding Patterns in Normal, Dysplastic and *Helicobacter pylori* Infected Gastric Mucosa. *Exp. Oncol.* **2017,** *39* (2), 138–140.

60. Weiser, M.M.; Douglas, A.P. Alternative Mechanism for Gluten-toxicity in Celiac Disease. *Lancet* **1976,** *307*, 567–569.

61. Yan, C.; Yersin, A.; Arfin, R. Single Molecular Dynamic Interactions between Glycophorin-A and Lectin as Probed by Atomic Force Microscopy. *Biophys. Chem.* **2009,** *144* (1–2), 72–77.

62. Yoshioka, H.; Inada, M.; Ogawa, K.; Ohshio, G.; Yamane, H; Hamashima, Y.; Miyake, T. Lectin Histochemistry of Ulcerative Colitis and Crohn's Disease. *J. Exp. Pathol.* **1989,** *4* (2), 69–78.

63. Yuan, M.; Itzkowitz, S.H. Comparison of T-antigen Expression in Normal, Premalignant and Malignant Human Colonic Tissue Using Lectin and Antibody Immunocytochemistry. *Cancer Res.* **1986,** *46* (9), 1841–1847.

64. Zhang, H.; Yadavalli, V.K. Functionalized Self-assembled Monolayers for Measuring Single Molecule Lectin Carbohydrate Interactions. *Analy. Chim. Acta* **2009,** *649* (1), 1–7.

CHAPTER 8

Therapeutic Efficacy of Black Pepper in Gastrointestinal Disorders

MRINMOY SARKAR and POOJA CHAWLA

ABSTRACT

Dried fruit of black pepper (*Piper nigrum*) is used as medicine for gastrointestinal disorders. Bioactive compound piperine has various pharmacological actions, such as digestive agent, antidiarrheal, anticancer, stomachic, tonic, carminative, antispasmodic, etc. Piperine also stimulates (1) the pancreatic and intestinal enzymes to aid on the digestive system and (2) the secretion of bile acid-rich bile to help in fat digestion and absorption. This chapter highlights the sources, phytochemistry, and various beneficial effects on gastrointestinal tract.

8.1 INTRODUCTION

Black pepper is a well-known spice with piperine being the main alkaloid that is responsible for its pungency in flavor. Black pepper is composed of various alkaloids, carbohydrates, and starch, etc.[40,53] Piperine is used to stimulate hunger and increase salivary secretions.[22] Black pepper has comprehensive medicinal properties against various diseases, such as increasing digestion, shortening gastrointestinal tract (GIT) holding time, protect damage due to oxidation, lowering oxidative degradation of lipids, gastroprotective, masking drug biotransforming reactions, bioavailability improvement of various pharmaceuticals, antimutagenic, antitumor, etc.[65]

This chapter explores the therapeutic efficacy of *Piper nigrum* (Black pepper) in the management of gastrointestinal (GI) disorders.

8.2   PHARMACOGNOSTIC CHARACTERISTICS OF BLACK PEPPER

Black pepper (*P. nigrum*) is one of the most well-known spices, which are extensively used in tropical regions of Indonesia, China, India, Brazil, Vietnam, etc. Vietnam is the bulkiest producer of black pepper in the world. The world production of black pepper was about 546,000 tons in 2016.[76] Black pepper includes the dried and raw fruits. The unripe and green fruits are heated in boiling water to modify the black color by enzymatic browning.[76] The color of the fruit is blackish-brown having aromatic odor and pungency taste. Fruits are 3.5–6 mm in width.[19] Different parts of black pepper are shown in Figure 8.1.

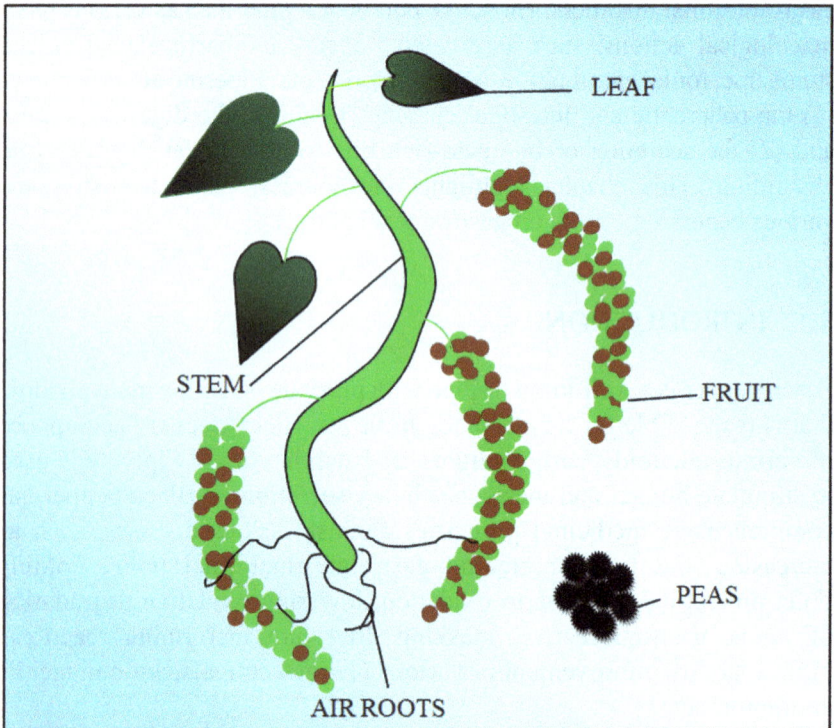

FIGURE 8.1   Different parts of black pepper plant.

With the help of a microscope, in the transverse and longitudinal section of black pepper, the pericarp portion can be easily described, which is thin and dark and the seed is compactly devoted to it (Fig. 8.2).

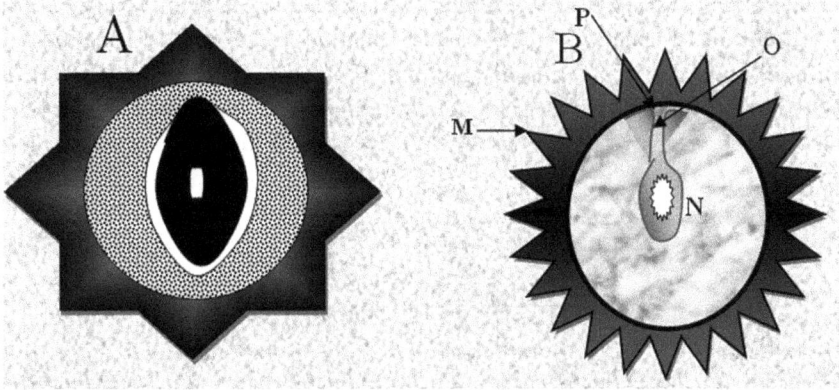

FIGURE 8.2   Black pepper: A. Transverse section, B. Longitudinal section; LEGEND: M – Perisperm, N – Endosperm, O – Embryo, P – Magnified.

Basically, seeds are rouletted and the inner pericarp portion is brown, made up of sclerenchyma. It consists of tiny endosperm and a small embryo is located nearby the apex of fruit but perisperm is the main part of the seed.[26] The main chemical constituents of black pepper are piperine (5%–9%), starch and piperidine (30%), resin (6%), and volatile oil (1%–2.5%). The volatile oil is yellow in color due to the presence of phellandrene and caryophyllene. The substitutes of *P. nigrum* are *Piper attenuatum*, *Piper brachystachyum,* and *Piper longum.*[34]

8.3   ETHNOPHARMACOLOGICAL CONSIDERATIONS OF BLACK PEPPER

Black pepper is one of the main flavoring agents in Turkish meals. Black pepper with honey has aphrodisiacal property. It is recommended for the removal of cough and influenza.[56] In the botanical family Piperaceae, black pepper and long pepper are well-cognizant species in the family as well as most likely avowed spices in the world. In the conventional medicine system, it is used for remittent fever and it improves the secretion of bile. It is also advised for GIT disorders, such as, dyspepsia, flatulence, constipation and hemorrhoids.[23,63]

Inflammatory bowel disease (IBD) is combined with long-standing swelling of the intestinal tract, and piperine has been indicated to be efficient for anti-inflammatory effects.[27] In Ayurveda, there is a very useful formulation "*Trikatu*," which contains black pepper, ginger, long pepper in co-equal ratios. The archaic evidenced *Ayurvedic Materia Medica* in which these three herbs refer to as vital constituents of many prescriptions and formulations used for extensive diseases. With the help of experimental data, it was proved that "*Trikatu*" increased the bioavailability of various drugs, such as, tetracycline, sulfadiazine, and vasicine.[31]

8.4   PHYTOCHEMISTRY OF BLACK PEPPER

Piperine in black pepper acts as a GIT active agent and increases the digestive power due to the action of pancreatic enzyme after appearing in the gut. There are different bioactive agents in the black pepper, such as piperine, pipericide, chavicine, sarmentosine, and piperonylamine. Among all these compounds, piperine shows the best pharmacological effects.

The pungent taste of black pepper is due to the presence of piperine.[40] Not only piperine, but also piperanine, piperylin-A, piperolein-B, pipericine, and piperettine possess some degree of pungency. Some alkaloids are obtained by extraction from black pepper. Figure 8.3 shows some chemical constituents derived from black pepper.[57]

Black pepper contains various antioxidant active chemicals, such as ascorbic acid, myristic acid, palmitic acid, beta carotene, lauric acid, and piperine.[40] Piperine oil contains about 25 sesquiterpene hydrocarbons, such as beta-caryophyllene, alpha-cis-bergamotene, beta-elemene, alpha-santalene, etc.

Fourteen compounds have been recognized in black pepper and six of them are hydrocarbons, five are esters and the other two together with piperine are enzymes. It is important to note that all the hydrocarbons described so far have been aliphatic and no aromatic hydrocarbons have yet been recognized from the chosen fractions mentioned here. These aliphatic hydrocarbons are composed of open chain, single-, bi-, and tri-cyclic compounds, saturated and unsaturated hydrocarbons.[59]

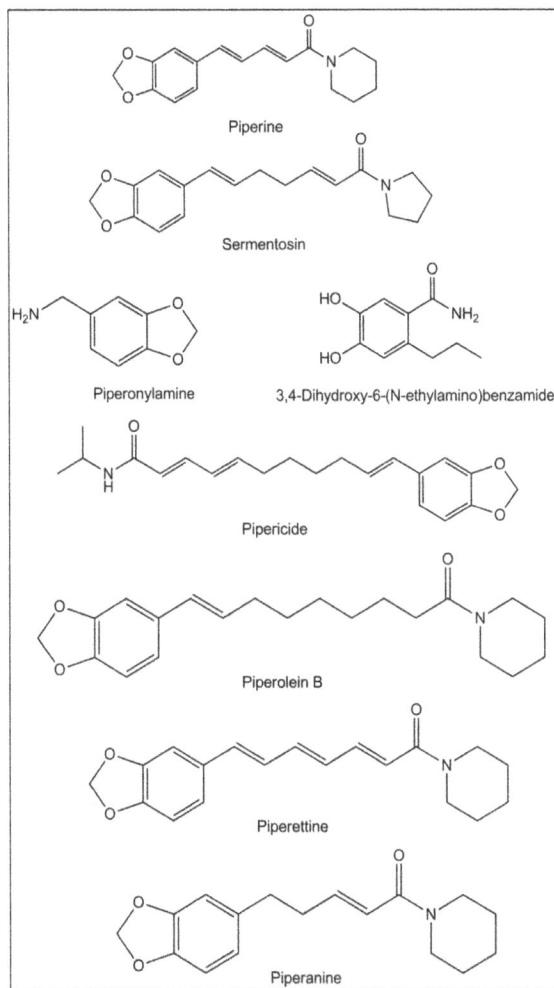

FIGURE 8.3 Chemical constituents derived from black pepper.

8.5 MECHANISMS OF ACTION OF BLACK PEPPER

- The black pepper can lower the cytokine concentrations thus promoting inflammation (TNF-α, PGE2, and IL-1b,) and can improve cytokine concentrations reducing inflammation (IL-10).[69]
- The black pepper inhibits enzymes CYP3A4 thus improving the intestinal absorption of drugs/substances in the intestine.[32]

- The black pepper functions as a radical scavenger of hydroxyl and superoxide ions thus producing its antioxidant effects.[42]
- The studies report that piperine with 8–32 mg/kg p.o. dose have a potential prostaglandin blocking effect in castor oil, $MgSO_4$ and arachidonic acid commenced diarrhea.[10]
- The black pepper can help to combat neurodegenerative disease mood, cognitive function, and fighting,[37,45] and increased muscle metabolism through increased activity of ATPase.[44] The mechanism to enhance the muscle metabolism can be explained by modulating efflux mechanisms, by modulating metabolizing enzymes, and thermogenesis.

8.5.1   Modulating Efflux Mechanisms

Piperine inhibits transport of drugs mediated by P-glycoprotein. Some studies have reported that dietary piperine influences the levels of metabolizing enzyme CYP3A4 and P-gp thus altering the levels of orally taken drugs.[14] Oral dose of 112 μg/kg for 14 days led to aggravated intestinal P-gp levels with decreased hepatic P-gp, with practically no effect on renal P-gp levels in rats.[25]

8.5.2   Modulating Metabolizing Enzymes

Piperine has been reported to alter the glucuronidation level by reducing the endogenous content of UDP-glucuronic acid and by preventing transferase activity.[51,61] Piperine blocks UDP-glucose dehydrogenase (UDP-GDH) function in intestine and liver by allosteric inhibition (Fig. 8.4).

8.5.3   Thermogenesis

Bioperine (a thermonutrient) can improve nutrient absorption by increasing thermogenesis involving autonomous nervous system through the alpha and beta-adrenergic receptors in the GIT. Beta receptors promote food-persuaded thermogenesis involving cyclic adenosine 3', 5' monophosphate (cAMP). As a "second messenger," the role of cAMP is well established into the hormonal and enzymatic functions. Once thermogenesis takes place in our body, there is a significant increase in the requirement for fresh nutrients to maintain the metabolism.[7]

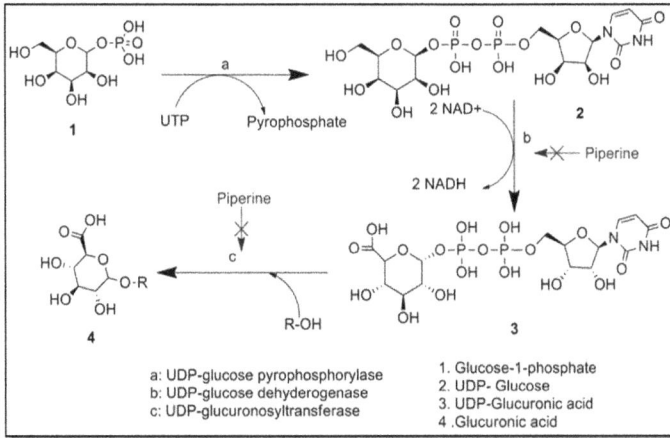

FIGURE 8.4   Effect of piperine on metabolizing enzymes.

8.6   THERAPEUTIC EFFECTS OF PIPERINE ON GIT DISORDERS

8.6.1   Carminative

Pepper has a high degree of stimulating and carminative characteristics, resulting in reflex saliva flow, with enhanced gastric juice secretion and increased appetite. GI movements are increased, resulting in gas eructation and colic relief. The black pepper can dilate the skin's surface vessels in adequate doses, causing a sensation of warmth, followed by diaphoresis and some temperature reduction. They are widely used as condiments because of these properties, particularly in warm climates. Also called stacks, black pepper is used as a remedy for hemorrhoids. A pepper oleoresin is prepared by acetone extraction and piperine separation.[40]

8.6.2   Aid in Digestion

Especially piperine, the pungent compound of *P. nigrum*. increases saliva production and gastric secretions. In addition, peppercorn intake improves salivary amylase output and activation. The development of digestive enzymes is likely to cause the liver to secrete bile by ingestion of *P. nigrum,* which further helps to digest food substances. Researchers have examined different bile secretion animal models after the absorption of piperine. Orally administered piperine can enhance the release of bile acid from the liver considerably.

The impact on the enzymes of the small intestinal mucosa of pepper-corn consumption in food products and oral administration of active genus piper compounds (such as piperine, piperamides, piperamines, and pipene) has been recorded. The addition of piperine to food products improves the activity of lipase, pancreatic amylase, chymotrypsin, and protease. Black pepper and its substances are widely used as traditional remedies against stomach problems. Black pepper is commonly recognized as instrumental in preventing and curing GI issues. By promoting histamine H2 receptors, piperine increases the formation of HCl by the stomach, which is helpful in digestion.[15]

8.6.3   Gastric and Antiulcer Activities

Piperine is a piperidine alkaloid with a pungent flavor and it has been studied in rats or mice in association with stomach mucosal harm induced by pressure, indomethacin, ethanol or pylorus ligature. This material shielded the stomach from ulceration by reducing the quantity of intravenous and oral gastric juice, acidity and pepsin-A function with respective dosage of 1.5 and 25 mg/kg, respectively.[18]

Like other NSAIDs, indomethacin also asserts its action by lowering the amount of serum and gastric tissue prostaglandins (PGE_2).[1,21] This therapeutic action of indomethacin and other NSAIDs carries with them harmful toxic effects in organs especially the stomach, where this PGE_2 executes its defensive action. PGE_2 induces the secretion of mucous and bicarbonate and facilitates the blood flow of mucous membranes and promotes angiogenesis. The serum rate of PGE_2 has been defended in piperine preadministered rats, further restoring the probability of using this alkaloid as an antiulcer drug.[21]

Figure 8.5 shows a schematic diagram illustrating the step-by-step development of gastric ulcer and the points at which piperine can assert its protective action. The figure clearly describes the oxidative stress caused by indomethacin that is the main contributor to the disruption and ulceration of the stomach tissue. Piperine preadministration by its antioxidant properties and defensive effects on the amount and type of gastroprotective mucin secretion results in defense against all harmful effects of indomethacin. Therefore, piperine can be used as an antiulcer drug and black pepper can be included in the regular diet of indomethacin patients and related NSAID treatments.[21]

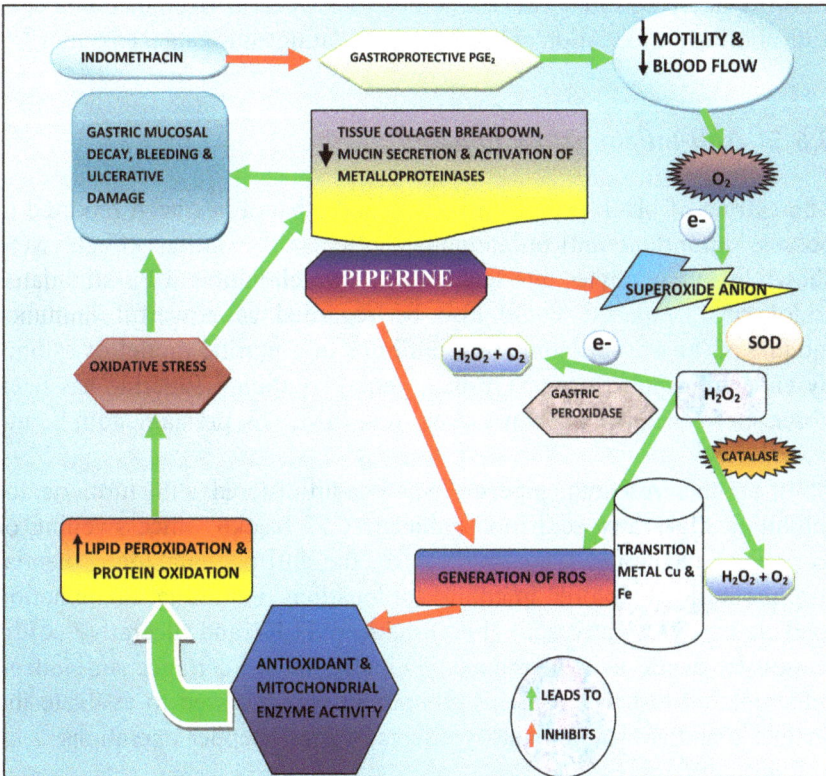

FIGURE 8.5 The possible mechanism of protection by piperine against indomethacin-induced oxidative stress-mediated gastric ulcer.

8.6.4 Antioxidant Activity

Different herbs and spices including pepper consist of number of effective constituents, such as terpenoids, flavonoids, minerals, and phytoestrogens.[3] Piperine is one of them with significant antioxidant activity that could decrease oxidative tissue damage, which was induced with excessive fatty acid food.[72] In addition, it also reduces the amount of reactive thiobarbituric acid by maintaining the levels of different enzymes, such as glutathione, catalase, glutathione peroxidase, superoxide dismutase, and glutathione-S-transferase.[72] In liver, piperine may enhance the biotransformation enzyme function.[60]

The antioxidant effects of piperine were further endorsed by the studies showing decreased lung metastatic outbreak in B16F-10 melanoma cells with altering peroxidation of lipid and stimulating antioxidant enzymes.[50,66]

8.6.5 Anti-Inflammatory Impact

The extract of black pepper in hexane and ethanol has been reported to possess important anti-inflammatory effects.[64,67] Similar effects were shown by synoviocytes interleukin (IL),[11] which inhibits LPS-stimulated endotoxins.[9] Piperine could also be regarded as powerful immuno-modulator, airway inflammation inhibitor in a murine model of asthma by enhancing pulmonary TGF-beta gene evolution.[33] Piperine has been observed to decrease the concentration in MMP-13, prostaglandin E, and IL-6.[11]

In another research, piperine was coadministered with turmeric for inhibiting high fatty acid food-induced "C57 black6" mice swelling or to prevent metabolic syndrome.[43] Also, the anti-inflammatory potential of piperine was explored in colorectal locations, inhibiting inflammation mediated by free fatty acid (FFA)-induced TLR4 and ulcerative colitis caused by acetic acid in rodents.[23] Finally, in the carrageenan-induced inflammation test in mice, this compound was assessed to evaluate the analgesic and anti-inflammatory effects of black pepper operations at an oral dose of 6 mg/kg/day.[75]

8.6.6 Antidiarrheal Activity

Several researchers have recorded the antidiarrheal property of pepper. Interestingly, local people, herbal practitioners, and herbal companies formulate the peppercorn especially for diarrhea for all ages in most developing countries. Antidiarrheal activity has already been recorded in experimental mice. In addition, the piperine minimizes the antidiarrheal activity caused by the addition of different chemical activators and oil in the experimental animal model. Some reports have shown that piperine could release the castor oil-induced small intestine inflammation in mice. Piperine sequentially prevents the accumulation of small intestine liquid in such an induced scenario. In addition, the decrease in fluid secretion and accumulation was controlled by capsaicin-sensitive nerve cells, but the caps-azepine-sensorial TRPV1 receptors were less efficient in the scenario caused by castor oil.[3]

Black pepper can be used in constipation and diarrhea. Black pepper's main active constituent is piperine and the mode of action involves the concentration-dependent and atropine-sensitive stimulant impact, loperamide and nifedipine-like spontaneous contractions, naloxone-sensitive effect inhibition, Ca^{2+} channel blocking activity, relaxing impact, and contractions induced by K^+ (80 mM). These mechanisms generate cholinergic (spasmodic) and opioid agonist and Ca^{2+} inhibitor (antispasmodic).[35,41]

8.6.7 Colitis

Assessment of piperine action mechanism for DSS (dextran sulfate sodium)-induced colitis resulted in the growth of siRNA-mediated PXR (pregnane X receptor) knock down in mouse colonies and also resulted in the function of PXR in the protection of colonic mucosa. Piperine therapy avoided loss of body weight, diarrhea, histological injury, and expression of inflammatory mediators on DSS-induced colitis in mice. DSS injury was exacerbated, and protection by piperine against DSS colitis was inhibited with the downregulation of PXR.[6,27]

8.6.8 Anticancer Activity

After oral administration, antitumor activity of piperine was identified in decreasing the incidence of certain types of GI cancer.[68] Ethanolic extraction of black pepper has been efficient to treat lung cancer by modifying the oxidative degradation of lipids.[3] Piperine allowsthe inhibition of cell cycle at the G1/S phase, blocking the HUVECs (human umbilical vein endothelial cells) proliferation and migration.[62] Piperine may hinder angiogenesis in animal models, suppressing tubular synthesis and protein kinase β phosphorylation.[62] Anticancer efficiency of piperine was observed for the treatment of "castrate-resistant prostate cancer" in combination with docetaxel.[43] Piperine reduces this drug's liver metabolization rate by inhibiting hepatic CYP3A4.[38]

Furthermore, it has been proved that supplementary piperine could also increase the reduction efficacy of the immune system impacts of docetaxel in xenograft animal models except serious adverse reactions.[38] Piperine is active in cell lines of prostate cancer, causing death of cells by activating PARP-1 and caspase-3 proteins.[9] Piperine interferes with the androgen receptor expression in prostate cancer cells, considerably lowering the identification of the prostate-specific antigen.[55]

8.6.9   Bioavailability Enhancer

Bioavailability of various phytochemicals (such as curcumin, catechins, and ubedicarenone) has been reported to be improved, due to following mechanisms[2]:

- Proficiency to improve the swift absorption.
- Defense from chemical reactions of GIT.
- Defense against oxidative damage.

In this respect, by enhancing absorption, piperine improves oral bioavailability of carbamazepine and phenytoin.[47] The piperine (@ 20 mg) shows synergistic effect in the presence of phenytoin.[48] The coadministration of coenzyme Q10 with piperine has proven to be statistically significant ($P = 0.0348$; 30%) superior plasma AUC in comparison with the standard coenzyme Q10.[8] Studies reported that piperine remarkably increases the oral manifestation of fexofenadine in rats by blocking P-gp-mediated cellular efflux during absorption in intestine.[36] Similarly, piperine has improved the bioavailability of nimesulide. Intense mice toxicological reports showed a decrease in the lethal dose (LD_{50}) of the combination relative to nimesulide alone.[24]

Furthermore, piperine (@ 20 mg/kg) has also been reported to improve the efficacy of ampicillin and norfloxacin.[29] Piperine also improves the rate and absorption of essential phytochemicals, for example, biologically active components present in green tea and curcumin. Curcumin has been commonly used throughout Asia as a food additive and herbal medicine.

The mixture of piperine with curcumin showed enhanced mobility, enhanced neurotransmission, and blocking effects of monoamine oxidase (MAO-A). In the intestinal mucosa, curcumin along with piperine can block CYP3A, CYP2C9, SULT, and UGT metabolism.[73] Black pepper can improve the beneficial effects of phytochemicals in other dietary spices. The ability of black pepper to improve bioavailability makes it a much-desired spice.

8.6.10 Antimicrobial Activity

In addition to traditional medicine, black pepper is an effective antimicrobial agent against resistant pathogenic strains[4]. It has been reported to be the most efficient antimicrobial agent against Gram-positive pathogenic species, such as, *Staphylococcus aureus, Streptococcus faecalis,* and *Bacillus cereus*. However, efficiency is low toward Gram-negative strains (*Pseudomonas aeruginosa, Escherichia coli*, and *Salmonella typhi*).[20]

The extracts of black pepper in aqueous solution possess the permeability in Gram-positive microbes due to antimicrobial activity. Several experiments have examined the antimicrobial and antifungal functions of various black pepper-derived alkaloids, including tannins, flavonoids, and glycosides. When formulated as nanoparticles with metals, extracts of pepper can act as a deterrent to the growth of plant pathogenic species.[49]

Pharmacokinetic analysis study stated that a single daily dose of piperine for 7 days was able to reduce the absorption half-life ($P < 0.05$), extended the elimination half-life ($P < 0.01$), resulting in a best AUC drug concentration ($P < 0.05$) in comparison to phenytoin alone. Therefore, piperine on multifarious dose administration, changes the pharmacokinetic factors of the antiepileptic.[12] *P. nigrum* enhanced sleep time for pentobarbitone, enhanced blood pressure and caused conditional avoidance in dogs.[31] Piperine also increases the impact of additives, such as beta carotene, curcumin, and resveratrol.[30,58,70]

8.7 SIDE EFFECTS AND TOXICITY

It has been proved in mice models that piperine (2.5 mg/kg) may decrease thyroid hormone concentration as much as conventional antithyroid drug,[46] hence making it useful for individuals with hyperthyroidism. However, it could be dangerous to reduce thyroid concentrations in healthy persons. Low concentrations can lead to symptoms of tiredness, joint pain and shortness of breath.[74]

When our body is under attack from an invader like bacteria, piperine is known to bring about an activation of T cells by rushing dendritic cells toward the lymphatic system. Piperine prevents dendritic cells from maturing in mice and makes them less capable of reaching the lymph nodes.[54]

Piperine has been associated with damage of sperms in mice by increasing the amounts of damaging radicals in the epididymis. It is also known to decrease the motility and count of sperms in rats when administered at a dose of 10 mg/kg.[17] Further, it acts as an abortifacient by inhibiting the attachment of fertilized eggs to the uterus. In mice, the number of implanted eggs was halved through injections of piperine.[16] This compound can increase the bioavailability of toxins through the same processes that enhance the bioavailability of supplements and drugs. Rats treated with piperine have assimilated more aflatoxin B1 (a fungal toxin responsible for cancer and damage to hepatic tissues).[5]

One research examined the motion of food and liquids in mice and rats through the digestive system. Piperine at low doses (1–1.3 mg/kg of body weight) improved the transit time required by the digestive system for solids to move. There was no liquid shift.[10] Slowing food passage decreases starvation, therefore piperine might assist in regulating hunger and weight.[13] Taking large quantities of black pepper or supplements can cause adverse side effects, such as throat burning or stomach burning.[39]

Some of the naturally occurring carcinogens are strongly linked in composition to piperine. Such agents exemplified by safrole, methyl eugenol, and estragole are essential components of frequently used spices and essential oils of plants. Researchers have warned against the mutagenic ability of pepper, while testing a number of spices via Ames test.[65]

8.8   PHARMACOKINETIC PROFILE

Piperine's pharmacokinetic profile has shown 97% absorption regardless of dosing mode, while 3% of piperine is excreted in fecal matters with no excretion in urine. The peak amount of piperine was discovered 6 hours after oral or i.v. in the stomach and small intestine. Administration and only traces of piperine in liver, serum, and spleen stayed within 24 h. There was enhanced excretion of uronic acids, phenols, and conjugated sulfates. The significant steps in its disposal appeared to be the methylenedioxy groups of piperine, glucuronidation, and sulfation.[31]

A homogenization cycle was prepared to determine the ADME (absorption, distribution, metabolism, excretion) of piperine. For this purpose, lipidic nanospheres and their pegylated versions were prepared and tested pharmacologically using male Albino mice. The pharmacokinetic study of piperine lipid nanospheres indicated high bioavailability and was known to exhibit a biexponential decline. The apparent volume of distribution and clearance of tested formulations was lower than piperine.[71]

8.9 SUMMARY

This chapter is an effort to understand the pharmacology of piperine in black pepper and its therapeutic effects on GI disorders. Not only black pepper has GIT effects, but it also has bioenhancing property and wide therapeutic use for neurological disorders, cancer, arthritis, bronchitis, vitiligo, weight loss, and menstrual pain, etc.

KEYWORDS

- antidiarrheal
- black pepper
- *Piper nigrum* L
- piperine
- carminative
- antispasmodic
- digestive

REFERENCES

1. Adhikary, B.; Yadav, S. K.; Roy, K.; Bandyopadhyay, S. K.; Chattopadhyay, S. Black Tea and Theaflavins Assist Healing of Indomethacin-Induced Gastric Ulceration in Mice by Antioxidative Action. *Evidence-Based Complem. Altern. Med.* **2011,** *2011,* 546–560.

2. Agbor, G.A.; Vinson, J. A.; Oben, J. E.; Ngogang, J. Y. Antioxidant Effect of Herbs and Spices on Copper Mediated Oxidation to Lower Low-Density Lipoprotein. *Chinese J. Nat. Med.* **2010,** *8* (2), 114–120.

3. Ahmad, N.; Fazal, H.; Abbasi, B.H.; Farooq, S.; Ali, M.; Khan, M. A. Biological Role of *Piper nigrum* L. (Black pepper): A Review. *Asian Pacific J. Trop. Biomed.* **2012,** *2* (3), S1945–S1953.

4. Aldaly, Z. T. Antimicrobial Activity of Piperine Purified from *Piper nigrum. J. Basrah Res.* **2010,** *36*, 54–61.

5. Allameh, A.; Saxena, M.; Biswas, G.; Raj, H. G.; Singh, J.; Srivastava, N. Piperine, A Plant Alkaloid of the Piper Species, Enhances the Bioavailability of Aflatoxin B1 in Rat Tissues. *Cancer Lett.* **1992,** *61* (3), 195–199.

6. Alves de Almeida, A. C.; de-Faria, F. M. Recent Trends in Pharmacological Activity of Alkaloids in Animal Colitis: Potential Use for Inflammatory Bowel Disease. *Evidence-Based Complem. Altern. Med.* **2017,** *2017*, article ID: 8528210.

7. Anjali, M. R.; Chandran, M.; Krishnakumar, K. Piperine as a Bioavailability Enhancer: A Review. *Asian J. Pharm. Analy. Med. Chem.* **2017,** *5* (1), 44–48.

8. Badmaev, V.; Majeed, M.; Prakash, L. Piperine Derived from Black Pepper Increases the Plasma Levels of Coenzyme Q10 Following Oral Supplementation. *J. Nutr. Biochem.* **2000,** *11* (2), 109–113.

9. Bae, G. S.; Kim, M. S.; Jung, W. S. Inhibition of Lipopolysaccharide-Induced Inflammatory Responses by Piperine. *Eur. J. Pharmacol.* **2010,** *642* (1–3), 154–162.

10. Bajad, S.; Bedi, K. L.; Singla, A. K.; Johri, R. K. Antidiarrheal Activity of Piperine in Mice. *Planta Medica* **2001,** *67* (3), 284–287.

11. Bang, J. S.; Choi, H. M.; Sur, B. J. Anti-Inflammatory and Antiarthritic Effects of Piperine In Human Interleukin 1β-Stimulated Fibroblast-Like Synoviocytes and in Rat Arthritis Models. *Arthritis Res. Therap.* **2009,** *11* (2), 1–9.

12. Bano, G.; Amla, V.; Raina, R. K.; Zutshi, U.; Chopra, C. L. The Effect of Piperine on Pharmacokinetics of Phenytoin in Healthy Volunteers. *Planta Medica* **1987,** *53* (6), 568–569.

13. Benini, L.; Todesco, T.; Dalle Grave, R. Gastric Emptying in Patients with Restricting and Binge/ Purging Subtypes of *Anorexia Nervosa. Am. J. Gastroenterol.* **2004,** *99* (8), 1448–1454.

14. Bhardwaj, R. K.; Glaeser, H.; Becquemont, L.; Klotz, U. Piperine, A Major Constituent of Black Pepper, Inhibits Human P-Glycoprotein and CYP3A4. *J. Pharmacol. Exp. Therap.* **2002,** *302* (2), 645–650.

15. Butt, M. S.; Pasha, I.; Sultan, M. T. Black Pepper and Health Claims: A Comprehensive Treatise. *Crit. Rev. Food Sci. Nutr.* **2013,** *53* (9), 875–886.

16. Daware, M.B.; Mujumdar, A.M.; Ghaskadbi, S. Reproductive Toxicity of Piperine in Swiss Albino Mice. *Planta Medica* **2000,** *66* (3), 231–236.

17. D'cruz, S.C.; Mathur, P.P. Effect of Piperine on the Epididymis of Adult Male Rats. *Asian J. Androl.* **2005,** *7* (4), 363–368.

18. de Sousa Falcão, H.; Leite, J.; Barbosa-Filho, J. Gastric and Duodenal Antiulcer Activity of Alkaloids: A Review. *Molecules* **2008,** *13* (12), 3198–3223.

19. Evans, W. C. *Trease and Evans: Pharmacognosy*, 14th ed.; Saunders Elsevier: New York, 2002, pp 363–364.

20. Ganesh, P.; Kumar, R.S.; Saranraj, P. Phytochemical Analysis and Antibacterial Activity of Pepper (*Piper nigrum* L.) Against Some Human Pathogens. *Centr. Eur. J. Exp. Biol.* **2014,** *3* (2), 36–41.

21. Ghosal, N.; Firdaus, S.B.; Paul, S.; Naaz, S. Amelioration of Gastro-toxic Effect of Indomethacin by Piperine in Male Wistar Rats: Novel Therapeutic Approach. *J. Pharm. Res.* **2016,** *10* (5), 240–254.

22. Gorgani, L.; Mohammadi, M. Piperine-The Bioactive Compound of Black Pepper: From Isolation to Medicinal Formulations. *Comprehen. Rev. Food Sci. Food Safe.* **2017,** *16* (1), 124–140.

23. Gupta, R.A.; Motiwala, M.N.; Dumore, N.G.; Danao, K.R.; Ganjare, A.B. Effect of Piperine on Inhibition of FFA Induced TLR4 Mediated Inflammation and Amelioration of Acetic Acid Induced Ulcerative Colitis in Mice. *J. Ethnopharmacol.* **2015,** *164*, 239–246.

24. Gupta, S.K.; Bansal, P.; Bhardwaj, R.K. Comparative Anti-Nociceptive, Anti-Inflammatory and Toxicity Profile of Nimesulide and Piperine Combination. *Pharmacol. Res.* **2000,** *41* (6), 657–662.

25. Han, Y.; Tan, T. M. C.; Lim, L. Y. In Vitro and In Vivo Evaluation of the Effects of Piperine on P-Gp Function and Expression. *Toxicol. Appl. Pharmacol.* **2008,** *230* (3), 283–289.

26. https://chestofbooks.com/health/materia-medica-drugs/Textbook-Materia-Medica/Black-Pepper-Piper-Nigrum.html/Description; Accessed on August 17, **2019.**

27. Hu, D.; Wang, Y.; Chen, Z.; Ma, Z. The Protective Effect of Piperine on Dextran Sulfate Sodium Induced Inflammatory Bowel Disease and its Relation with Pregnane-X Receptor Activation. *J. Ethnopharmacol.* **2015,** *169*, 109–123.

28. Hu, Z.; Yang, X.; Ho, P. C. L. Herb-drug interactions. *Drugs* **2005,** *65* (9), 1239–1282.

29. Janakiraman, K.; Manavalan, R. Studies on Effect of Piperine on Oral Bioavailability of Ampicillin and Norfloxacin. *Afr. J. Trad., Complem. Altern. Med.* **2008,** *5* (3), 257–262.

30. Johnson, J. J.; Nihal, M.; Siddiqui, I. A. Enhancing Bioavailability of Resveratrol by Combining it with Piperine. *Mol. Nutr. Food Res.* **2011,** *55* (8), 1169–1176.

31. Johri, R. K.; Zutshi, U. Ayurvedic Formulation 'Trikatu' and its Constituents. *J. Ethnopharmacol.* **1992,** *37*, 85–91.

32. Kesarwani, K.; Gupta, R. Bioavailability Enhancers of Herbal Origin: An Overview. *Asian Pacific J. Trop. Biomed.* **2013,** *3* (4), 253–266.

33. Kim, S. H; Lee, Y. C. Piperine Inhibits Eosinophil Infiltration and Airway Hyper responsiveness by Suppressing T-Cell Activity and Th2 Cytokine Production in the Ovalbumin-Induced Asthma Model. *J. Pharm. Pharmacol.* **2009,** *61* (3), 353–359.

34. Kokate, C. K.; Purohit, A. P.; Gokhale, S. B. (Eds.). *Pharmacognosy*, Vol. 464; Nirali Prakashan: Pune, India, 2008; pp 14.21–14.24.

35. Lambert, J. D.; Hong, J.; Kim, D. H.; Mishin, V. M.; Yang, C. S. Piperine Enhances the Bioavailability of the Tea Polyphenol (-)-Epigallocatechin-3-Gallate in Mice. *J. Nutr.* **2004,** *134* (8), 1948–1952.

36. Jin, M. J.; Han, H. K. Effect of Piperine, A Major Component of Black Pepper on the Intestinal Absorption of Fexofenadine and its Implication on Food–Drug Interaction. *J. Food Sci.* **2010,** *75* (3), H93–H96.

37. Lee, S. A.; Hong, S. S.; Han, X. H. Piperine from the Fruits of *Piper Longum* with Inhibitory Effect on Monoamine Oxidase and Antidepressant-Like Activity. *Chemical and Pharmaceutical Bulletin* **2005,** *53* (7), 832–835.

38. Makhov, P.; Golovine, K.; Canter, D. Co-Administration of Piperine and Docetaxel Results in Improved Anti-tumor Efficacy via Inhibition of CYP3A4 Activity. *Prostate* **2012,** *72* (6), 661–667.

39. McNamara, F. N.; Randall, A.; Gunthorpe, M. J. Effects of Piperine, the Pungent Component of Black Pepper at the Human Vanilloid Receptor (TRPV-1). *Br. J. Pharmacol.* **2005,** *144* (6), 781–790.

40. Meghwal, M.; Goswami, T. K. Chemical Composition, Nutritional, Medicinal and Functional Properties of Black Pepper: A Review. *Open Access Sci. Rep.* **2012,** *1* (2), 1–5.

41. Mehmood, M. H.; Gilani, A. H. Pharmacological Basis for the Medicinal Use of Black Pepper and Piperine in Gastrointestinal Disorders. *J. Med. Food* **2010,** *13* (5), 1086–1096.

42. Mittal, R.; Gupta, R. L. In Vitro Antioxidant Activity of Piperine. *Methods Find. Exp. Clin. Pharmacol.* **2000,** *22* (5), 271–274.

43. Miyazawa, T.; Nakagawa, K.; Kim, S. H. Curcumin and Piperine Supplementation of Obese Mice Under Caloric Restriction Modulates Body Fat and Interleukin-1β. *Nutr. Metabol.* **2018,** *15* (1), 1–9.

44. Nogara, L.; Naber, N.; Pate, E.; Canton, M.; Reggiani, C.; Cooke, R. Piperine's Mitigation of Obesity and Diabetes can be Explained by its Up-Regulation of the Metabolic Rate of Resting Muscle. *Proc. Natl. Acad. Sci.* **2016,** *113* (46), 13009–13014.

45. Pal, A.; Nayak, S.; Sahu, P. K.; Swain, T. Piperine Protects Epilepsy Associated Depression: A Study on Role of Monoamines. *Eur. Rev. Med. Pharmacol. Sci.* **2011,** *15* (11), 1288–1295.

46. Panda, S.; Kar, A. Piperine Lowers the Serum Concentrations of Thyroid Hormones, Glucose and Hepatic 5′-D Activity in Adult Male Mice. *Hormone Metabol. Res.* **2003,** *35* (9), 523–526.

47. Pattanaik, S.; Hota, D.; Prabhakar, S.; Kharbanda, P.; Pandhi, P. Pharmacokinetic Interaction of Single Dose of Piperine With Steady-State Carbamazepine in Epilepsy Patients. *Phytotherap. Res. Int. J. Devoted Pharmacol. Toxicol. Eval. Nat. Prod. Derivatives* **2009,** *23* (9), 1281–1286.

48. Pattanaik, S.; Hota, D.; Prabhakar, S.; Kharbanda, P.; Pandhi, P. Effect of Piperine on the Steady-State Pharmacokinetics of Phenytoin in Patients with Epilepsy. *Phytotherap. Res. Int. J. Devoted Pharmacol. Toxicol. Eval. Nat. Prod. Derivatives* **2006,** *20* (8), 683–686.

49. Paulkumar, K.; Gnanajobitha, G.; Vanaja, M. *Piper Nigrum* Leaf and Stem Assisted Green Synthesis of Silver Nanoparticles and Evaluation of its Antibacterial Activity Against Agricultural Plant Pathogens. *Sci. World J.* **2014** *2014,* article ID: 829894

50. Pradeep, C.R.; Kuttan, G. Effect of Piperine on the Inhibition of Lung Metastasis Induced B16F-10 Melanoma Cells in Mice. *Clin. Exp. Metast.* **2002,** *19* (8), 703–708.

51. Reen, R. K.; Jamwal, D. S. Impairment of UDP-Glucose Dehydrogenase and Glucuronidation Activities in Liver and Small Intestine of Rat and Guinea Pig In Vitro by Piperine. *Biochem. Pharmacol.* **1993,** *46* (2), 229–238.

52. Rezaee, M. M.; Kazemi, S.; Kazemi, M. T. The Effect of Piperine on Midazolam Plasma Concentration in Healthy Volunteers, A Research on the CYP3A-Involving Metabolism. *DARU J. Pharm. Sci.* **2014,** *22* (1), 8–12.

53. Rezvanian, M.; Ooi, Z. T.; Jamal, J. A. Pharmacognostic and Chromatographic Analysis of Malaysian *Piper Nigrum* Linn. Fruits. *Ind. J. Pharm. Sci.* **2016,** *78* (3), 334–343.

54. Rodgers, G.; Doucette, C. D.; Soutar, D. A.; Liwski, R.S.; Hoskin, D.W. Piperine Impairs the Migration and T Cell-Activating Function of Dendritic Cells. *Toxicol. Lett.* **2016,** *242*, 23–33.

55. Samykutty, A.; Shetty, A. V.; Dakshinamoorthy, G. Piperine, A Bioactive Component of Pepper Spice Exerts Therapeutic Effects on Androgen Dependent and Androgen Independent Prostate Cancer Cells. *PloS One* **2013,** *8* (6), article ID: e65889.

56. Sekeroglu, N.; Kaya, D.A.; Inan, M.; Kirpik, M. Essential Oil Contents and Ethnopharmacological Characteristics of Some Spices and Herbal Drugs Traded in Turkey. *Int. J. Pharmacol.* **2006,** *2* (2), 256–261.

57. Shityakov, S.; Bigdelian, E.; Hussein, A. A. Phytochemical and Pharmacological Attributes of Piperine: A Bioactive Ingredient of Black Pepper. *Eur. J. Med. Chem.* **2019,** *176*, 149–161.

58. Shoba, G.; Joy, D.; Joseph, T.; Majeed, M. Influence of Piperine on The Pharmacokinetics of Curcumin in Animals and Human Volunteers. *Planta Medica* **1998,** *64*, 353–356.

59. Siddiqui, B. S.; Gulzar, T.; Mahmood, A. Phytochemical Studies on the Seed Extract of *Piper Nigrum* Linn. *Nat. Prod. Res.* **2005,** *19* (7), 703–712.

60. Singh, A.; Rao, A. R. Evaluation of the Modulatory Influence of Black Pepper (*Piper nigrum,* L.) on the Hepatic Detoxication System. *Cancer Lett.* **1993,** *72* (1–2), 5–9.

61. Singh, J.; Dubey, R. K.; Atal, C. K. Piperine-Mediated Inhibition of Glucuronidation Activity in Isolated Epithelial Cells of the Guinea-Pig Small Intestine: Evidence That Piperine Lowers the Endogenous UDP-Glucuronic Acid Content. *J. Pharmacol. Exp. Therap.* **1986,** *236* (2), 488–493.

62. Singh, S.; Awasthi, M.; Pandey, V. P.; Dwivedi, U. N. Natural Products as Anticancerous Therapeutic Molecules with Special Reference to Enzymatic Targets Topoisomerase, COX, LOX and Aromatase. *Curr. Protein Peptide Sci.* **2018,** *19* (3), 238–274.

63. Smith, S. H. In the Shadow of a Pepper-Centric Historiography: Understanding the Global Diffusion of Capsicums in the Sixteenth and Seventeenth Centuries. *J. Ethnopharmacol.* **2015,** *167*, 64–77.

64. Sosa, S.; Balick, M. J.; Arvigo, R. Screening of the Topical Anti-Inflammatory Activity of Some Central American Plants. *J. Ethnopharmacol.* **2002,** *81*, 211–215.

65. Srinivasan, K. Black Pepper and its Pungent Principle-Piperine: A Review of Diverse Physiological Effects. *Critical Reviews in Food Science and Nutrition* **2007,** *47* (8), 735–748.

66. Sunila, E. S.; Kuttan, G. Immunomodulatory and Antitumor Activity of *Piper Longum* Linn. and Piperine. *J. Ethnopharmacol.* **2004,** *90*, 339–346.

67. Tasleem, F.; Azhar, I.; Ali, S. N.; Perveen, S.; Mahmood, Z. A. Analgesic and Anti-Inflammatory Activities of *Piper nigrum* L. *Asian Pacific J. Trop. Med.* **2014,** *7*, S461–S468.

68. Tharmalingam, N.; Kim, S. H.; Park, M.; Woo, H. J.; Kim, H. W.; Yang, J. Y.; Rhee, K. J.; Kim, J. B. Inhibitory Effect of Piperine on Helicobacter pylori Growth and Adhesion to Gastric Adenocarcinoma Cells. *Infect. Agents Cancer* **2014**, *9* (1), 1–10.

69. Umar, S.; Sarwar, A. H. M. G. Piperine Ameliorates Oxidative Stress, Inflammation and Histological Outcome in Collagen Induced Arthritis. *Cell. Immunol.* **2013**, *284* (1–2), 51–59.

70. Veda, S.; Srinivasan, K. Influence of Dietary Spices on the In Vivo Absorption of Ingested B-Carotene in Experimental Rats. *Br. J. Nutr.* **2011**, *105* (10), 1429–1438.

71. Veerareddy, P. R.; Vobalaboina, V. Pharmacokinetics and Tissue Distribution of Piperine Lipid Nanospheres. *Int. J. Pharm. Sci.* **2008**, *63* (5), 352–355.

72. Vijayakumar, R.S.; Surya, D.; Nalini, N. Antioxidant Efficacy of Black Pepper (*Piper Nigrum* L.) and Piperine in Rats with High Fat Diet Induced Oxidative Stress. *Redox Rep.* **2004**, 9 (2), 105–110.

73. Volak, L. P.; Ghirmai, S.; Cashman, J. R. Curcuminoids Inhibit Multiple Human Cytochromes P450, UDP-Glucuronosyltransferase, and Sulfotransferase Enzymes, Whereas Piperine is a Relatively Selective CYP3A4 Inhibitor. *Drug Metabolism and Disposition* **2008**, *36* (8), 1594–1605.

74. Wheeler, M. H.; Lazarus, J. H. (Eds.) *Diseases of the Thyroid: Pathophysiology and Management*; Chapman & Hall: New York, 1994; p 314.

75. Yasir, A.; Ishtiaq, S.; Jahangir, M.; Ajaib, M.; Salar, U.; Khan, K. M. Biology-Oriented Synthesis (BIOS) of Piperine Derivatives and Their Comparative Analgesic and Antiinflammatory Activities. *Med. Chem.* **2018**, *14* (3), 269–280.

76. Zhu, F.; Mojel, R.; Li, G. Structure of Black Pepper (*Piper Nigrum*) Starch. *Food Hydrocoll.* **2017**, *71*, 102–107.

CHAPTER 9

Curative Properties of Chamomile in Gastrointestinal Disorders

MRINMOY SARKAR and POOJA CHAWLA

ABSTRACT

Traditionally chamomile is a herbal medicinal plant in Egypt, Greece, Rome, Germany, Western Europe, and Northern Africa, belong to the family of *Asteraceae* and categorized into two types, German (*Matricaria recutita*) and Roman (*Chamaemelum nobile*) Chamomile. The chamomile flowers exhibit curative properties to alleviate colic in children, help in digestion, treat gastritis, minimize the ulcerative colitis, diminish inflammation/intestinal cramps, and simplify bowel movement. It is very useful in treatment of diverticular disorder and has a positive effect on an upset stomach, dispelling gas and muscle relaxation.

9.1 INTRODUCTION

The human gastrointestinal (GI) system consists of exocrine supplementary gland, nose, esophagus, uterus, stomach, small intestine, large intestine, salivary glands, liver, gallbladder, and pancreas. The main function of this system is food assimilation and waste product excretion. The enteric nervous system (ENS: a large intrinsic network of neurons in the gastro-intestinal tract (GIT) wall) and several hormones have extensive control mechanisms.[38]

GI tract diseases are common, painful, or complex and can affect the mucosa, musculature, and neural intervals from the esophagus into the colon, which present themselves as ulceration, swelling, congestion, vomiting, constipation, and abdominal pain. Abnormalities in gastroesophageal reflux (GERD) and irritable bowel syndrome (IBS) cause life-threatening conditions, such as inflammatory bowel disease (IBD). Symptoms of certain GI disorders get escalated under stressful conditions.[22]

Various natural plants including chamomile have been exploited to treat GIT disorders since ancient times. Another part of the *Asteraceae* family is a dried floral head having up to 1.5% blue essential oil with principal constituents, such as chamazulene and (-)-α-bisabolol. The floral tips contain flavonoids, apigenin-7 glycosides with antispasmodic effects to prevent peristalsis. This medicinal plant has been used in severe GIT problems (such as spasms, severe gastritis, ulcers, and dyspepsia) due to its carminative and spasmolytic effects.[37]

This chapter discusses beneficial effects of perennial herbaceous plant chamomile on the GIT related disorders.

9.2 PHARMACOGNOSTIC CHARACTERISTICS OF CHAMOMILE PLANT

Chamomile plants are categorized into two types: (1) German (*Matricaria recutita*) and (2) Roman (*Chamaemelum nobile*) Chamomile. The flower is primarily cultivated in southern England, Germany, France, Belgium, Hungary, Poland, Bulgaria, Egypt, and Argentina.[16]

This perennial herbaceous plant has twelve to twenty terminal ligulate flowers and abundant central vasiform florets in the capitulum (10–17 mm) (Figure 9.1). *Matricaria* has a hollow receptacle without paleae, one to three rows of lanceolate bracts with a frightening brownish-grey border that covers the capitulum. There are five stamens with anthers. Several tiny shiny, yellow trichomes are distributed over each portion of blooms and bracts.[27] The herb has an enticing scent of pleasure.[35] It is propagated by means of vegetative propagation, for which loamy soil and optimum climate conditions are necessary. Flowers collection begins by manual labor in June and continues until September. In thin layers, they are exposed to direct sunlight, otherwise in drying rooms with artificial heat at temperatures not exceeding 40°C. Dried flowers are classified by sieving into small, medium, and large.[49]

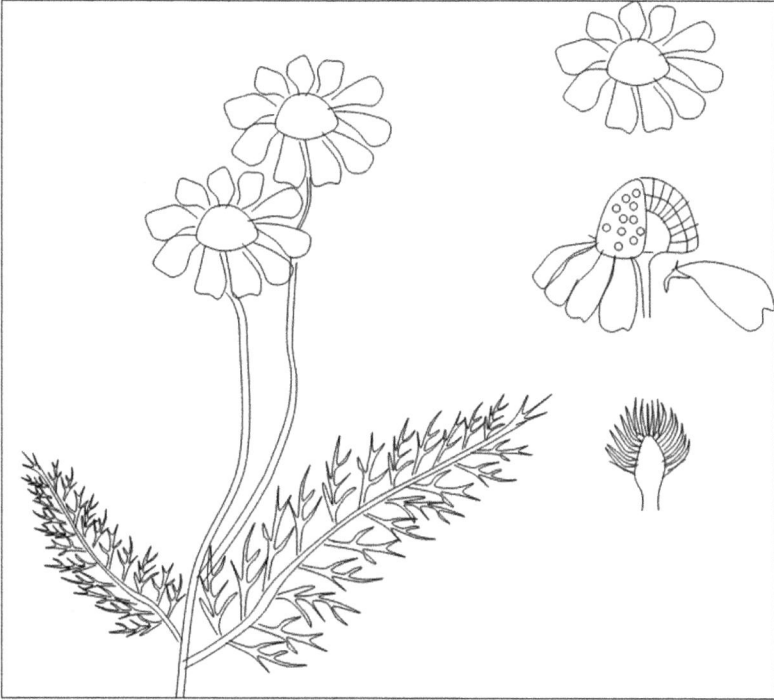

FIGURE 9.1 Typical chamomile plant.[26]

9.3 ETHNOPHARMACOLOGY OF CHAMOMILE

Chamomile smells like apple; for this reason, it is named "chamomile" in Greek meaning "ground apple." It was applied by ancient Egyptians to treat the "ague," which is known as an acute fever associated with malaria in Egypt. In a traditional manner, chamomile has been used to aid digestion, keep breathing fresh, boost the immunity, and have a good sleep. It is also used as an excitant for common use, hypersensitivity alleviation, complications in the menstrual cycle for women, inflammation in bronchial tubes, worms, and insect bite and irritation.[12,55]

From the ancient time, chamomile flowers are used daily to treat xerosis and erythema due to climatic conditions in Roman, Greek, and Egypt.[6] Chamomile has been commonly used: (1) for diagnosis of digestive system disorders in traditional Tunisian medicine[51]; (2) as a hypnotic and tranquillizer in Iranian traditional medicine[1]; and (3) a key component in several medicinal preparations that are conventional, and in unani and homoeopathy.[52] This herb has been grown in Lucknow in India for around 200 years, and in Punjab for around 300 years ago during the Mughal Empire.

German chamomile flowers are intensely aromatic with a bitter flavor. Its extract is used as a herbal tea for relieving flatulence, neuroleptic and as a body stimulant purpose, for abdominal cramps and infections. The extract can also be used as a mask for mucous membranes and for treating skin inflammation and bacterial skin disease.[39]

9.4   PHYTOCHEMICAL CONSIDERATIONS OF CHAMOMILE PLANT

Chamomile contains a large number of bioactive compounds, such as flavonoids, sesquiterpenes, polyacetylene, and coumarins.[50] The coumarins are illustrated in chamomile by active constituents, such as herniarin, umbelliferone, and other minor compounds.[40] The (Z)- and (E)-2-β-d-glucopyranosyloxy-4-methoxycinnamic acids (GMCA: glucoside ancestor of herniarin) are endemic compounds in chamomile.[36] Chamomile extract[23] contains different bioactive phenolic compounds, such as chlorogenic acid and caffeic acid (phenylpropanoids), herniarin and umbelliferone (coumarin), luteolin and luteolin-7-O-glucoside (flavones), apigenin, apigenin-7-O-glucoside, naringenin, quercetin, and rutin (flavonols) (Fig. 9.2).

Over 120 bioactive constituents with effective therapeutic action have been isolated as secondary metabolites in chamomile flowers. Among these, there are 28 terpenoids, 36 flavonoids, and 52 other biocompounds.[47,48,59]

The α-bisabolol and cyclic ethers having antimicrobial activity and umbelliferone are fungistatic, while antiseptic properties are found in chamazulene and α-bisabolol.[43] An instinctive source of blue oil (essential oil) is German chamomile, and this oil is extracted from flowers and flower heads.

Interestingly, this blue oil consists only of by-products of sesquiterpene (75%–90%). The oil comprises of polyenes up to 20%. Main components of this essential oil extract are terpene alcohol (farnesol), (E)-β-farnesene (4.9%–8.1%), α-bisabolol (4.8%–11.3%), chamazulene (2.3%–10.9%), α-bisabolol oxides-A (25.5%–28.7%) and α-bisabolol oxides-B (12.2%–30.9%); these have been recognized for their anti-inflammatory, antiseptic,

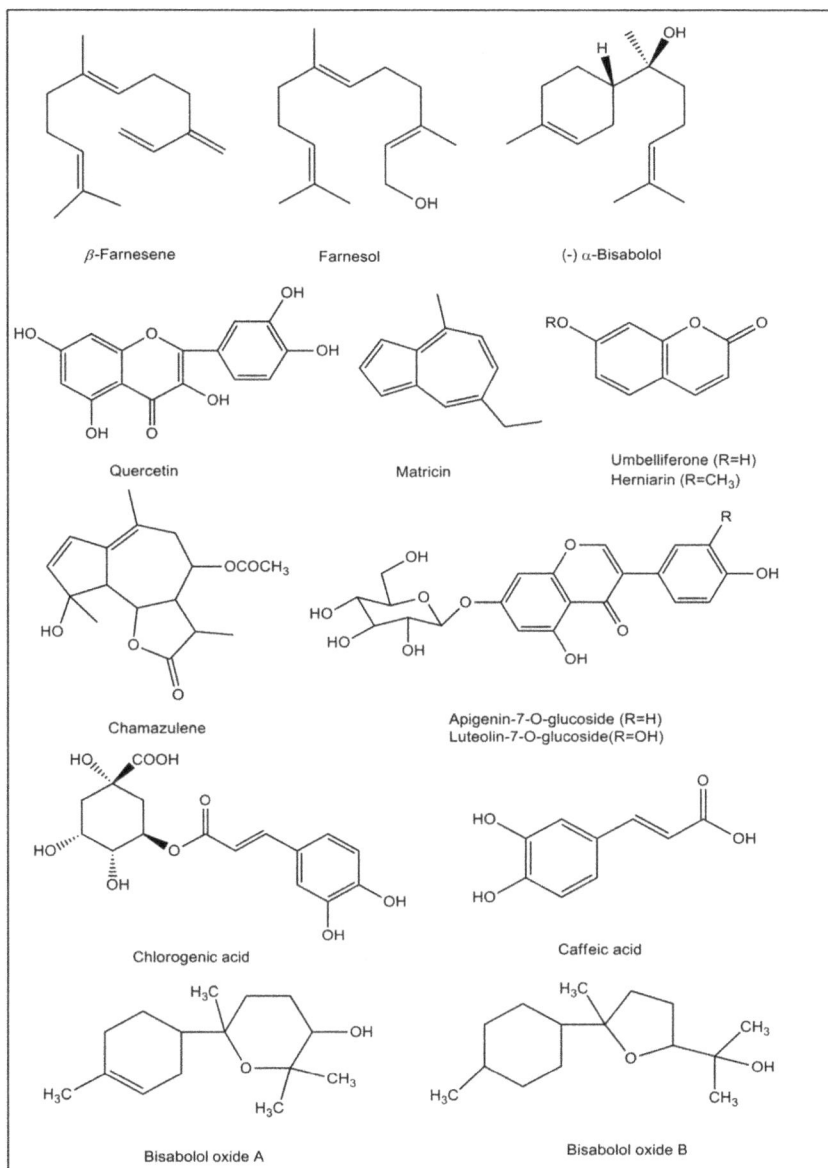

FIGURE 9.2   Selected phytochemical compounds in chamomile plant.

antiphlogistic, and spasmolytic characteristics.[33,58] However, the amount of chamazulene is less in Roman chamomile consisting of angelic acid esters, tiglic acid, farnesene, and α-pinene.[55]

Bisabolol has been reported to decrease the quantity of proteolytic enzyme "pepsin" by the stomach except for any alterations in the amount of stomach acid, as a result of which it was prescribed for the treatment of stomach and upper intestinal disorders.[45]

9.5   MECHANISMS OF ACTION

- By blocking or decreasing the conjugation of nitric oxide (NO), it may aid in relieving migraine-related headaches. Therefore, the prevention of nitric oxide synthase (NOS) is an aim in the management of migraine.[46] The hydrophilic compounds of chamomile (polyphenolic compounds, that is, flavonoids (such as apigenin)) can block inducible nitric oxide synthase (iNOS) development in activated macrophages and may result in a ban on NO release and synthesis.[7] This effect has been seen with use of basic chamomile oil along chamazulene.
- In the aqueous extract of chamomile, it appears that flavonoids (particularly lyapigenin 7-O-glucoside) have potential blocking activity on the RAW 264.7 macrophages of endogenous prostaglandin E2 (PGE2). It is a COX-2 antagonist with efficacy against inflammation and pain relief.[54]
- Meningeal or dural trigeminal nociceptor neuroinflammation results in peripheral sensitization.[13] Traditionally, chamomiles have been effective against inflammation, pain, neuralgia, etc.[12] Its polyphenolic components (basically apigenin) have additional anti-inflammatory activity, which is much more potent as compared to hydrocortisone and have no adverse effects.[10] The reason behind this activity is blocking of THP1 macrophages by pro-inflammatory biomarkers.[14] Assuming the impact of inflammation on neurovascular units (NVU) at the site of pain as a unique concept in migraine pathogenesis, chamomile migraine pain relief may clinch the topical anti-inflammatory impact.[56]

9.6   THERAPEUTIC ACTIVITIES OF CHAMOMILE ON GIT DISORDERS

The description of various phytochemical nutrients found in chamomile is given in Tables 9.1 and 9.2.

TABLE 9.1   Different Types of Nutrients in Chamomile.

Nutrient	Amount (in flowers), g	Determination method	Ref.
Moisture	22.2	Loss on drying	[8,11]
Ash content	9.8	Muffle furnace	[32]
Calcium	14.02	Titrimetric method	[17]
Fat	20.4	Soxhlation	[29]
Protein	0.87	Kjeldahl method	[30]
Vitamin C	16.47	Titrimetric method	[28]

TABLE 9.2   Screening of Phytochemicals in Chamomile.

Phytochemical	Present (in flowers)	Determination method	Ref.
Alkaloids	No	Mayer's test	[4,64]
Flavonoids	Yes	Alkaline Reagent Test	[34,41,64]
Glycosides	No	Keller-Killiani test	[4]
Phytosterol	Yes	Libermann-Burchard's test	[3,11]
Saponin	No	Foam Test	[11,64]
Tanin	Yes	Gelatin Test	[4,11]
Terpenoids	Yes	Salkowski Test	[3,11]

9.6.1   Promotes Digestion

Chamomile is considered a potent digestive relaxant helpful in alleviating various GIT problems, such as stomach pain, gastroesophageal reflux disease (GRD), digestive problems, dysentery, sitophobia, motion sickness, nausea, vomiting, and so on. The oil extracted from flowers of chamomile (with antispasmodic and anodyne constituents) can reduce pediatric dysentery and colic; it can alleviate prefix associated with pain and anxiety, cramping, constipation, and stomach pains. Various beneficial effects are due to natural relaxing properties of chamomile. Since the brain and intestine interact directly through X-cranial nerve, comfortable (calm) mind can also help to cure leaky intestines, which can lead to the lower prefix of long situations, such as IBS and other gut-SIBO problems. It also makes it a better choice for pregnant mothers to recline the GI tract and to serve as a herbal preparation to avoid vomiting.[25]

9.6.2   Spasmolytic Activity of Chamomile

Chamomile has carminative, spasmolytic and anti-peristalsis effects, due to presence of flavonoids (such as apigenin-7-glycoside) in the essential oil. Thus, chamomile is used in severe digestive spasms, acute gastritis, ulcers, and dyspepsia.[37]

9.6.3   Use in Pediatrics for Gastrointestinal Tract Problem

Mothers have been using chamomile for centuries to relax crying children, minimize fever, cure ear-aches, and soothe upset stomach. Because of its ability to help children with attention-deficit/hyperactivity disorder, it is often called the "kid calmer," thus proving beneficial for infants and children. A study was carried out on 79 children with severe, uncomplicated diarrhea to evaluate the efficacy of chamomile extract and apple pectin formulation. After treating with chamomile and pectin for three days, diarrhea was found to stop earlier as compared with placebo group. Therefore, chamomile can be utilized safely as a natural diarrheal treatment to treat upset stomach in children.[55]

9.6.4   Effects on Irritable Bowel Syndrome

Patients (aged 12 years and older) with signs of severe diarrhea caused by acute gastrointestinal inflammatory disorder (GAID), IBD, and IBS were treated with a mixed herbal formulation comprising of chamomile. The extracts studied were similar to the traditional treatments in routine care at the end of the study.[2] Initial research indicated that chamomile inhibits slow-wave movement in the small intestine.[57]

9.6.5   Chamomile Tea as Immune Booster

Chamomile tea intake has been believed to boost the immune system and to combat cold-related infections. Health beneficial effects of chamomile plant were established through a study with 14 volunteers, who had consumed 5 glasses of chamomile liquid extract per day for two successive weeks. Regular urine samples were taken and analyzed throughout the study for both after and before consuming the plant extract. Results showed that, in urine, the cabalistic increase of hippurate and glycine along with antibacterial mobility was correlated with chamomile extract.[60] Chamomile was able to ease the hypertensive symptoms in another study, and significantly reduced systolic blood pressure and increased the urine production. There is a need for further studies before a more conclusive link can be established for health efficacy with chamomile.[62]

9.6.6   Anti-colic Activity

Apple pectin in combination with chamomile tea reduced the duration of pediatric dysentery and relieved the condition-related symptoms.[21] Two clinical tests assessed chamomile's effectiveness in treating colic in pediatric patients. The tea was administered in conjunction with different plants (German chamomile, caraway, lemon balm). Sixty-eight healthy children, who had been suffering from colic (2–8 weeks of age) diseases, accepted the herbal tea or placebo (glucose, flavoring) in an expected, randomized, double-blind, placebo-controlled study. Each infant was offered up to 150 mL/dose with each bout of colic, no more than three times a day. Parents confirmed that tea reduced colic in 57% of infants after 7 days of treatment compared to 26% in placebo treatment. No side effects were observed in other categories, such as number of night-time wakefulness.[19]

9.6.7   Treatment of Ulcers

Mercantile herbal formulations with anti-ulcerogenic property was prepared by the extraction process from candytuft, lemon balm, chamomile, fennel, peppermint, liquorice, garden angelica, milk thistle, and nipplewort in combination. This is related to lower acid intake, increased mucin secretion, enhanced E2 release of prostaglandin, and reduced leukotrienes.[34] Inflammation is related to many issues of GIT, such as heartburn, acid reflux, diverticulosis, and IBD. Preclinical test data indicated that chamomile can prevent *Helicobacter pylori*, which is responsible for ulcers in the stomach, due to reduction in smooth muscle spasms.[61]

9.6.8   Effect on Mucositis

Mouth ulcers are associated with a number of etiologies.[20] Stomatitis is the main dose-limiting toxicity for chemotherapy regimens dependent on 5-fluorouracil (5-FU) bolus. There was a double-blind, placebo-controlled clinical trial with 164 volunteers. At the time of their first 5-FU-based chemotherapy phase, patients were admitted into the study and randomized for 14 days of accepted chamomile liquid formulation three times in a day.[18] In case of stomatitis, no significant difference was observed among the clinical trial volunteers. No toxicity was reported. The same outcome was acquired in this condition by other chamomile trials. The pre-study theory was not assisted by evidence of clinical studies that chamomile could decrease stomatitis induced by 5-FU. Whether chamomile is beneficial in this case, the findings remain unclear.

9.6.9   Gastrointestinal Disorders

Traditionally, chamomile has been applied in several GIT disorders, along with digestion problems, "convulsion" or enteralgia, stomach ache, flatulence, stomach lesion, and digestional nuisance. *Matricaria* helps to decreased flatulency, mollifying the stomach issues, and calm the intestinal brawns, which help in passing the food through the intestines.[41]

A licensed herbal mixer of myrrh, coffee, charcoal, and chamomile flower extracts was tested for clinical effectiveness, protection, and tolerance in patients with signs of acute diarrhea. This study indicated that this mixture was efficient, well tolerated, and harmless for patients with acute diarrhea symptoms. The results are similar to the modern medicinal treatment.[60] The presence of volatile components and active ingredients in chamomile extract (such as terpenoids, flavonoids, quercetin, rutin, quercitrin, and gallic acid) are mainly responsible for healthcare compliance and healing effects in various GI conditions.

9.6.10   Anti-inflammatory Action

The anti-inflammatory effect has been associated with presence of flavonoids in chamomile. A decrease in the development of TNF-α in mice treated with apigenin-7-glucoside (APG), after lipopolysaccharide (LPS) treatment, supported the anti-inflammatory effect. The effect of chamomile on systemic inflammation was investigated in a clinical trial. There was enhanced mechanical joint function and decreased knee and lower back pain, but no major anti-inflammatory effects were observed.[14] The efficacy of chamomile extract as mouth rinse was tested in a clinical trial, and it was revealed that herbal mouth rinses were beneficial because they had antimicrobial and anti-inflammatory properties. Mainly the flavonoid compound (APG) was responsible for anti-inflammatory effects.[5]

9.6.11 Antimicrobial Activity

The chamomile fractions contain enantiopure (-)α-bisabolol as terpene and activated (-)α-bisabolol showed Gramnegative antibacterial activity. Gram-negative bacteria was tested for the antibacterial activity of chamomile fractions. Studies have established its antibacterial activity through its key essential oils, including coumarin, flavonoids, phenolic acids, and fatty acids.[53]

9.6.12 Antioxidant Activity

The antioxidant effects of ethanolic extracts of chamomile have been studied. The antioxidant property was confirmed by high rosmarinic acid concentration.[9] The level of bioactivity of this plant's aqueous extract revealed that after first week, microencapsulated extract of this plant was able to increase the antioxidant activity. The study on antioxidant properties of chamomile, milk thistle, and halophilic bacteria[44] confirmed that different concentrations of these natural components can inhibit the upregulation of free radicals produced by H_2O_2 in human skin fibroblasts in vitro and thus possess antioxidant activities.

The antioxidant function of extract of chamomile flower[15] had shown that CuO nanoparticles (CuO–NPs) have concentration-dependent antioxidant activity by breaking the DNA structure. Leaves and flowers of chamomile and marigold have been associated with their antioxidant activity; and extract from flower heads and chamomile leaves are the richest source of antioxidant activity.[41]

9.7   INTERFERENCES AMONG HERBS AND DRUGS

Due to the presence of coumarins in chamomile, aspirin and other anti-platelet drugs (such as ticlopidine, clopidogrelcan) can interfere with chamomile that can potentially lead to bleeding. In combination with warfarin, chamomile tea caused internal bleeding. The enzyme CYP1A2 is metabolized in the skin. Along with tricyclic antidepressants (amitriptyline, clomipramine, imapramine), clozapine, beta-blocker (propanolol), and theophylline, chamomile had been found to have a blocking effect on CYP1A2 and can increase the risk of toxicity by increasing the levels of these drugs in the blood. Tacrineis, a centrally functioning acetylcholinesterase antagonist, is used to prevent Alzheimer's disease and dementia-related symptoms. Chamomile being the blocker of CYP1A2 in the presence of tacrine may lead to toxicity and elevate the volume of blood.[31]

9.8   SIDE EFFECTS AND TOXICITY

There are some allergic effects of chamomile probably due to its adulterants "Dog chamomile," which have extremely allergic and bad-tasting properties.[10] Safety dose of chamomile is 3–4 g of tea thrice daily and 270 mg as a medicine, twice daily.[63] Chamomile is usually safe for consumption, although it should be used with caution in patients with ragweed hypersensitivity and other members of the composite family. Allergic reactions of chamomile are uncommon, and there have been no records on possible toxic action by compounds in chamomile.[12] People in critical situations (such as endometriosis, fibroids, or breast/uterine/ovarian cancers) must avoid the use of chamomile. It should be kept in mind that chamomile items are considered as a light uterine stimulants, and therefore in case of pregnancy, physician must be consulted before taking chamomile tea (mild chamomile tea should not cause any problems).[24]

9.9   SUMMARY

Today it is well known that medicinal plant chamomile particularly for GIT issues is the most versatile therapy. In this chapter, authors have discussed the various beneficial effects of chamomile on GIT including the mechanism of action. Preclinical studies and in-depth research are must to know the efficacy of this plant.

KEYWORDS

- **anti-inflammatory**
- **antiphlogistic**
- **chamomile**
- ***Chamomilla recutita***
- **digestion**
- ***Matricaria chamomilla***

REFERENCES

1. Adib-Hajbaghery, M.; Mousavi, S. N. The Effects of Chamomile Extract on Sleep Quality Among Elderly People: Clinical Trial. *Complemen. Therap. Med.* **2017,** *35,* 109–114.
2. Albrecht, U.; Müller, V.; Schneider, B.; Stange, R. Efficacy and Safety of Herbal Medicinal Product Containing Myrrh, Chamomile and Coffee Charcoal for the Treatment of Gastrointestinal Disorders: A Non-Interventional Study. *BMJ Open Gastroenterol.* **2014,** *1* (1), article ID: e000015.
3. An, S.; Zhao, L. P.; Shen, L. J; Wang, S. USP18 Protects Against Hepatic Steatosis and Insulin Resistance Through Its Deubiquitinating Activity. *Hepatology* **2017,** *66* (6),1866–1884.
4. Ayoola, G. A.; Coker, H. A.; Adesegun, S. Phytochemical Screening and Antioxidant Activities of Some Selected Medicinal Plants Used for Malaria Therapy in Southwestern Nigeria. *Trop. J. Pharm. Res.* **2008,** *7* (3),1019–1024.
5. Batista, A. L.; Lins, R. D.; De Souza Coelho, R. Clinical Efficacy Analysis of The Mouth Rinsing With Pomegranate And Chamomile Plant Extracts in The Gingival Bleeding Reduction. *Complem. Therap. Clin. Pract.* **2014,** *20* (1), 93–98.
6. Baumann, L.S. Less-known botanical cosmeceuticals. *Dermatol. Therap.* **2007,** *20* (5), 330–342.
7. Bhaskaran, N.; Shukla, S.; Srivastava, J. K.; Gupta, S. Chamomile: An Anti-Inflammatory Agent Inhibits Inducible Nitric Oxide Synthase Expression by Blocking RelA/p65 Activity. *Int. J. Mol. Med.* **2010,** *26* (6), 935–940.
8. Bouraoui, M.; Richard, P.; Fichtali, J. A Review of Moisture Content Determination in Foods Using Microwave Oven Drying. *Food Res. Int.* **1993,** *26* (1), 49–57.

9. Caleja, C.; Ribeiro, A.; Barros, L. Cottage Cheeses Functionalized With Fennel and Chamomile Extracts: Comparative Performance Between Free and Microencapsulated Forms. *Food Chem.* **2016,** *199*, 720–726.

10. Charousaei, F.; Dabirian, A.; Mojab, F. Using chamomile solution or a 1% topical hydrocortisone ointment in the management of peristomal skin lesions in colostomy patients: results of a controlled clinical study. *Ostomy-Wound Manage.* **2011,** *57* (5), 28–32.

11. Chauhan, E. S.; Aishwarya, J. Nutraceutical Analysis of *Marticaria recutita* (Chamomile) Dried Leaves and Flower Powder and Comparison Between Them. *Int. J. Phytomed.* **2018,** *10* (2), 111–114.

12. Chauhan, E.S.; Jaya, A. Chamomile an Ancient Aromatic Plant—A Review. *J. Ayurveda Med. Sci.* **2017,** *2* (4), 251–255.

13. Dodick, D.; Silberstein, S. Central Sensitization Theory of Migraine: Clinical Implications. Headache. *J. Head Face Pain* **2006,** *46*, S182–S191.

14. Drummond, E. M.; Harbourne, N. Inhibition of Proinflammatory Biomarkers in THP1 Macrophages By Polyphenols Derived From Chamomile, Meadowsweet and Willow Bark. *Phytotherap. Res.* **2013,** *7* (4), 588–594.

15. Duman, F.; Ocsoy, I.; Kup, F.O. Chamomile Flower Extract-Directed Nanoparticle Formation For its Antioxidant and DNA Cleavage Properties. *Mater. Sci. Engg.—C* **2016,** *60*, 333–338.

16. Evans, W. C. *Trease and Evans: Pharmacognosy*, 9th ed.; Saunders Elsevier: New York, 2002; pp 294–296.

17. Ferguson, E.; Vaughan, A.; Swale, J. A. Method for the Estimation of Total Calcium in Serum or Heparinized Plasma. *Clin. Chim. Acta* **1976,** *67* (3), 281–286.

18. Fidler, P.; Loprinzi, C. L.; O'Fallon, J. R. Prospective evaluation of a chamomile mouthwash for prevention of 5-FU-induced oral mucositis. *Cancer: Interdiscipl. Int. J. Am. Cancer Soc.* **1996,** *77* (3), 522–525.

19. Gardiner, P. Complementary, Holistic, and Integrative Medicine: Chamomile. *Pediatr. Rev.* **2007,** *28* (4), article ID: e16; online.

20. Gonsalves, W. C.; Wrightson, A. S.; Henry, R. G. Common Oral Conditions in Older Persons. *Am. Fam. Phys.* **2008,***78* (7), 845–852.

21. Gould, L.; Reddy, C. R.; Gomprecht, R. F. Cardiac Effects of Chamomile Tea. *J. Clin. Pharmacol. New Drugs* **1973,** *13* (11), 475–479.

22. Greenwood, B.; Johnson, A. C.; Grundy, D. Gastrointestinal Physiology and Function. In *Gastrointestinal Pharmacology*; Springer: Cham, 2017; pp 1–16.

23. Gupta, V.; Mittal, P.; Bansal, P.; Khokra, S. L.; Kaushik, D. Pharmacological Potential of *Matricaria recutita*-A Review. *Int. J. Pharm. Sci. Drug Res.* **2010,** *2* (1), 12–16.

24. https://draxe.com/nutrition/chamomile-benefits/; Precautions and Possible Chamomile Side Effects; (Accessed on October 22, 2019).

25. https://nccih.nih.gov/health/chamomile/ataglance.htm/SupportsDigestiveHealth/; (Accessed on October 21, 2019).

26. https://prairiestarbotanicals.com/products/chamomile; (Accessed on October 18, 2019).

27. https://thepharmacognosy.com/chamomile-flower/; Macroscopical and Microscopical Characters of Chamomile Flower; (Accessed on October 18, 2019).

28. https://www.canterbury.ac.nz/media/documents/scienceoutreach/vitaminc_iodine.pdf/Titration; (Accessed on October 20, 2019).

29. https://www.fsis.usda.gov/wps/wcm/connect/dd881c92-c19b-4530-b6ee931c368b 8904/CLG_FAT_03.pdf?MOD=Ajperes/AnalyticalProcedure/; (Accessed on October 20, 2019).
30. https://www.itwreagents.com/uploads/20180114/A173_EN.pdf/NitrogenDetermination by Kjeldahl Method/; (Accessed on October 20, 2019).
31. https://www.verywellhealth.com/chamomile-possible-drug-interactions-89174; (Accessed on October 22, 2019).
32. Ismail, B.P. Ash Content Determination. In *Food Analysis Laboratory Manual*; Springer: Cham, 2017; pp 117–119.
33. Jakovlev, V.; Isaac, O.; Thiemer, K.; Kunde, R. Pharmacological Investigations with Compounds of Chamomile, II: New Investigations on the Antiphlogistic Effects of (-)-Alpha-Bisabolol and Bisabolol Oxides. *Planta Medica* **1979**, *35* (2), 125–132.
34. Jarrahi, M. Effects of *Matricaria* Extract on Cutaneous Burn Wound Healing in Albino Rats. *Nat. Prod. Res.* **2008**, *22* (5), 422–427.
35. Kalia, A. N. *Textbook of Industrial Pharmacognosy*; CBS Publishers & Distributors Pvt.: New Delhi, 2011; p 255.
36. Kanamori, H.; Terauchi, M.; Fuse, J. I.; Sakamoto, I. Simultaneous and Quantitative Analysis of Glycoside. *Shoyakugaku Zasshi* **1993**, *47*, 34–38.
37. Kelber, O.; Bauer, R.; Kubelka, W. Phytotherapy in Functional Gastrointestinal Disorders. *Digest. Dis.* **2017**, *35* (S1), 36–42.
38. Kibble, J.D.; Halsey, C.R. Medical Physiology: The Big Picture. *Singapore Med. J.* **2009**, *50* (8), 833–840.
39. Kobayashi, Y.; Takahashi, R.; Ogino, F. Antipruritic Effect of the Single Oral Administration of German Chamomile Flower Extract and its Combined Effect with Antiallergic Agents in DDY Mice. *J. Ethnopharmacol.* **2005**, *101* (1–3), 308–312.
40. Kotov, A. G.; Khvorost, P. P.; Komissarenko, N. F. Coumarins of *Matricaria recutita*. *Chem. Nat. Comp.* **1991**, *27* (6), 753–760.
41. Kováčik, J.; Babula, P.; Hedbavny, J.; Klejdus, B. Hexavalent, Chromium Damages Chamomile Plants by Alteration of Antioxidants and Its Uptake Is Prevented by Calcium. *J. Hazard. Mater.* **2014**, *273*, 110–117.
42. Kroll, U.; Cordes, C. Pharmaceutical Prerequisites for a Multi-Target Therapy. *Phytomedicine* **2006**, *13*, 12–19.
43. Maday, E.; Szöke, É.; Muskáth, Z.; Lemberkovics, E. Study on the Production of Essential Oils in Chamomile Hairy Root Cultures. *Eur. J. Drug Metabol. Pharmacokinetics* **1999**, *24* (4), 303–308.
44. Mamalis, A.; Nguyen, D. H.; Brody, N.; Jagdeo, J. The Active Natural Anti-Oxidant Properties of Chamomile, Milk Thistle and Halophilic Bacterial Components in Human Skin In Vitro. *J. Drugs Dermatol.: JDD* **2013**, *12*(7), 780–784.
45. Mills, S.Y. *The Essential Book of Herbal Medicine (Arkana)*; Penguin Books: New York, 1994; p 706.
46. Olesen, J. The Role of Nitric Oxide in Migraine, Tension-Type Headache and Cluster Headache. *Pharmacology & Therapeutics* **2008**, *120* (2), 157–171.
47. Pino, J. A.; Bayat, F.; Marbot, R.; Aguero, J. Essential Oil of *Chamomilla recutita* (L.) Rausch. from Iran. *J. Essent. Oil Res.* **2002**, *14* (6), 407–408.

48. Pirzad, A.; Alyari, H.; Shakiba, M. R.; Zehtab-Salmasi, S.; Mohammadi, A. Essential Oil Content and Composition of German Chamomile (*Matricaria Chamomilla* L.) at Different Irrigation Regimes. *J. Agron.* **2006,** *5* (3), 451–455.

49. Rangari, V. D. Pharmacognosy & Phytochemistry. *Career Pub.* **2009,** *1,* 66–75.

50. Schilcher, H. *Die Kamille: Handbuchfürärzte, Apotheker Und Andere Naturwissenschaftler* (Chamomile: Handbook for Doctors, Pharmacists and Other Scientists). Wiss. Verl. (Knowledge Loss): Stuttgart, 1987; pp. 59–61.

51. Sebai, H.; Jabri, M. A.; Souli, A.; Rtibi, K.; Selmi, S.; Tebourbi, O.; El-Benna, J.; Sakly, M. Antidiarrheal and Antioxidant Activities of Chamomile (*Matricaria recutita* L.) Decoction Extract in Rats. *J. Ethnopharmacol.* **2014,** *152* (2), 327–332.

52. Singh, O.; Khanam, Z.; Misra, N.; Srivastava, M. K. *Matricaria chamomilla* L.: An Overview. *Pharmacognosy Rev.* **2011,** *5* (9), 82–90.

53. Son, Y. J.; Kwon, M.; Ro, D. K.; Kim, S. U. Enantioselective Microbial Synthesis of the Indigenous Natural Product (-)-A-Bisabolol by a Sesquiterpene Synthase From Chamomile (*Matricaria recutita*). *Biochem. J.* **2014,** *463* (2), 239–248.

54. Srivastava, J.K.; Pandey, M.; Gupta, S. Chamomile: Novel and Selective COX-2 Inhibitor With Anti-Inflammatory Activity. *Life Sci.* **2009,** *85* (19–20), 663–669.

55. Srivastava, J. K.; Shankar, E.; Gupta, S. Chamomile: A Herbal Medicine of the Past With a Bright Future. *Mol. Med. Rep.* **2010,** *3* (6), 895–901.

56. Stanimirovic, D.B.; Friedman, A. Pathophysiology of the Neurovascular Unit: Disease Cause or Consequence? *J. Cerebr. Blood Flow Metabol.* **2012,** *32* (7), 1207–1221.

57. Storr, M.; Sibaev, A.; Weiser, D.; Kelber, O. Herbal Extracts Modulate the Amplitude and Frequency of Slow Waves in Circular Smooth Muscle of Mouse Small Intestine. *Digestion.* **2004,** *70* (4), 257–264.

58. Tubaro, A.; Zilli, C.; Redaelli, C. Evaluation of Antiinflammatory Activity of Chamomile Extract After Topical Application. *Planta Medica* **1984,** *50* (4), 359–364.

59. Tyihak, E.; Sarkany-Kiss, J.; Verzar-Petri, G. Phytochemical Investigation of Apigenin Glycosides of *Matricaria chamomilla*. *Pharmazie* **1962,** *17,* 301–304.

60. Wang, Y.; Tang, H.; Nicholson, J. K. Metabonomic Strategy for the Detection of the Metabolic Effects of Chamomile (*Matricaria recutita* L.) Ingestion. *J. Agric. Food Chem.* **2005,** *53* (2), 191–196.

61. Wu, J. Treatment of Rosacea with Herbal Ingredients. *J. Drugs Dermatol.: JDD* **2006,** *5* (1), 29–32.

62. Zeggwagh, N.A.; Moufid, A.; Michel, J.B.; Eddouks, M. Hypotensive Effect of *Chamaemelum nobile* Aqueous Extract In Spontaneously Hypertensive Rats. *Clin. Exp. Hypertension* **2009,** *31* (5), 440–450.

63. Zick, S. M.; Wright, B. D.; Sen, A.; Arndt, J. T. Preliminary Examination of the Efficacy and Safety of a Standardized Chamomile Extract for Chronic Primary Insomnia: A Randomized Placebo-Controlled Pilot Study. *BMC Complem. Altern. Med.* **2011,** *11* (1), 78–84.

64. Zohra, S.F.; Meriem, B.; Samira, S.; Muneer, M.A. Phytochemical Screening and Identification of Some Compounds from Mallow. *J. Nat. Prod. Plant Resour.* **2012,** *2* (4), 512–516.

CHAPTER 10

Pharmacology and Therapeutics of Dandelion in Gastrointestinal Disorders

DILIPKUMAR PAL and SUPRIYO SAHA

ABSTRACT

Dandelion, *Taraxacum officinale*, is a highly nutritious plant with a rich source of vitamin, fiber, minerals, and antioxidants. This chapter affirms that dandelion is effective as an antifibrotic agent with anti-hepatocellular carcinoma activity by inhibition of PI3K/AKT/mTOR pathway and high fat-induced hepatic steatosis, acute and chronic gastritis, and other digestive disorders. Furthermore, the anti-ulcer and antidiabetic activities of dandelion against ethanol and carbon tetrachloride-induced hepatocellular injury with NF-κβ modulation and α-glucosidase enzyme have shown promising anti-lipid peroxidative and anti-inflammatory effects. In addition, dandelion effectively suppresses the viability of stomach cancer by targeting the cells of lncRNA-CCAT1. This literature review clearly indicates the medicinal value of dandelion against various digestive disorders.

10.1 INTRODUCTION

Every eight out of 10 persons are suffering from stomach and intestine diseases.[23] Nowadays, an average person only walks for 5000 steps per day, which is too low, and they eat lot of fast food (oily and contain high calories and less antioxidants). These features collectively hamper the health of an individual.

The gastric juice and pancreatic enzymes collectively regulate various digestive disorders, such as *diabetes mellitus*, gastroesophageal reflux disease (GRD), jaundice, irritable bowel syndrome (IBS), constipation, cancer of different organs, generation of free radicals, hepatitis, liver cirrhosis, stomach pain, and so on.[13-17]

Dandelion is a perennial herb with long roots and green rose-like arranged leaves. Persians were the first to recognize dandelion that was named as tarasque, around 900 A.D.[18] Almost 100 years later, the name was changed into *Taraxacum*. The most common dandelion is *Taraxacum officinale* (TO).[19] Normally, dandelion is characterized with around 20-cm long leaf, yellow, orange, or white color flower and stems or leaves with white milky latex.[8]

The aim of the chapter is to provide detailed information on the efficacies of dandelion against various gastrointestinal disorders.

10.2 DIFFERENT SPECIES AND CHEMICAL CONSTITUENTS OF DANDELION

More than two hundred macro- and microspecies of dandelions exist in nature. *TO* and *T. erythrospermum* (*TE*) are the most abundant species of dandelion (Fig. 10.1). In this chapter, only *TO* is discussed.

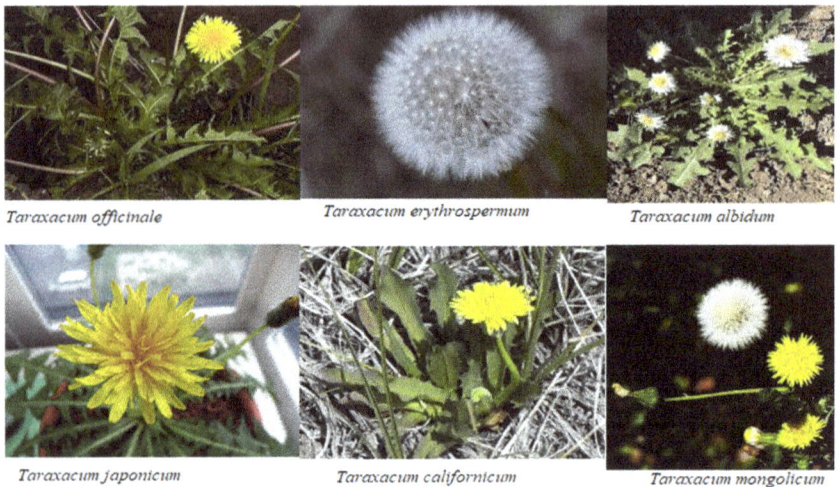

Taraxacum officinale   *Taraxacum erythrospermum*   *Taraxacum albidum*

Taraxacum japonicum   *Taraxacum californicum*   *Taraxacum mongolicum*

FIGURE 10.1   Different species of dandelion.

- Japan[24]: *T. albidum* (*TA*) and *T. pamiricum* (*TP*).
- Paphos, California, China, Colorado, Island, Russia, northern part of North America, Turkey, Scotland, and Korea[24]: *T. aphrogenes (TA), T. californicum (TC), T. centrasiaticum (TC), T. ceratophorum (TC), T. holmboei (TH), T. kok-saghyz (TK), T. laevigatum (TL), T. mirabile (TM), T. pankhurstianum (TP), and T. platycarpum (TP).*

The principal bioactive components in dandelion are[12]: taraxacin, taraxacerin, taraxafolin, coumarin analogue, indole alkaloid, β-carboline alkaloid, and choline (as vitamin B complex) along with vitamin A and vitamin C.

10.3 POTENTIAL OF DANDELION FOR PREVENTION OF METABOLIC DISORDERS

10.3.1 Effect of T. Officinale for Prevention of Fibrosis

Domitrovic et al.[7] extracted and evaluated the effect of aqueous ethanolic extract of *TO* roots on fatal liver condition generated by carbon tetrachloride application, such as, abnormal levels of aspartate aminotransferase (AsAt), alanine aminotransferase (AlAt), alkaline phosphatase (AP), both copper- and zinc-induced superoxide dismutase (SoD) and hydroxyproline amino acid (correlated with collagen breakdown), followed by histopathology of liver to quantify the specimen of collagen and the presence of glial fibrillar acidic protein; spinal muscular atrophic condition was identified. The data indicated that administration of extract (@600 mg/kg body weight) on mice resulted in:

- The weight gain was normalized to 3.11 from 1.46 g.
- The level of AsAt was not much altered with extract application (36.7 and 38.2 unit/L before and after administration).
- The level of AlAt was slightly decreased (18.3–15.7 unit/L).
- The AP level was increased (to 87.9 from 80.4 unit/L).
- The antioxidative nature of SoD was increased (from 0.72 to 1.01 mg protein).
- The hydroxyproline content was decreased (from 729 to 226 g/g liver).

The histopathology was observed to contain regular structure of hepatic cells on treatment with the extract (600 mg/kg body weight) with very minimal presence of atrophic condition. These data confirmed the importance of dandelion extract in minimizing the liver damage.[7]

10.3.2 Dandelion (Taraxacum officinale) Polysaccharides Exert Anti-hepatocarcinoma Activity

Ren et al.[22] evaluated the anticancer property of dandelion polysaccharide on hepatocarcinoma cells (HepG2 and Huh7). To quantify the amount of protein, western blot technique was used with β-actin, phosphor-PI3K, and phosphor- mTOR antibodies followed by cell counting assay using 50, 100, 200, 400, and 800 mg/L of polysaccharide dose, incubated for 0, 1, 2, and 4 days. The polysaccharide concentration (200 mg/L) with 2 days of incubation was selected for cell cycle analysis, ribonucleotides assessment, and evaluation of the growth of tumor. Oral toxicity was assessed by using BALB/c mice with a dose of 200, 400, 800, and 1600 mg/kg/day for a fortnight. Then the immunohistochemistry of mice tumor was conducted after incubation with rabbit Ki67 primary antibody. These data stated favorable effects of dandelion polysaccharide on hepatocellular carcinoma. The outcomes revealed that dandelion polysaccharide (200 mg/L) dose statistically:

- inhibited the abnormal growth and increased programmed cell death process and
- also minimized the growth of tumor formation with the prevention of inter-signaling pathway (phosphoinositide-3-kinase/protein kinase B/mechanistic target of rapamycin pathway) at G0/G1 phase without any cell toxicity.

10.3.3 Anti-ulcer and Antioxidative Properties of Leaf Extract of Taraxacum officinale

Berezi et al.[2] evaluated the anti-ulcer and oxidative stress (OS) inhibiting properties of the aqueous leaf extract of dandelion (final concentration of 250 and 500 mg/kg). By doing so, oral acute toxicity was performed with increasing dose up to 5000 mg/kg body weight followed by estimation of ulceration index by assessing the presence of edema and hemorrhage in damaged tissue.

The antioxidative activity of the extract was observed by measuring glutathione (Gl) and catalase (Cat) levels (correlated with greater OS, accumulation of toxins); and inhibition of ulcer generation was evaluated by the ability of mucus (protecting layer) generation, programmed by administration of ibuprofen and ethanol. The outcomes revealed that dandelion extract (500 mg/kg body weight) showed the importance of *TO* extract to prevent ulcer generation by:

- greater minimization of ulcer progression (55.22% and 67.79%); and
- proportional outcome was observed after 1 and 2 weeks followed by greater level of Gl (42.97 unit/mg protein), Cat (275.93 unit/mg protein), and mucus formation (124.40 and 178.47 mg).

10.3.4   Effect of Extract of Taraxacum officinale on Liver Cirrhosis

Al-Malki et al.[1] evaluated the effects of aqueous *TO* extract on carbon tetrachloride-induced liver damage, levels of serum AsAt, AlAt, AP, gamma glutamyl transferase (GaGlT), lactate dehydrogenase (LaD), urea, albumin, and anticholinesterase (AchE) followed by histopathological examination of the infected rat liver using hematoxylen and eosin stain. These data indicated the importance of *TO* extract on liver damage. The outcomes revealed that:

- the reduced levels of components after 14 and 28 days: AlAt (from 147.5 to 128 international unit/L), AsAt (from 276 to 116 international unit/L), GaGlT (from 274.3 to 264.6 international unit/L), LaD (from 677.4 to 215.3 international unit/L), AchE (from 34.6 to 19.2 unit/L), and urea (from 47.3 to 16.4 unit/L);
- with increasing amount of albumin, a prominent sign of reduced inflammation was observed with dandelion application after 42 days.

10.3.5   Effect of Extract of Taraxacum officinale on Inhibition of α-Glucosidase

Choi et al.[4] evaluated the antihyperglycemic activity of *TO* extract on the inhibition of α-glucosidase enzyme using acarbose as standard molecule. There were 28 compounds (C_1 to C_{28}): three novel butyrolactones and three butanoates (taraxiroside A-F), along with 22 known compounds.

Among them, inhibitory concentration$_{50}$ of taraxiroside A-F was observed between 145.3 and 181.3 µM; whereas C_7 and C_{12} were observed with greater inhibition of glucosidase enzyme with concentration of 61.2 and 39.8 µM, which was greater with 179.9 µM inhibitory concentration value as compared to standard. These statements clearly indicate the importance of phytoconstituents in *TO* for the management of diabetes.

10.3.6   Protective Effect of Taraxacum officinale on Nonalcoholic Fatty Liver Disease

Davaatseren et al.[5] evaluated the protective effect of aqueous extract of *TO* on high-fat-diet administered hepatic steatosis (fat deposition on liver). In this feature, two *TO* extracts (2 and 5 g/kg) were used to determine the level of triglyceride, total cholesterol, insulin, fasting blood sugar, and insulin resistance. For this experiment, C57BL/6 mice with normal diet, high fat diet, high fat diet with 2 g/kg extract and high fat diet with 5 g/kg diet were considered. The outcomes revealed that values of these parameters were decreased after the extract application (2 g/kg of body weight), such as:

- triglycerides (from 78.49 to 61.15 mg/dL);
- total cholesterol (from 94.8 to 93 mg/dL);
- insulin (from 2.27 to 1.29 mg/dL);
- fasting glucose sugar (from 201 to 168 mg/dL); and
- insulin resistance (from 33.43 to 16.47).

Further, the extract inactivated the uptake of glucose and fatty acid uptake and oxidation process by inhibiting the work of adenosine monophosphate activated protein kinase enzyme.

These data confirmed the effects of *TO* extract (2 g/kg of body weight) against the nonalcoholic fatty liver disease.

10.3.7   Effects of Leaf Extract of Taraxacum officinale on the Oxidation Stress (OS) and Lipid Peroxidation

Hue et al.[9] evaluated the ethanolic extract of *TO* leaves for its antioxidative property using DPPH scavenging process, superoxide radical process, hydroxyl radical process, and inhibition of NO (nitric oxide) production induced by lipopolysaccharide (LiPS) in RAW 264.7 cells. These data correlates with the effectivity of *TO* extract on the inhibition of OS and peroxidation of lipid. The outcomes revealed that:

- total phenolic content and inhibition of superoxide radical of *TO* extract were observed with 195.4 and 417.0 µg/mg, respectively;
- gradually increased inhibition of superoxide generation (extract @ 50 µg/mL = 22.4%, 100 µg/mL = 44.2% and 150 µg/mL = 63.6%); and
- the inhibition of NO production by RAW 264.7 cells showed that 86% inhibition was observed with 500 µg/mL concentration and maximum cell viability (CV) (109.2) was observed with 250 µg/mL concentration.

10.3.8   Antihyperlipidemic and Antioxidative Effects of Roots and Leaf Powder of Taraxacum officinale

Choi et al.[3] evaluated the antihyperglycemic and reducing power properties of *TO* root and leaf powder (1%) by assessing the evaluation of serum liver markers, such as triglyceride, total cholesterol, high density lipoprotein (HDL), low-density lipoprotein (LDL), AsAt, AlAt, Gl, Glutathione-S-transferase (GSt), Cat, SoD, and thiobarbituric acid reactive substances (TARS), followed by histopathological changes in the aorta of rabbit. These data confirmed the antihyperlipidemic and antioxidative nature of *TO* root and leaf powder. The outcomes revealed that:

- body and liver weight were decreased by *Taraxacum officinale* root extract;
- level of AsAt was decreased by leaf powder;
- AlAt was decreased by root powder of *TO*;
- the amount of HDL and LDL was reduced, and there was marked reduction in atheromatous plaque formation.

10.3.9   Anti-inflammatory Activity of Ethanolic Extract of Taraxacum officinale

Jeon et al.[10] evaluated the anti-inflammatory activity of ethanolic extract of *TO* using diphenyl-picrylhydrazyl reducing power assay and its antiangiogenic activity using chicken chorioallantoic assay and carrageenan-induced inflammation assay method. This data confirmed the anti-inflammatory effects. The ethanolic extract of *TO* showed:

- greater inhibition of free radical generation with elimination from RoS generation;
- a marked decrease in cell protein debris (exudate); and
- minimization of nitric acid production and leukocyte level.

10.3.10   Cytotoxic Effects of Taraxacum officinale against Hepg2 Cell Lines

Koo et al.[11] evaluated the toxicity of aqueous extract of *TO* (0, 0.02, 0.2, 2.0 mg/mL) against tumor necrosis factor-alpha (secreted from HepG2 (hepatocellular carcinoma)) cell line. These data confirmed the cell toxicity of *TO* against hepatocellular cancer. It was observed that 0.2 mg/mL of *Taraxacum officinale* showed:

- greater amount of factor-alpha (after 1 day 130 picogram/mL and after 2 days 186 picogram/mL) and
- also increased the amount of interleukin-1alpha (after 1 day 47 picogram/mL and 2 days 66 picogram/mL).

10.3.11   Polysaccharides from Taraxacum officinale Exert Hepatoprotective Activity

Park et al.[21] isolated two polysaccharides (TOP1 and TOP2) from *TO*, and these were evaluated against carbon tetrachloride-induced liver damage by calculating the liver markers (such as AsAt, AlAt, copper-zinc SoD, manganese SoD, Gl); and they also evaluated the cell toxicity behavior of polysaccharides of tumor necrosis factor-alpha and interleukin-1β. The outcomes revealed that:

- TOP2 showed greater response to inhibit AsAt and AlAt;
- antioxidative properties were improved as values of copper-zinc SoD, manganese SoD, Gl were increased;
- the cell toxicity of the polysaccharides showed decreased level of inflammatory mediators (such as cytokines tumor necrosis factor-alpha and interleukin-1β); and

- the anti-inflammatory activity and other mentioned parameters justi-fied the protective nature of the polysaccharides against liver disease.

10.3.12 Extract of Taraxacum officinale Inhibits Oxidation Stress and Nitric Oxide Production

Park et al.[20] evaluated the anti-inflammatory nature of methanolic and aqueous extract of *TO* against LiPS-induced RAW 264.7 macrophages and antioxidative was evaluated by measuring the amount of luteolin, chicoric acid, and total phenolic content. The outcomes revealed that increasing concentration of *TO* (methanolic and water extracts) showed:

- greater antioxidative properties by the values of SoD, Cat, gluta-thione peroxidase (GlP), and glutathione reductase (GlR) along with greater inhibition of NO production with inhibitory concentra-tion$_{50}$ of 79.9 mL and 157.5 µg/mL, respectively; and
- the decreasing concentration of NO production and increasing concentration of Glu with increasing concentration of extracts are directly correlated with the anti-inflammatory effects.

10.3.13 Anti-inflammatory Activity of Taraxacum officinale

Xue et al.[25] evaluated the inhibition of inflammatory responses of dande-lion extract (50% ethanolic, 50% ethanolic with 1% formic acid, 80% ethanolic, 80% ethanolic with 1% formic acid). They found that:

- Total phenolic content and flavonoid (gallic acid, chlorogenic acid, caffeic acid, syringic acid, ferulic acid, trans-cinnamic acid, vanillic acid, coumaric acid, chicoric acid, rutin, and quercetin) were higher with 50% ethanolic without/with 1% formic acid and leaf was the primary source.
- Leaf extract (400 µg/mL) and chicoric acid were observed with greater inhibition against human colorectal carcinoma (HT-29) cell lines and inflammasome activity.

These data confirmed the effectivity of dandelion as an anti-inflamma-tory agent.

10.3.14   Protective Activity of Taraxacum mongolicum (TM) against LiPS-Activated Inflammation

Yang et al.[27] evaluated the percent CV of organic acid component (OAC) of *TM* (concentration gradient of 100, 200, 400, 800, 1600, and 3200 µg/mL) on normal human bronchial epithelial cell lines. It was observed that:

- Cell viability was increased above 800 µg/mL.
- The inhibition of cytokines and interleukins and reduction in caspase expression were directly correlated with dose.
- The OAC of *TM* could inhibit the inflammatory response through toll-like receptor-4/IκB kinase nuclear receptor and block the phosphorylation of IκB kinase enzyme.

These data confirmed the activity of *TM* against LiPS-induced inflammation.

10.3.15   Acute and Chronic Gastroprotective Nature of Extract of Taraxacum corneaum nakai (TCN)

Yang et al.[26] suggested the gastroprotective nature of *TCN* using the high and low dose. In this way, total phenolic compounds and flavonoids were quantified (total polyphenol: 99.9 mg, total flavonoid: 20.7 mg, chlorogenic acid: 1.44 mg, caffeic acid: 12.8 mg, and rutin: 8.81 mg). It was observed that:

- Ethanol and hydrochloric acid caused the formation of gastric lesion and formation of gastric acid.
- High dose of *TCN* minimized the redness and swelling of gastric parietal cells with moderate change in the gastric acid production.

This information confirmed the importance of *TCN* as gastroprotective agent.

10.3.16   In Vitro and In Vivo Hepatoprotective Effects of Taraxacum officinale

You et al.[28] evaluated the gastroprotective of aqueous extract of *TO* roots on (300 mM) ethyl alcohol induced liver damage. In this experiment, serum markers (such as AsAt, AlAt, AP, LaD, Cat, GSt, GlP, GlR, and Gl) were measured. Outcomes showed that:

- values of AsAt, AlAt, AP, and LaD were decreased;
- Cat, GSt, GlP, GlR, and Gl were increased;
- the CV against HepG2 cell line was increased with aqueous extract;

These data confirmed the protective nature of *TO* against alcohol-induced liver damage.

10.3.17   Antiproliferative Activity of Extract of Taraxacum officinale on Gastric Cancer Cell Line

Zhu et al.[29] evaluated the aqueous extract of dandelion on two gastric cell lines (SGC7901 and BGC823) along with one gastric epithelium cell line (GES-1) as the control. CV and colony formation assay were evaluated after the ribonucleic acid isolation using trizol reagent. The outcomes revealed that:

- CV was dose-dependent and was suppressed in both cell lines.
- The concentration (3 mg/mL) of the extract showed greater antiproliferative effect and inhibition of the cancerous cell invasion to the secondary phase.
- Total anticancer activity of the extract was mediated through long non-coding RNA-colon cancer-associated transcript1.

This showed the anticancer therapy of the aqueous extract of dandelion.

10.3.18   Effect of Taraxacum officinale on Ulcerative Colitis

Ding et al.[6] evaluated the effect of aqueous root extract of dandelion on ulcerative colitis (which was the major response of inflammatory bowel syndrome (IBS)). In this evaluation, human colonocyte (NCM460) and human colonic epithelium cell line were selected and progressed in Dulbecco's modified eagle medium and dandelion root extracts (1, 3, 6 mg/mL) were applied for assessment of anti-cancer effect. Dextran sodium sulphate (2%) was used to induce colitis condition on mice followed by evaluation of CV assay, induction of programmed cell death, cytokine measurement, and also evaluation of the serum liver markers, such as RoS,

SoD, and the ratio of Gl and Gl-disulfide. The outcomes revealed that the extract showed:

- increased CV along with minimization of programmed cell death and OS;
- reduced ratio of glutathione along with its disulfide form in dextran induced colonic cells;
- in histopathologic evaluation, there was a marked decrease in inflammatory responses after addition of extract on 2% dextran induced inflammation.

These data are surely correlated with the anti-ulcerative colitis effect of dandelion.

10.4   FUTURE SCOPE

Out of more than 200 species of dandelion found in nature, authors of this chapter discussed only *Taraxacum officinale*, *T. erythrospermum*, *T. mongolicum*, *T. formosanum,* and *T. coreanum* for their health benefits. Therefore, other species should also be explored if they are beneficial to control GI diseases. Folkloric use of dandelion indicates that this plant is highly used as a blood purifier, and to treat urinary tract infections (along with uvaursi), to increase appetite, and to relieve from gallstones. Therefore, if this knowledge is cultured scientifically, then many other diseases could be cured with the use of "Dandelion."

10.5   SUMMARY

The activity profile of dandelion showed that dandelion is highly recommended for the prevention of fibrosis and liver damage, minimization of oxidative stress, and LiPS-induced NO production. It also showed good health benefits on antiproliferative nature on gastric cancer, colon cancer, ethanol-induced liver cirrhosis, non-alcoholic fatty liver disease, diabetics, acute and chronic gastritis, and stomach cancer (with target cell of lncRNA-CCAT1). These data clearly state the medicinal value of dandelion against various digestive disorders.

KEYWORDS

- celiac disease
- dandelion
- irritable bowel syndrome
- stomach cancer
- ulcer

REFERENCES

1. Al-Malki, A. L.; Abo-Golayel, M. K.; Abo-Elnaga, G.; Al-Beshri, H. Hepatoprotective Effect of Dandelion (*Taraxacum officinale*) Against Induced Chronic Liver Cirrhosis. *J. Med. Plants Res.* **2013,** *7* (20), 1494–1505.

2. Berezi, E. P.; Uwakwe, A. A.; Monago-Ighorodje, C. C.; Nwauche, K. T. Anti-ulcer and Antioxidant Defenses of *Taraxacum officinale* (Dandelion) Leaf Extracts Against Ethanol Induced Gastric Ulcer in Rats. *World J. Pharm. Sci.* **2017,** *7* (1), 35–50.

3. Choi, U. K.; Lee, O. H.; Yim, J. H.; Cho, C. W. Hypolipidemic and Antioxidant Effects of Dandelion (*Taraxacum officinale*) Root and Leaf on Cholesterol-Fed Rabbits. *Int. J. Mol. Sci.* **2010,** *11* (1), 67–78.

4. Choi, J.; Yoon, K.D.; Kim, J. Chemical Constituents from *Taraxacum officinale* and their α-glucosidase Inhibitory Activities. *Bioorg. Med. Chem. Lett.* **2018,** *28* (3), 476–481.

5. Davaatseren, M.; Hur, H. J.; Yang, H. J. *Taraxacum officinale* (dandelion) Leaf Extract Alleviates High-Fat Diet-Induced Nonalcoholic Fatty Liver. *Food Chem. Toxicol.* **2013,** *58,* 30–36.

6. Ding, A.; Wen, X. Dandelion Root Extract Protects NCM460 Colonic Cells and Relieves Experimental Mouse Colitis. *J. Nat. Med.* **2018,** *72* (4), 857–866.

7. Domitrovic, R.; Jakovac, H.; Romic, Z.; Rahelic, D.; Tadic, Z. Antifibrotic Activity of *Taraxacum officinale* Root in Carbon Tetrachloride-Induced Liver Damage in Mice. *J. Ethnopharmacol.* **2010,** *130* (3), 569–577.

8. Fatima, T.; Bashir, O.; Naseer, B.; Hussain, S. Z. Dandelion: Phytochemistry and Clinical Potential. *J. Med. Plants Stud.* **2018,** *6* (2), 198–202.

9. Hue, C.; Kitts, D. D. Dandelion (*Taraxacum officinale*) Flower Extract Suppresses Both Reactive Oxygen Species and Nitric Oxide and Prevents Lipid Oxidation in vitro. *Phytomedicine* **2005,** *12* (8), 588–597.

10. Jeon, H. J.; Kang, H. J.; Jung, H. J.; Kang, Y. S. Anti-inflammatory Activity of *Taraxacum officinale*. *J. Ethnopharmacol.,* **2008,** *115* (1), 82–88.

11. Koo, H. N.; Hong, S. H.; Song, B. K.; Kim, C. H.; Yoo, Y. H.; Kim, H. M. *Taraxacum officinale* Induces Cytotoxicity through TNF-α and IL-1α Secretion in Hep G2 cells. *Life Sci.* **2004,** *74* (9), 1149–1157.

12. Leu, Y. L.; Shi, L. S.; Damu, A. G. Chemical Constituents of *Taraxacum formosanum*. *Chem. Pharm. Bull. (Tokyo)* **2003**, *51* (5), 599–601.
13. Pal, D.; Saha, S. Current Status and Prospects of Chitosan-Metal Nanoparticles and Their Applications as Nanotheranostic Agents. Chapter 5; In *Nanotheranostics*; Rai, M., Jamil, B., Eds.; Springer Nature: Cham, Switzerland, **2019**; pp 79–114.
14. Pal, D.; Kumar, S.; Saha, S. Antihyperglycemic Activity of Phenyl and Ortho-hydroxy Phenyl Linked Imidazolyl Triazolo Hydroxamic Acid Derivatives. *Int. J. Pharm. Pharma. Sci.* **2017**, *9* (12), 247–251.
15. Pal, D.; Nayak, A. K.; Saha, S. Cellulose Based Hydrogel. Chapter 10; In *Natural Bio-active Compounds, Volume 1: Production and Applications*; Akhtar, M. S., Ed.; Springer Nature Singapore Pvt. Ltd.: Singapore, 2019; pp 285–332.
16. Pal, D.; Nayak, A. K.; Saha, S. Interpenetrating Polymer Network Hydrogels of Chitosan: Applications in Controlling Drug Release. Chapter 5; In *Cellulose-Based Superabsorbent Hydrogels. Polymers and Polymeric Composites: A Reference Series*; Mondal, Md. I. H., Ed.; Springer Nature: Cham, 2018; pp 1–41.
17. Pal, D.; Nayak, A. K.; Hasnain, M. S.; Saha, S. Pharmaceutical Applications of Chondroitin. Chapter 5; In *Natural Polymers for Pharmaceutical Applications: Volume 3: Animal-Derived Polymers*; Nayak, A.K., Hasnain, Md Saquib, Pal, D., Eds.; Apple Academic Press: Burlington, ON, 2019; p 31.
18. Pal, D.; Saha, S. Chondroitin: Natural Biomarker with Immense Biomedical Applications. *RSC Adv.* **2019**, *9* (48), 28061–28077.
19. Pal, D.; Saha, S.; Nayak, A.K.; Hasnain, M.S. Marine-Derived Polysaccharides: Pharmaceutical Applications. Chapter 1; In: *Natural Polymers for Pharmaceutical Applications: Volume 2: Marine and Microbiologically Derived Polymers*; Nayak, A. K., Hasnain, Md Saquib, Pal, D., Eds.; Apple Academic Press: Burlington–ON, 2019; pp 1–42.
20. Park, C.M.; Park, J.Y.; Noh, K.H.; Shin, J.H.; Song, Y.S. *Taraxacum officinale* Weber Extracts Inhibit LPS-Induced Oxidative Stress and Nitric Oxide Production via the NF-κB Modulation in RAW 264.7 cells. *J. Ethnopharmacol.* **2011,** *133* (2), 834–842.
21. Park, C.M.; Youn, H.J.; Chang, H.K.; Song, Y. S. TOP1 and TOP2, Polysaccharides from *Taraxacum officinale*, Attenuate CCl_4-Induced Hepatic Damage through the Modulation of NF-κB and its Regulatory Mediators. *Food Chem. Toxicol.* **2010,** *48* (5), 1255–1261.
22. Ren, F.; Li, J.; Yuan, X.; Wang, Y.; Wu, K.; Kang, L. Dandelion Polysaccharides Exert Anticancer Effect on Hepatocellular Carcinoma by Inhibiting PI3K/AKT/mTOR Pathway and Enhancing Immune Response. *J. Funct. Food* **2019**, *55*, 263–274.
23. Richards, A.J. Sectional Nomenclature in Taraxacum (Asteraceae). *Taxon* **1985**, *34* (4), 633–644.
24. Schutz, K.; Carle, R.; Schieber, A. Taraxacum: A Review on its Phytochemical and Pharmacological Profile. *J. Ethnopharmacol.* **2006**, *107* (3), 313–323.
25. Xue, Y.; Zhang, S.; Du, M.; Zhu, M. J. Dandelion Extract Suppresses Reactive Oxidative Species and Inflammasome in Intestinal Epithelial Cells. *J. Funct. Food* **2017**, *29*, 10–18.
26. Yang, H.J.; Kim, M.J.; Kwon, D.Y.; Kang, E.S.; Kang, S.; Park, S. Gastroprotective Actions of *Taraxacum coreanum* Nakai Water Extracts in Ethanol-Induced Rat Models of Acute and Chronic Gastritis. *J. Ethnopharmacol.* **2017,** *208*, 84–93.

27. Yang, N.; Tian, G.; Zhu, M.; Li, C. Protective Effects of Organic Acid Component from *Taraxacum mongolicum* Hand.-Mazz. Against LPS Induced Inflammation: Regulating the TLR4/IKK/NF-κB Signal Pathway. *J. Ethnopharmacol.* **2016,** *194*, 395–402.

28. You, Y.; Yoo, S.; Yoon, H.G.; Park, J. In vitro and In vivo Hepatoprotective Effects of the Aqueous Extract from *Taraxacum officinale* (Dandelion) Root Against Alcohol-Induced Oxidative Stress. *Food Chem. Toxicol.* **2010,** *48*, 1632–1637.

29. Zhu, H.; Zhao, H.; Zhang, L.; Xu, J.; Zhu, C.; Zhao, H.; Lv, G. Dandelion Root Extract Suppressed Gastric Cancer Cells Proliferation and Migration through Targeting lncRNA-CCAT1. *Biomed. Pharmcotherap.* **2017,** *93*, 1010–1017.

PART III

Plant-Based Remedies in the Treatment of Gastrointestinal Diseases

CHAPTER 11

Role of *Aloe vera* in Irritable Bowel Disease

DILIPKUMAR PAL and SOUVIK MUKHERJEE

ABSTRACT

Based on literature review, the efficacy of *Aloe vera* has been validated for the treatment of irritable bowel syndrome. This plant has high therapeutic effects on human health due to presence of aloe-emodin, acemannan, aloeride, ethyl chromones, flavonoids, saponin, amino acids, vitamins, and minerals. Leaves containing jelly substances have been able to reduce the secretion of autacoid E2 and interleukin-18 (IL-18) in the colon tissue layer. An in vivo study shows that the extract of this plant could reduce tumor necrosis factor-α levels and the expression of IL-1β messenger RNA.

11.1 INTRODUCTION

Several medicinal plants including *Aloe vera* (Fig. 11.1) and their derivatives have been used in the traditional medicine therapy to treat irritable bowel syndrome (IBS) (Fig. 11.2) and various other diseases[8,78] in living beings; and to overcome undesirable side-effects of synthetic drugs.[4,76]

Symptoms of the irritable bowel disease (IBD) include diarrhea, anemia, bleeding, and weight loss.[35] This disease is divided into two major groups: ulcerative colitis (UC) and Crohn's disease (CD).[5] UC is characterized by flowing mucosal inflection of the colon[71–75] and is mostly observed in ileocecal valve. Current therapy (azathioprine and cyclosporine) for IBD is also available commercially but these treatments have several side effects.[7,77] Drug delivery to the relevant section(s) along with the gastrointestinal (GI) tract has also become a primary challenge to this issue.[9,79–83] In this respect, second-generation agents have improved with drug administration, increased competence, and diminished drug reactions.

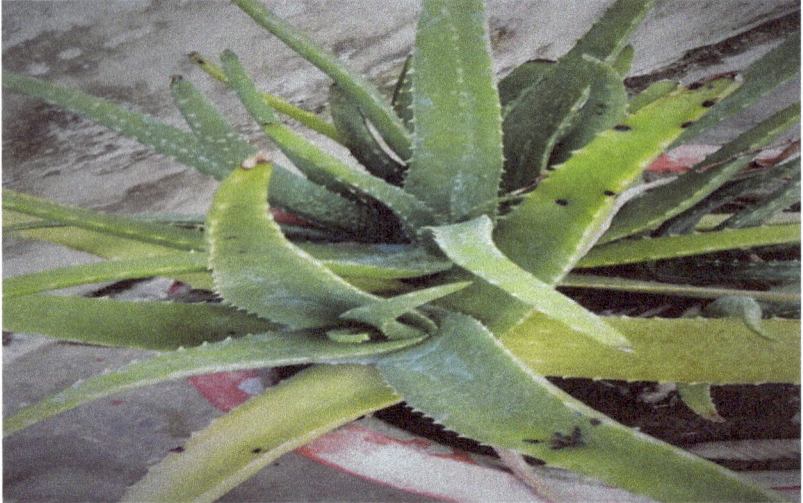

FIGURE 11.1   *Aloe vera* plant.

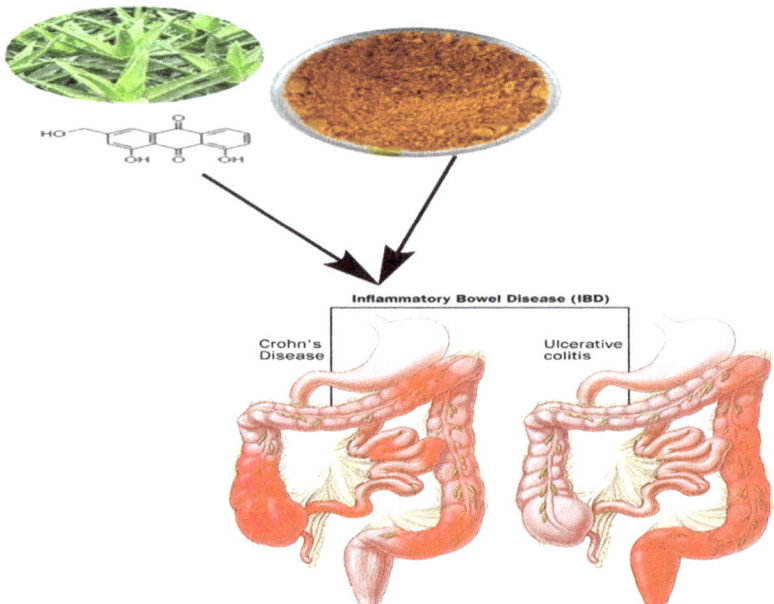

FIGURE 11.2   *Aloe vera* and inflammatory bowel disease (IBD).

11.1.1 Pathophysiology of Irritable Bowel Disease

UC and CD are sustained idiopathic anarchy of the alimentary tract with a summary of proposed pathogenic events as shown in Figure 11.3. In comparison, the inflammation reaction in UC resembles attitudes of that arbitrated through T Helper cell-2 (TH2) route.[17,84–87] Currently, this approximately overly simplified classification has been amended in light of the depiction of T Helper cell-17 (TH17).[11] Significant pathogenesis has materialized genetic analysis of CD mutations in the gene with infrequent CD in whites. It is projected to work as an intracellular sensor for bacterial bug by perceiving peptidoglycans,[29,88,89] thereby providing crucial performance in the legitimate immune system to bacterial bug.[33,90–95] Consistent with this model, other investigations have pinpointed bacterial antigens, together with interleukin-18 and a flagellin protein as preeminent superantigens that can prompt the T Helper cell-1 (TH1) reaction in CD.[37,96]

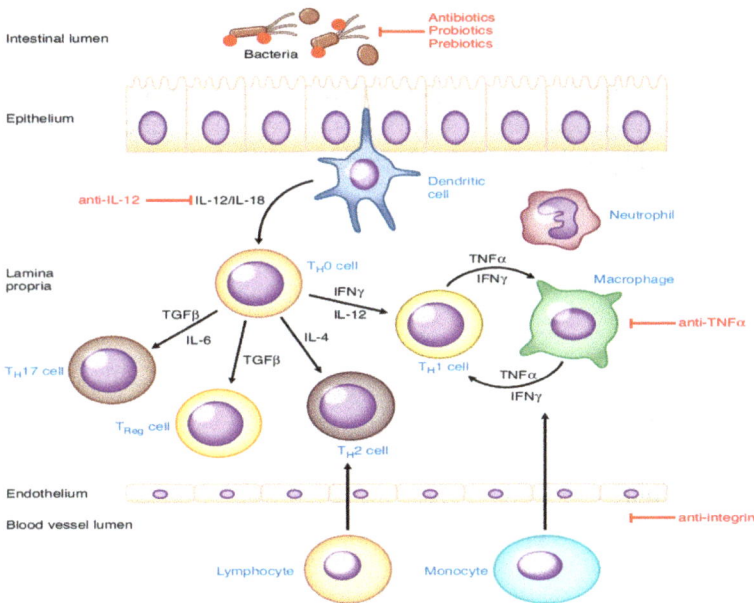

FIGURE 11.3 Pathogenesis of IBD.

This chapter enumerates its ethnopharmacology, chemistry, clinical and preclinical studies focusing on the utilization of the plant when there is the situation of vital afflictions.

11.2   BOTANICAL AND GEOGRAPHICAL DISTRIBUTION OF
ALOE VERA

The biological source of this plant is *Aloe barbadense* with about 300 species belonging to the family Liliaceae.[97] Plant is cultivated in Caribbean islands, Europe, and India (North-West Himalayan region).[2,34] The taste of each diversity of plant is repulsive and bitter.[21,54] The juice from leaves is water-soluble substance and leaves consist of 98% water and are succulent.[1] These plants have juicy leaves and spines at the margins that are cut during March and April.[50,53] This plant leaves are fleshy and thick, green to grey-green to reddish-brown to reddish black to brownish-black to dark brown,[51,98–100] with some species exhibiting white flecks on their upper and lower stem faces.[20,55] Margins of leaves are serrated and have tiny-size white teeth.[10,52] The plant flowers in summer season.[49]

11.3   PHYTOCHEMISTRY OF *ALOE VERA*

Aloe vera contains about 200 potentially chemical constituents, such as vitamins, enzymes, minerals, sugars, lignin, saponins, salicylic acids, and amino acids. Phytochemicals in aloe species are[13–16,64–70]:

- 3-furanmethanol,
- Acemannan,
- Aloe-emodin,
- Aloechrysone,
- Aloeride,
- Aloesaponol,
- Aloetic acid,
- Alosone,
- oxylipin,
- Anthracene compounds and their derivatives,
- Anthraquinones,
- babaloin,
- Chrysamminic acid,
- Chrysophanic acid,
- Cinnamic acids and their derivatives,
- Dihydro-coumarone,
- Ethyl chromones,

- Feroxidin,
- Flavonoids,
- Flavonoids,
- Galacturonic acid,
- Homonataloin,
- Iso-babaloin,
- Isoxanthorin,
- Laccaic acid,
- Nataloe emodin,
- Nataloe-emodin-
- 2-O-glucoside
- Plicataloside,
- Pluridone,
- Saponin, etc.

11.4   ETHNOPHARMACOLOGY OF *ALOE VERA*

It is used for a broad spectrum of traditional medicine purposes world-wide.[60,101–104] It is used as a curative, laxative, and purgative agents[28,39–41]; for the recuperating[47,56–59,61] of various skin confusion, mouth defilements, wounds; and is consumed as disinfectant and cell duplication possession.[3,42] For example, Indian Ayurvedic medicine recommends the use of leaves and defecates of *Aloe vera* as an anthelmintic[48] and cathartic agent[30,43]; and for the treatment of stomach and digestive complaints.[27] This plant is also used in old Chinese medicinal system for analogous actions[18,44,45]; and in Central America and Caribbean Islands.[62,63] Today, this plant been incorporated into modern Western complementary and alternative medicine systems.[19] It is also commonly utilized for the treatment of sunburn and when absorbed orally, it serves a routine analeptic.[6,46] Other medicinal activities include rheumatic (RHT) and joint inflammation (IFL) and gout; and cancer and hyperglycemic conditions.[12,105–108]

11.5   MECHANISM OF ACTION OF *ALOE VERA* PLANT IN INFLAMMATORY BOWEL DISEASE (IBD)

An inflammation is an ordinary reaction by our body.[26] It is not an isolated phenomenon, but is associated with complex system of metabolic incidents provoked by various expressions, such as redness of eye, heat, and pain.[24,25] The inflammation techniques are apprised of suppuration of different biomolecules.[22] Aloe vera plant has shown to reduce IBD and IBS. Water extract of this plant can subdue cytolytic T-lymph can lower the cytokine (CK) production. Equivalently, the plant comprising lectins are also excited to CK yielding. Also, these compounds significantly depress the expression of pro-inflammation-CK.[23]

11.6 PRECLINICAL AND CLINICAL TRIALS

It is validated that *Aloe vera* plays significant role in intestinal inflammatory conditions that has led to the development of different natural formulations. It is important to note that most botanical drugs are going through tight testing so as to recognize these pharmaceutical agents, in an attempt to maintain standard of herbal drugs.[31,36,38]

11.7 SUMMARY

This chapter on medicinal properties of *Aloe vera* plant has enlightened the curative importance of this accessible genus of plant. The species and various extracts of this plant possess significant anticancer, antidiabetic, antiseptic, antihypertensive, and anti-inflammatory potential. More recently, *Aloe vera* gel has been used widely as oral preparation to treat IBD.

KEYWORDS

- *Aloe vera*
- inflammatory bowel disease
- inflammatory bowel symptoms
- preclinical study
- prostaglandin E2

REFERENCES

1. Alvarado-Morales, G.; Minjares-Fuentes, R. Application of Thermosonication for *Aloe vera* (*Aloe barbadensis* Miller) Juice Processing: Impact on the Functional Properties and the Main Bioactive Polysaccharides. *Ultrasonic Sonochem.* **2019,** *1*, 125–133.
2. Amir, H.M.; Grace, O.M.; Wabuyele, E.; Manoko, M. L. Ethnobotany of *Aloe vera* L. in Tanzania. *SA J. Bot.* **2019,** *12* (2), 330–335.
3. Asghari, R.; Ahmadvand, R. Salinity Stress and its Impact on Morpho-Physiological Characteristics of *Aloe vera*. *Pertanika J. Trop. Agric. Sci.* **2018,** *41* (1), 33–45.
4. Atreya, I.; Atreya, R.; Neurath, M.F. NF-κB in Inflammatory Bowel Disease. *J. Intern. Med.* **2008,** *263* (6), 591–596.
5. Arunkumar, S.; Muthuselvam, M. Analysis of Phytochemical Constituents and Antimicrobial Activities of *Aloe vera* L Against Clinical Pathogens. *World J. Agric. Sci.* **2009,** *5* (5), 572–576.
6. Akinyele, B.O.; Odiyi, A.C. Comparative Study of the Vegetative Morphology and the Existing Taxonomic Status of *Aloe vera* L. *J. Plant Sci.* **2007,** *2* (5), 558–563.
7. Ali, II.; Umut, G.; Semih, Y.; Mehmet, Y.D. Cytotoxicity of *Aloe vera* Gel Extracts on *Allium cepa* Root Tip Cells. *Turkish J. Bot.* **2012,** *36*, 263–268.
8. Ahlawat, K.S.; Khatkar, B.S. Processing, Food Applications and Safety of *Aloe vera* Products: A Review. *J. Food Sci. Technol.* **2011,** *48* (5), 525–533.
9. Atherton, P. Aloe vera: Magic or Medicine. *Nursing Standard* **1998,** *12* (41), 49, 52–54.
10. Atherton, P. Aloe vera Revisited: Review of Aloe Gel. *Br. J. Phytotherap.* **1984,** *4*, 176–183.
11. Boudreau, M.D.; Beland, F.A. Evaluation of the Biological and Toxicological Properties of *Aloe barbadensis* (Miller), *Aloe vera*. *J. Environm. Sci. Health* **2006,** *24*, 103–154.
12. Bajpai, S. Biological Importance of Aloe vera and its Active Constituents. In *Synthesis of Medicinal Agents from Plants*; Tiwari, A., Tiwari, S., Eds., Vol. 2; Elsevier: Cambridge, USA, **2018;** pp 177–203.
13. Baumgart, D.C.; Carding, S. R. Inflammatory Bowel Disease: Cause and Immuno-biology. *Lancet* **2007,** *369* (95), 1627–1640.
14. Baumgart, D.C.; Sandborn, W.J. Inflammatory Bowel Disease: Clinical Aspects and Established and Evolving Therapies. *Lancet* **2007,** *369* (95), 1641–1657.
15. Byeon, S.; Pelley, R.; Ullrich, S.E.; Waller, T.A.; Bucana, C.D; Strickland, F.M. *Aloe barbadensis* Extracts Reduce the Production of Interleukin-10 After Exposure to Ultraviolet Radiation. *J. Invest. Dermatol.* **1988,** *110*, 811–817
16. Bai, W.; Xiao, J. (Eds.). *Third International Symposium on Phytochemicals in Medicine and Food*, 4th ed.; Springer: New York, 2019; pp 1–3.
17. Borges, A. R.; Chan, A. R.; Cetina, M. L. In vitro Evaluation of Anthraquinones from *Aloe vera* (*Aloe barbadensis* Miller) Roots and Several Derivatives Against Strains of Influenza Virus. *Indus. Crops Prod.* **2019,** *13* (2), 468–475.
18. Bruneton, J. *Pharmacognosy, Phytochemistry, Medicinal Plants*, 3rd ed.; Lavoisier Press: New York, 1995; pp 18–25.
19. Chithra, P.; Sajithlal, G.; Chandrakasan, G. Influence of *Aloe vera* on the Glycos-aminoglycan's in the Matrix of Healing Dermal Wounds in Rats. *J. Ethnopharmacol.* **1998,** *59*, 179–186.

20. Dash, B.K.; Sultana, S.; Sultana, N. Antibacterial Activities of Methanol and Acetone Extracts of Fenugreek (*Trigonella foenum*) and coriander (*Coriandrum sativum*). *Life Sci. Med. Res.* **2011**, *27*, 1–8.
21. Davis, R.H.; Donato, J.J.; Hartman, G.M.; Hass, R.C. Anti-Inflammatory and Wound Healing Activity of a Growth Substance in *Aloe vera*. *Am. Podiatr. Med. Assoc.* **1994**, *84*, 77–81.
22. Davis, K.; Philpott, S.; Kumar, D.; Mendall, M. Randomized Double-blind Placebo-Controlled Trial of *Aloe vera* for Irritable Bowel Syndrome. *Int. J. Clin. Prac.* **2006**, *60* (9), 1080–1086.
23. Davis, R.H. Method of Using *Aloe vera* as a Biological Vehicle. *US Patent* **1998**, *66* (1), 112–118.
24. De Souza, G.C.; Haas, A.P.; Von Poser, G.L. Ethnopharmacological Studies of Antimicrobial Remedies in the South of Brazil. *J. Ethnopharmacol.* **2004**, *90* (1), 135–143.
25. Dubey, S.; Sao, S. Antimicrobial Activity of Crude Stem Extracts of Some Medicinal Plants Against Skin Disease Causing Microbes from Chhattisgarh Region. *J. Ethnopharmacol.* **2010**, *14* (1), 138–143.
26. Egbuna, C.; Ifemeje, J.C.; Kumar, S.; Sharif, N. Marine Sources, Industrial Applications, and Recent Advances. *Phytochem.* **2018**, *3*, 120–130.
27. Evans, W.C. (Ed.). *Trease and Evans: Pharmacognosy*, 11th ed.; Elsevier Health Sciences: New York, 2009; pp 1138–1145.
28. Enas-Ali, K.M. Anti-diabetic, Anti-hypercholestermic and Antioxidative Effect of *Aloe vera* Gel Extract in Alloxan Induced Diabetic Rats. *Aust. J. Basic Appl. Sci.* **2001**, *5* (11), 1321–1327.
29. Fani, M.; Kohanteb, J. Inhibitory Activity of Aloe vera Gel on Some Clinically Isolated Cariogenic and Periodontopathic Bacteria. *J. Oral Sci.* **2012**, *54*, 15–21
30. Fujino, S.; Andoh, A.; Bamba, S. Increased Expression of Interleukin 17 in Inflammatory Bowel Disease. *GUT* **2003**, *52* (1), 65–70.
31. Furukawa, F.; Nishikawa, A.; Chihara, T.; Shimpo, K.; Beppu, H.; Kuzuya, H. Chemo Preventive Effects of *Aloe Arborescence* on N-nitrosobis (2-oxopropyl) Amine-induced Pancreatic Carcinogenesis in Hamsters. *Cancer Lett.* **2002**, *178*, 117–122.
32. Fenig, E.; Nordenberg, J.; Beery, E.; Sulkes, J.; Wasserman, L. Combined Effect of Aloe - Emodin and Chemotherapeutic Agents on the Proliferation of an Adherent Variant Cell Line of Merkel Cell Carcinoma. *Oncology* **2004**, *11*, 213–217.
33. Gao, Y.; Kuok, K.I.; Jin, Y.; Wang, R. Biomedical Applications of *Aloe vera*. *Crit. Rev. Food Sci. Nutr.* **2019**, *59*, 244–256.
34. Gupta, M.; Mazumdar, U.K.; Pal, D.; Bhattacharya, S.; Chakrabarty, S. Studies on Brain Biogenic Amines in Methanolic Extract of *Cuscuta reflexa* Roxb. and *Corchorus olitorius* Linn. Seed Treated Mice. *Acta Poloniae Pharm.* **2003**, *60* (3), 207–210.
35. Gupta, S. Review on Traditional Medicinal Plants and Their Usage. *J. Med. Plants* **2018**, *6* (3), 131–135.
36. Hamman, J.H. Composition and Applications of *Aloe vera* Leaf Gel. *Molecules* **2008**, *13* (8), 1599–1616.
37. Hutter, J.A.; Salmon, M.; Stavinoha, W.B. Anti-inflammatory C-glucosyl Chromone from *Aloe Barbadensis*. *J. Nat. Prod.* **1996**, *59*, 541–543.
38. Heggers, J.; Kucukcelebi, A.; Listengarten, D. Beneficial Effect of Aloe on Wound Healing in an Excisional Wound Model. *J. Altern. Complem. Med.* **1996**, *2*, 271–277.

39. Heinrich, M.; Barnes, J.; Prieto-Garcia, J.; Gibbons, S.; Williamson, E.M. *Fundametals of Pharmacognosy and Phytotherapy.* 2017, Elsevier.

40. Heng, H.C.; Zulfakar, M.H.; Ng, P.Y. Pharmaceutical Applications of *Aloe vera*. *Indon. J. Pharm.* **2018,** *29* (3), 101–105.

41. Hęś, M.; Dziedzic, K.; Górecka, D.; Jędrusek, Golińska, A.; Gujska, E. *Aloe vera* (L.) Webb. Natural Sources of Antioxidants: A Review. *Plant Foods Human Nutr.* **2019,** *12* (1), 13–19.

42. Ishii, Y.; Tanizawa, H.; Takino, Y. Studies of *Aloe vera*: Mechanism of Cathartic Effect. *Biol. Pharma. Bull.* **1994,** *17*, 651–663.

43. Ibrahim, A.S. *Use of Molecular Biology for Studying the Mode of Action of Some Medicinal Plant Extracts as Anticancer Agents*; Master Degree Thesis; Calcutta University, Kolkata, India, 2019; pp 2–8.

44. Jha, A.K.; Kumari, N.; Kumari, P.; Prasad, K. Phytochemical Synthesis of ZnO Nanoparticles: Antimicrobial and Anticancer Activity. *J. Bionanosci.* **2018,** *12* (6), 836–841.

45. Joseph, B.; Raj, S.J. Pharmacognostic and Phytochemical Properties of *Aloe vera* linn : An Overview. *Int. J. Pharma. Sci. Rev. Res.* **2010,** *4* (2), 106–110.

46. Kar, S.K.; Bera, T.K. Phytochemical Constituents of *Aloe vera* and Their Multifunctional Properties: A Comprehensive Review. *Int. J. Pharma. Sci. Res.* **2018,** *9* (4), 1416–1423.

47. Khor, B.; Gardet, A.; Xavier, R.J. Genetics and Pathogenesis of Inflammatory Bowel Disease. *Nature* **2011,** *474* (7351), 307–317.

48. Kokate, C.K.; Purohit, A.P.; Gokhale, S.B. (Eds.). *Text Book of Pharmacognosy*, 13th ed.; Nirali Prakashan: New Delhi, 2003; pp 58–66.

49. Kundu, S.; Salma, U.; Sutradhar, M.; Mandal, N. Update on the Medicinal Uses, Phytochemistry and Pharmacology of *Leucas aspera*, a Medicinally Important Species. *Int. J. Agric. Innov. Res.* **2018,** *6* (4), 39–44.

50. Kilic, N. The Effect of *Aloe vera* gel on Experimentally Induced Peritoneal Adhesions in Rats. *Revue de MÃdecineVÃtÃrinaire* **2005,** *156* (7), 409–413.

51. Kim, H.S.; Lee, B.M. Inhibition of Benzo [a] Pyrene-DNA Adduct Formation by *Aloe Barbadensis* Miller. *Carcinogenesis* **1997,** *18*, 771–776.

52. Kanojia, S.; Zaidi, A.; Pandey, N. Nutritive Value and Chemical Attributes of *Aloe vera* Jam. *Pharma. Biol.* **2018,** *3* (2), 16–20.

53. Loots, D.T.; vander, W.; F.H, Botes, L. Aloe ferox Leaf Gel Phytochemical Content, Antioxidant Capacity and Possible Health Benefits. *J. Agric. Food Chem.* **2007,** *55* (17), 6891–6896.

54. Langmead, L.; Makins, R.J.; Rampton, D.S. Anti-inflammatory Effects of *Aloe vera* Gel in Human Colorectal Mucosa In Vitro. *Aliment. Pharmacol. Therap.* **2004,** *19*, 521–527.

55. Langmead, L.; Feakins, M.; Goldthorpe, S. Randomized, Double-blind, Placebo-Controlled Trial of Oral *Aloe vera* Gel for Active Ulcerative Colitis. *Aliment Pharmacol. Therap.* **2004,** *19, 739*–747.

56. Muthukumaran, P.; Divya R.; Indhumathi, E.; Keerthika, C. Total Phenolic and Flavonoid Content of Membrane Processed *Aloe vera* Extract: A Comparative Study. *Int. Food Res. J.* **2018,** *25* (4), 212–220.

57. Marshall, J.M. Aloe vera gel: What is the Evidence? *Pharma. J.* **1990,** *24*, 360–362.

58. Mamun-Rashid, A.N.M.; Islam, M.R.; Dash, B.K. In Vitro Antibacterial Effect of Bushy Mat grass (*Lippia alba* Mill.) Extracts. *Res. J. Med. Plant* **2012,** *6,* 334–340.
59. Maxwell, O.A.; Chinwe, U.V.; Obinna, EI. Evaluation of Therapeutic Uses of *Aloe barbadensis* miller Plant. *Int. J. Pharma. Sci.* **2009,** *1* (1), 59–70.
60. Nimse, S.B.; Pal, D. Free Radicals, Natural Antioxidants and Their Reaction Mechanisms. *RSC Adv.* **2015,** *5* (35), 27986–27990.
61. Nwaoguikpe, R.N.; Braide, W. The Effect of *Aloe vera* Plant (*Aloe barbadensis*) Extracts on Sickle Cell Blood. *Afr. J. Food Sci. Technol.* **2010,** *1* (3), 58–63.
62. Pal, D.K.; Dutta, S. Evaluation of the Antioxidant Activity of the Roots and Rhizomes of *Cyperus rotundus* L. *Ind. J. Pharma. Sci.* **2006,** *68* (2), 131–138.
63. Pal, D.K.; Mandal, M.; Senthilkumar, G.P.; Padhiari, A. Antibacterial Activity of *Cuscuta reflexa* Stem and *Corchorus olitorius* Seeds. *Fitoterapia* **2006,** *77* (7–8), 589–591.
64. Pal, D.K. Comparative Analysis of In Vitro Antioxidant Activity of Two Selected Plants with a Reference to Antidiabetic Profile. *Asian J. Chem.* **2013,** *25* (4), 2165–2169.
65. Pal, D.K.; Mazumdar U.K.; Gupta, M. Fractionation of Stigmasterol Derivative and Study of the Effects of *Celsia coromandeliane* Aerial Parts Petroleum Ether Extract on Appearance of Puberty and Ovarian Steroidogenesis in Immature Mice. *Pharma. Biol.* **2012,** *50* (6), 747–753.
66. Pal, D.K.; Mishra, P.; Sachan, N.; Ghosh, A.K. Biological Activities and Medicinal Properties of *Cajanus cajan* (L) Millsp. *J. Adv. Pharma. Technol. Res.* **2011,** *2* (4), 207–211.
67. Pal, D.K.; Saha, S; Singh, S. Importance of Pyrazole Moiety in the Field of Cancer. *Int. J. Pharm. Pharma. Sci.* **2012,** *4,* 98–104.
68. Pal, D.K.; Saha, S. Hydroxamic Acid–A Novel Molecule for Anticancer Therapy. *J. Adv. Pharma. Technol. Res.* **2012,** *3* (2), 92.
69. Pal, D.K.; Sahoo, M.; Mishra, A.K. Analgesic and Anticonvulsant Effects of Saponin Isolated from the Stems of *Opuntia vulgaris* Mill in Mice. *Eur. Bull. Drug Res.* **2005,** *13,* 91–97.
70. Park, M.Y.; Kwon, H.J.; Sung, M.K. Dietary Aloin, Aloesin, or Aloe-gel Exerts Anti-Inflammatory Activity in a Rat Colitis Model. *Life Sci.* **2011,** *88* (11), 486–492.
71. Patel, D.K.; Patel, K.; Dhanabal, S.P. Phytochemical Standardization of *Aloe vera* Extract by HPTLC Techniques. *J. Acute Dis.* **2012,** *1* (1), 47–50.
72. Peng, S.Y.; Norman, J.; Curtin, G.; Corrier, D.; McDaniel, H.R.; Busbee, D. Decreased Mortality of Norman *Murine Sarcoma* in Mice Treated with the Immunomodulator. *Mol. Biol.* **1991,** *3,* 79–87.
73. Prabhu, K.; Karar, P.K.; Hemalatha, S.; Ponnudurai, K. Comparative Micro Morphological and Phytochemical Studies on the Roots of Three *Viburnum* species. *Turkish J. Bot.* **2011,** *35,* 663–670.
74. Rahman, M.S.; Rahman, M.Z. Antimicrobial Activity of Some Indigenous Plants of Bangladesh. *Dhaka Univ. J. Pharma. Sci.* **2008,** *7,* 23–26.
75. Rahimi, R.; Mozaffari, S.; Abdollahi, M. On the Use of Herbal Medicines in Management of Inflammatory Bowel Diseases: A Systematic Review of Animal and Human Studies. *Digest. Dis. Sci.* **2009,** *54* (3), 471–480.
76. Raphael, E. Phytochemical Constituents of Some Leaves Extract of *Aloe vera* and *Azadirachta indica* Plant Species. *Global Adv. Res. J. Environ. Sci. Toxicol.* **2012,** *1* (2), 140–147.

77. Roberts, D.; Travis, E. Acemannan-Containing Wound Dressing Gel Reduces Radiation-Induced Skin Reactions in C3H Mice. *Int. J. Radiat. Oncol. Biol. Phys.* **1995,** *32* (4), 1047–1052.

78. Reynolds, T.; Dweck, A.C. *Aloe vera*, the Secret Plant. *J. Ethnopharmacol.* **1999,** *68,* 3–6.

79. Robinson, M. Medical Therapy of Inflammatory Bowel Disease for the 21st Century. *Eur. J. Surg.* **1998,** *582,* 90–98.

80. Rachid, A.; Rabah, D.; Farid, L. Ethnopharmacological Survey of Medicinal Plants Used in the Traditional Treatment of Diabetes Mellitus in the North Western and South Western Algeria. *J. Med. Plants Res.* **2012,** *6* (10), 2041–2050.

81. Radha, M.H.; Laxmipriya, N.P. Evaluation of Biological Properties and Clinical Effectiveness of *Aloe vera*: A Systematic Review. *J. Trad. Complemen. Med.* **2015,** *5* (1), 21–26.

82. Rahimi, R.; Mozaffari, S.; Abdollahi, M. On the Use of Herbal Medicines in Management of Inflammatory Bowel Diseases: A Systematic Review of Animal and Human Studies. *Digest. Dis. Sci.* **2009,** *54* (3), 471–480.

83. Rajasekaran, S.; Ravi K.; Sivagnanam, K.; Subramanian, S. Beneficial Effects of *Aloe vera* Leaf Gel Extract on Lipid Profile Status in Rats with Streptozotocin Diabetes. *Clin. Exp. Pharmacol. Physiol.* **2006,** *33* (3), 232–237.

84. Rajeswari, R.; Umadevi, M.; Rahale, CS.; Pushpa, R. *Aloe vera*: The Miracle Plant– Its Medicinal and Traditional Uses in India. *J. Pharmacognosy Phytochem.* **2012,** *1* (4), 118–124.

85. Singh, B.; Mohan, R.; Maurya, A.; Mishra, G. Phytoconstituents and Biological Consequences of: A Focused Review *Aloe vera. Asian J. Pharm. Pharmacol.* **2018,** *4* (1), 17–22.

86. Saeed, M.A.; Ahmad, I.; Yaqub, U.; Akbar, S. *Aloe vera*: A Plant of Vital Significance. *Quart. Sci. Vis.* **2004,** *9* (12), 1–13.

87. Sonia, M.; Damak, M. In Vitro Antioxidant Activities of *Aloe vera* Leaf Skin Extracts. *J. de la SociÂtÃ Chimique de Tunisie (Chem. Soc. Tunisia)* **2008,** *10,* 101–109.

88. Steenkamp, V.; Stewart, M.J. Medicinal Applications and Toxicological Activities of Aloe Products. *Pharma. Biol.* **2007,** *45* (5), 411–420.

89. Sydiskis, R.J. Owen, D.G.; Lohr, J.L.; Rosler, K.H.; Blomster, R.N. Inactivation of Enveloped Viruses by Anthraquinones Extracted from Plants. *Antimicrob. Agents* **1991,** *35, 2463*–2466

90. Schmidt, J.M.; Greenspoon, J.S. *Aloe vera* Dermal Wound Gel is Associated with a Delay in Wound Healing. *Obsterian Gynecol.,* **1991,** *78,* 115–117.

91. Strober, W.; Fuss, I.; Mannon, P. The Fundamental Basis of Inflammatory Bowel Disease. *J. Clin. Invest.* **2007,** *117* (3), 514–521.

92. Srinivasan, N.; Palanisamy, K.; Mulpuri, S.; Jatropha: Phytochemistry, Pharmacology, and Toxicology. In *Jatropha, Challenges for a New Energy Crop,* 10th ed.; Springer India: New Delhi, 2019, pp 415–435.

93. Shen, Z.; Chauser-Volfson, E.; Gutterman, Y.I.; Hu, Z. Anatomy, Histochemistry and Phytochemistry of Leaves in *Aloe vera* var. chinensis. *Acta Bot. Sinica* **2001,** *43* (8), 780–787.

94. Sidek, H.J.; Azman, M.A.; Sharudin, M.S. (Eds.). *The Synergistic Antibacterial Effect of Azadirachtaindica Leaves Extract and Aloe barbadensis Gel against*

Bacteria Associated with Skin Infection, 1st ed.; Springer-Marapalia: Malaysia, **2018**; pp 581–591.

95. Serrano, M.; Valverde, J.M.; Guillén, F.; Castillo, S. Use of *Aloe vera* Gel Coating Preserves the Functional Properties of Table Grapes. *J. Agric. Food Chem.* **2006**, *54* (11), 3882–3886.

96. Samuelsson, G.; Bohlin, L. *Drugs of Natural Origin: A Treatise of Pharmacognosy*, 2nd ed.; CRC Press Inc: London, 2017; pp 420–439.

97. Tanwar, R.; Gupta, J.; Asif, S.; Panwar, R.; Heralgi R. *Aloe vera* and Its Uses in Dentistry. *Ind. J. Dent. Adv.* **2011**, *3* (4), 656–658.

98. Torres, J.; Ellul, P.; Langhorst, J.; Mikocka-Walus, A. Crohn's and Colitis Organization Topical Review on Complementary Medicine and Psychotherapy in Inflammatory Bowel Disease. *J. Crohn's Colitis* **2019**, *13* (6), 673–685.

99. Vera, A. Wound Healing, Oral and Topical Activity of *Aloe vera*. *J. Am. Podiatr. Med. Assoc.* **1989**, *79*, 559–562.

100. Visuthikosol, V.; Chowchuen, B.; Sukwanarat, V. Effects of *Aloe vera* Gel to Healing of Burn Wound: A Clinical Histologic Study. *J. Med. Assoc. Thailand* **1995**, *78*, 403–409.

101. Waris, Z.; Iqbal, Y.; Arshad, H.S. Proximate Composition, Phytochemical Analysis and Antioxidant Capacity of *Aloe vera*, *Cannabis sativa* and *Mentha longifolia*. *Pure Appl. Biol.* **2018**, *7* (3), 1122–1130.

102. West, D.P.; Zhu, Y.F. Evaluation of *Aloe vera* Gel Gloves in the Treatment of Dry Skin Associated with Occupational Exposure. *Am. J. Infect. Contr.* **2003**, *31*, 40–42.

103. Waris, Z.; Iqbal, Y.; Arshad, H.S.; Khan, A.A.; Ali, A.; Khan, M.W. Proximate Composition, Phytochemical Analysis and Antioxidant Capacity of *Aloe vera*, *Cannabis sativa* and *Mentha longifolia*. *Pure Appl. Biol.* **2018**; *7* (3), 1122–1130.

104. Wang, X.; Feng, L.; Zhou, T.; Ruhsam, M. Genetic and Chemical Differentiation Characterizes Top-geo herb and Non-top-geo herb Areas in the TCM Herb Rhubarb. *Sci. Rep.* **2018**, *8* (1), 1–4.

105. Xavier, R.J.; Podolsky, D.K. Unravelling the Pathogenesis of Inflammatory Bowel Disease. *Nature* **2007**, *448* (7152), 427–434.

106. Yeh, G.Y.; Eisenberg, D.M.; Kaptchuk, T.J.; Phillips, R.S. Systematic Review of Herbs and Dietary Supplements for Glycemic Control in Diabetes. *Diab. Care* **2003**, *26*, 1277–1294.

107. Yim, D.; Kang, S.S.; Kim, D.W.; Kim, S.H.; Lillehoj, H.S.; Min, W. Protective Effects of *Aloe vera*—based Diets in Eimeria Maxima-infected Broiler Chickens. *Exp. Parasitol.* **2011**, *127* (1), 322–325.

108. Zawahry, ME.; Hegazy, M.R.; Helal, M. Use of Aloe in Treating Leg Ulcers and Dermatoses. *Int. J. Dermatol.* **1973**, *12*, 68–73.

CHAPTER 12

Herbal Treatment for Irritable Bowel Syndrome

HASYA NAZLI EKIN and DIDEM DELIORMAN ORHAN

ABSTRACT

The clinical manifestations of irritable bowel syndrome (IBS) include abdominal pain, abdominal discomfort, and frequency and consistency of defecation. Rome-III and -IV criteria are currently used in the diagnosis of IBS. The symptoms of IBS patients can be improved through drug treatment, psychotherapy, and diet programs, and also through the use of extracts of medicinal plants, essential oils, and natural bioactive compounds. This chapter discusses the potential use of plants (such as *Aloe vera, Carum carvi, Cuminum cyminum, Curcu*ma sp., *Cynara scolymus, Hypericum perforatum, Mentha piperita,* and *Panax ginseng*) for the treatment of IBS.

12.1 INTRODUCTION

Functional gastrointestinal disorders are divided into six classes, which are: irritable bowel syndrome (IBS), functional diarrhea and constipation, opioid-induced constipation, functional abdominal bloating, tension, and non-specific functional bowel disorder.[28] The disorder is common in the world and generally affects young people and women.[21] The prevalence of IBS has been varied from region to region. In the world, South America has most common IBS (21%) compared to South Asia with lowest percentage of IBS patients (7%).[10] Women have two times higher risk of developing IBS symptoms compared to men. IBS is a chronic disorder identified by flatulence, bloating, pain in abdomen, changed bowel conditions (such as constipation, diarrhea, or both).[22,62] The etiology of the disorder has not been elucidated yet, but it is considered that the mechanism could be based on allergic, immunological, psychiatric, and toxic reactions.[43]

IBS generally cannot be diagnosed with serum biomarkers or tests. Generally, the test results have been shown as normal. As a result of these handicaps, some criteria have been determined for the diagnosis of IBS. Nowadays, Rome criteria are used based on clinical studies on IBS symptoms in the United Kingdom. When the process of the regulation of these criteria is examined, it is seen that it was designed based on the Manning criteria prepared as a result of the studies carried out by Manning in 1978.[38] At least two of six cardinal criteria (such as the looser stool of the starting of the pain, the mucus passage, relief of pain after intestinal movements, apparent distension, and lacking evacuation sensation, more frequent intestinal movements at the beginning of pain) should be seen in patients.[34] After the Manning criteria were revised in 1990, the Rome criteria were published. Rome criteria are more restrictive than the Manning criteria.

This chapter discusses: (1) diagnostic crtiteria for IBS (Rome I, II, III, IV), (2) synthetic and herbal drugs to alleviate pain due to IBS, and (3) medicinal plants, such as *Aloe vera, Carum carvi, Cuminum cyminum, Curcu*ma sp., *Cynara scolymus, Hypericum perforatum, Mentha piperita,* and *Panax ginseng* for the treatment of IBS.

12.2   DIAGNOSTIC CRITERIA FOR IBS

12.2.1   *Rome I Criteria, 1994*[13]

Following symptoms for 3 months or more:

- Abdominal pain or discomfort feelings
- Alteration of stool consistency
- Alteration of stool frequency
- Alteration of the form of stool (watery/loose or hard/lumpy stool)
- Alteration of the frequency of stool (>3 bowel movements per day or <3 per week)
- Alteration of the passage of stool (urgency, straining, tenesmus)
- Mucus passaging
- Relief feelings with defecation
- The feeling of bloating and abdominal tension, and
- Two or more of the above, at least 25% of days or conditions

12.2.2 *Rome II Criteria, 1999–2000*[32]

Abdominal pain or discomfort for at least 12 weeks (consecutive or not) in the previous 12 months, two of the three following symptoms must be present:

- Onset involved with a change in defecation frequency,
- Onset involved with a change in stool appearance, and
- Relief sensation after defecation.

12.2.3 *Rome III Criteria, 2006*[55]

Recurrent abdominal discomfort or pain related to two or more of the following symptoms for more than 3 days per month for three consecutive months:

- Onset involved with a change in defecation frequency,
- Onset involved with changes in stool appearance, and/or form.
- Relief sensation after defecation.

12.2.4 *Rome IV Criteria, 2016*[2,54]

In the last 3 months, repetitive abdominal pain for at least 1 day/week. It is associated with at least two of the following symptoms:

- Alteration of stool appearance,
- Alteration of stool frequency, and
- Increase in frequency of defecation.

12.3 MEDICATIONS SELECTED ACCORDING TO DOMINANT SYMPTOMS IN PATIENTS WITH IBS

Nowadays, the Rome IV criteria are utilized in the diagnosis of IBS. There is still no definite and permanent treatment for IBS. Generally, symptom-based treatment methods are applied for this disorder.[15] There are four main methods for the treatment of IBS,[9,15,40,48] and it is considered that all of these should be applied together to eliminate or reduce the complaints. For this purpose, a diet program, medication (conventional drug and phytothera-peutics), and psychotherapy program should be designed for the patients.

TABLE 12.1   Medications for the Treatment of Dominant Symptoms of IBS.

Medication group	Drug
5-HT3 antagonists	Alosetron
5-HT4 agonists	Tegaserod
Activators of chlorine channels	Lubiprostone
Antibiotics	Rifaximin
Antidiarrheal drug	Loperamide
Antispasmodic and antiflatulence	Simethicone, Alverine citrate
Antispasmodic	Dicyclomine, pinaverium, trimebutine, hyoscine-N-butylbromide, mebeverine, peppermint oil
Bile acid bindings	Cholestyramine
Bulk-forming agents	*Psyllium*, calcium, polycarbophil, oats
Guanylate cyclase 2C analogs	Linaclotide
Osmotic laxatives	Mg^{+2} citrate, polyethylene glycol solution, sorbitol
Probiotics	*Bifidobacterium infantis, Lactobacillus* sp.
Selective serotonin reuptake inhibitors	Citalopram, fluoxetine, escitalopram, paroxetine
Stool softener laxatives	Sodium docusate
Tricyclic antidepressants	Imipramine, doxepin, nortriptyline, amitriptyline, trimipramine

- Pain/abdominal discomfort: Antispasmodic and anxiolytic, selective serotonin reuptake inhibitor, tricyclic antidepressant, and 5-HT4 agonist.
- Flatulence: Antispasmodic and antiflatulence, antibiotic, and probiotics.
- IBS-constipation: Bulk-forming agents, 5-HT3 antagonists, osmotic laxatives, stool softener laxatives, activators of chlorine channels, selective serotonin reuptake inhibitors, and guanylate cyclase 2C analogs.
- IBS-diarrhea: Antibiotic, 5-HT3 antagonists, tricyclic antidepressant, antidiarrheal drugs, and bile acid bindings.

12.4   CURATIVE EFFECTS OF NATURAL PLANTS ON IRRITABLE BOWEL SYNDROME

Herbal medicines and plant-based products are being used worldwide to treat many diseases or to complement conventional drugs. This section includes discussions on the outcomes of clinical trials in IBS treatment using herbal products.

12.4.1   Aloe vera (L.) Burm. F.

A placebo-controlled, randomized, double-blind trial examined whether the *Aloe vera* gel has curative effects on IBS symptoms. Forty-one IBS patients were diagnosed with Rome II criteria, who received 50 mL of *A. vera* gel 4 times a day for 1 month. Bowel habit satisfaction, pain, IBS, and distension scores were used as the evaluation criteria. Findings exerted that *A. vera* gel was well-tolerated and had curative effects as indicated by criteria scores (bowel habit satisfaction, pain, and IBS scores). Despite all this, the results of this study are inadequate for the use of *A. vera* gel in the treatment of IBS. Further clinical studies on this natural product should be planned.[18]

Hutchings et al.[25] designed multicenter, cross-over placebo-controlled, double-blind, randomized clinical trials to test the effect of ingestion of *A. vera* gel on IBS patients. Participants were randomized to placebo, washout, *Aloe* or *Aloe*, wash-out, placebo group. 47 voluntary patients were grouped into different categories for the treatment. i.e., selected according to Rome II criteria. The clinical study comprised of four periods and was continued for 11 months. These four clinical test durations were: baseline (2 weeks), treatment period (5 months), wash-out (2 weeks), and second-treatment period (5 months). *A. vera* drink (60 mL) was taken orally twice daily, during both the treatment periods. Gastrointestinal symptoms rating scale, EuroQol (EQ5D) questionnaire, the irritable bowel syndrome quality of life questionnaire (IBSQOL), and Short Form-12 (SF-12). Quality of life questionnaire was used to assess the effect of the treatment protocol. This study displayed that *A. vera* drink was not very effective based on the criteria examined in IBS patients.

12.4.2   Carum carvi L.

The seeds of *C. carvi* contain high amounts of essential oil and are used both in the food industry and in traditional medicine (such as carminative, mild stomachic, and diuretic). The plant contains secondary metabolites with biological activities such as flavonoids, alkaloids, aliphatic compounds, monoterpenoids and sesquiterpenoids, steroids, and coumarins.[50]

Lauche et al.[33] compared the effects of a hot *C. carvi* essential oil poultice (CarO), a nonheated olive oil poultice, and a hot olive oil poultice (OlivH) to improve the quality of life (QOL) and relieve IBS symptoms in patients. For this purpose, a monocentric randomized controlled open-label cross-over trial was performed on 48 patients with IBS. *C. carvi* essential oil was prepared as a 2% solution in olive oil and then this solution was applied topically to the abdomen of the patients. This area was covered with a dry and moist towel. Finally, a hot pad is placed on the towel and waited for 20–30 min. In hot OlivH application, the solution did not contain *C. carvi* essential oil, but the procedures were the same. In the nonheated poultice (OlivC) application, the hot pad was not placed on the towel. These treatments were continued daily for 3 weeks. The EuroQol questionnaire (EQ-5D), IBS-symptom severity scale (IBS-SSS), the hospital anxiety and depression scale and score were used to evaluate the effect of all treatments. Hot CarO application was more effective and safer than the other two treatments. It has been suggested that the effect of this method is responsible for the placement of a hot pad.

12.4.3   *Cuminum cyminum L.*

Cuminum cyminum (cumin) has been used in traditional medicine as a bitter tonic, carminative, and purgative and as a spice due to its pleasant aromatic smell. Although cumin seeds are rich source of essential oil, yet the main components of essential oil are: α- and β-pinene, cumin aldehyde, 1,8-cineole, limonene, α-terpinene and γ-terpinene, *o*-cymene and *p*-cymene, and linalool and safranal.[27]

Cumin essential oil is commonly used in gastrointestinal disorders; and it was evaluated for its effects on IBS symptoms in a prospective study. Fifty patients in Kashan, Iran[1] were selected based on Rome II criteria, who took twice daily 10 drops of cumin extract containing 2% essential oil (cumin oral drop) for 4 weeks. Fifteen minutes after the meal, the extract was dissolved in a glass of warm water and was orally drank by the patient. Patients filled out the questionnaire about changes in IBS symptoms at 2nd and 4th weeks after the initiation and termination of treatment. For this evaluation, abdominal pain, changes in stool consistency, presence of mucosa in stool, painful defecation, nausea, and defecation frequency were considered as IBS-related symptoms. After the initiation and termination of treatment, some symptoms, such as abdominal pain, painful defecation, nausea, presence of mucosa in stool were significantly reduced. The stool consistency and defecation frequency, which are the IBS dominant partners, had also been considerably improved. Results exerted that cumin essential oil is effective in IBS patients.[1]

12.4.4 Curcuma L.

Curcuma longa species (turmeric) are used in traditional medicine for colds, cough, sinusitis, rheumatism, and skin diseases.[17] Rhizomes of the plant include important secondary metabolites (carbohydrates, proteins, essential oil, polypeptides, curcuminoids) with curative properties.[16]

Bundy et al.[8] examined the activity of a standardized turmeric extract on IBS symptoms in a randomized, partly blinded, two-dose, pilot study, placebo-controlled clinical trial. The study included 207 healthy volunteers suffering from IBS symptoms for at least 3 months: one group received 72 mg (one tablet) for 8 weeks and the second group received 144 mg (two tablets) for 8 weeks. The participants were chosen according to Rome II criteria. IBS pain, self-reported effectiveness, and symptom-associated quality of life (IBSQOL) were used to appraise the efficacy of the protocol. The 22 and 25% reduction in abdominal pain/discomfort score were found in one- and two-tablet groups, respectively. At the end of the therapy protocol, there were remarkable improvements in the IBSQOL scores from 5 to 36% in both groups. Also 70 and 67% of volunteers (in two- and one-tablet groups, respectively) described definite or partial healing in IBS complaints after the therapy. On the other hand, very minor side effects (such as dry mouth and flatulence nausea) were reported. These effects were observed in very few participants. This study showed that further clinical studies on the use of standardized turmeric extract to reduce IBS symptoms are needed.

The combinations with turmeric and other medicinal plants were tested in IBS patients. In a clinical trial (placebo-controlled and randomized), 121 patients defined with Rome III criteria were given a combination of fennel oil and curcumin oil for 30 days. At the end of this period, improvements in QOL and symptoms of the patients were evaluated. The patients with

IBS-SSS of 100–300 and abdominal pain score of 30–70 on 100 mm visual analog scale were included in the study. Patients were given a dose of two capsules (CU-FEO: Fennel essential oil 25 mg and Curcumin 42 mg) b.i.d. for a period of 3 months. After the treatment period, the number of patients (25.9%) without IBS symptoms was significantly higher compared with the placebo (6.8%). CU-FEO treatment led to positive improvements for each score of the IBSQOL. No adverse effects were reported during the treatment.[47]

Di Ciaula et al.[19] tested the effects of a standardized bio-optimized turmeric extract (Enterofytol®) to 25 mg fennel essential oil (*trans*-anethole) and 42 mg of curcumin in 211 patients from suffering IBS. For the first 30 days, patients used two capsules containing standardized extract before meal 3 times daily. After this period, whether the patients (complaints decreased or not due to treatment) were evaluated by face-to-face interviews. Then, the dose of the drug for 30 days was reduced to two tablets twice a day in patients with decreased complaints. At the end of 30 and 60 days, it was found that the patients had significant improvement in IBSQoL and a reduction in the IBS severity index. This report proposed that QOL and symptoms of patients (regardless of age, sex, and IBS subtypes) using this combination over a period of more than 2 months had improved.

Two supplements prepared from *Fumaria officinalis* and *C. xanthorrhiza* approved by the German Commission-E for the treatment of gastrointestinal disorders were assessed in a randomized, placebo-controlled, double-blind clinical trial for their effect on IBS treatment. *F. officinalis* tablets were standardized (containing at least 3.75% alkaloid) on the basis of alkaloid protopine as a marker. On the other hand, *C. xanthorrhiza* tablets contained 20 mg spray-dried extract but were not standardized. The participants in *C. xanthorrhiza* group ($n = 24$) were treated for 18 weeks (one tablet thrice a day), whereas participants in placebo ($n = 58$) and *F. officinalis* ($n = 24$) groups were treated for 18 weeks (two tablets thrice a day). The participants completed the questionnaire 4 weeks before the treatment protocol, initially, 6th, 12th, and 18th weeks during the treatment. Changes in IBS-related pain and distension scores were used as the main outcome parameters. As a result of the study, no clinical significant changes in patterns of leading IBS symptoms (pain, distension, defecation irregularity) were observed in patients in the placebo, *F. officinalis,* and *C. xanthorrhiza* groups. In *C. xanthorrhiza* group, only one patient had adverse reactions (constipation and distension) related to the treatment, whereas eight patients in *F. officinalis* group had adverse reactions (constipation, distension, nausea, epigastric pain, pruritus, and loss of hair).[6]

Tomasello et al.[58] conducted an open-label, prospective observational clinical study on 187 patients with IBS to assess the effect of a combination of chamomile, fennel, caraway, passionflower, melissa, and beta-galactosidase (Spasmicol®). This natural product, which was formulated as a chewable tablet, was administered to patients twice daily before the meals for 30 days. Evaluation after 30 days displayed that the natural product caused positive improvements in many IBS symptoms (decreasing in intestinal gas formation, abdominal pain, constipation, diarrhea, and intestinal distension). All these effects have been suggested to be caused by the synergistic effect of the components in the natural product, based on the fact that there are many scientific studies on the curative effect of each component on the intestinal mucosa, intestinal motility, and intestinal smooth muscle.

Lior et al.[35] organized a prospective, placebo-controlled, double-blind, crossover study to assess the effect of a mixture of curcumin, green tea, and selenomethionine on 12 randomly chosen patients with IBS based on Rome III criteria. The treatment process was assessed using IBS quality of life (QOL) and health-related QOL questionnaires. For 4 weeks, the patients received a dietary supplement containing green tea (25% epigallocatechin gallate and green tea extract [60% polyphenols]), curcumin (*C. longa* extract [the extract was standardized to 95% curcuminoids] and *C. longa* powder), and L-selenomethionine; and then placebo group patients received this dietary supplement for 4 weeks following a washout period of 2 weeks. Although this supplement had no effect on most of the evaluation parameters (abdominal pain, bloating, and effects of IBS on daily activity, symptoms, IBS-related quality of life and general health quality of life), yet there were positive effects on patients' satisfaction with intestinal habits during treatment.

12.4.5 Cynara scolymus L.

C. scolymus (Artichoke) is also used in nutraceuticals due to the rich polyphenol and inulin contents in the leaves of the plant. Artichoke leaves and heads are rich in polyphenolic compounds, such as flavonoids, isoflavones, anthocyanins, and catechins. Hepatoprotective, choleretic, antichole static, hypolipidemic, antioxidative, antimicrobial, and antispasmodic effects of the plant have been shown in various scientific studies.[3]

A study was conducted by Walker et al.[60] on post-marketing surveil-lance study on dyspeptic patients (n = 553) to evaluate the effect of Artichoke leaf extract on a sub-group with IBS symptoms (n = 279). The data of patients that have at least three of five IBS symptoms for Rome III criteria were evaluated. After 6 weeks of treatment, the abdominal pain, right-sided abdominal cramps, bloating, flatulence, and constipation complaints were reduced significantly ($p < 0.05$). Also, the tolerability of Artichoke leaf extracts was acceptable.[60]

The activity of standardized (1:5) aqueous full-spectrum *C. scolymus* (Artichoke) leaf extract was studied on 208 adults. The volunteers were divided into two groups: 320 mg extract (one capsule for each day) was given to the first group, and 640 mg extract (two capsules for each day) was given to the latter group for 2 months. At the beginning of the study, some of the volunteers had constipation, diarrhea or both (alternating diarrhea/constipation). As a result, while the percentage of volunteers that have diarrhea or constipation remained nearly the same as in the beginning, the percentage of volunteers that have alternating diarrhea or constipation was decreased by 26.4% after 2 months. Furthermore, after the treatment, nepean dyspepsia index (NDI), which indicates the dyspepsia and form from total score and 15 domain scores, was decreased in all scores (41% in the total score). Also, QOL scores were increased by 20%. In the study, there were no differences between the two doses in all scores.[7]

Antispasmodic activity of leaves of *C. scolymus* was demonstrated in a bioactivity-guided isolation study.[20] The plant dichloromethane fractions of methanol extract and the main compound, which is isolated from dichloromethane fractions, cynaropicrin were administered to the isolated Guinea pig ileum. As a consequence, cynaropicrin showed antispasmodic activity with 0.065 (0.049–0.086) mg/mL IC$_{50}$; and the antispasmodic activity on the smooth muscle of the plant was attributed to the cynaropicrin. The relief effect of the plant on IBS symptoms may be due to the antispasmodic activity of the plant.

One of the complaints of the IBS patients is dyspepsia.[59] The effect of *C. scolymus* leaf extract on dyspepsia was displayed in a randomized, double-blind, placebo-controlled trial (for 6 weeks on 244 patients).[24]

Consequently, recovery in dyspepsia symptoms was better in the group that used *C. scolymus* leaf extract, when compared with placebo ($p <$ 0.01). Also, QOL scores were higher in *C. scolymus* group than the placebo ($p < 0.01$). This study indicated that the healing of the symptoms in IBS patients was lower than the non-IBS patients. While the number of completely treated non-IBS patients ($n = 27$) was higher than placebo ($n = $ 14), the number of completely treated IBS patients ($n = 4$) was lower than placebo ($n = 9$).

12.4.6   *Hypericum perforatum L.*

H. perforatum has been used in the treatment of inflammation, hematoma, burns, wounds, and muscle pain in traditional folk medicine.[5] Phenylpropanoids, flavonol glycosides, biflavones, oligomeric proanthocyanidins, xanthones, napthodianthrones (hypericin), and prenylated phloroglucinols (hyperforin) are the main secondary metabolite groups.[31]

Depression and anxiety were found to be associated with IBS.[4,14,39] The effect of *H. perforatum* on depression and anxiety[26] was studied by Saito et al. on 70 IBS patients (selected based on Rome II criteria) with a randomized, placebo-controlled, and double-blind clinical trial. *H. perforatum* was given 450 mg twice a day to the patients, internally for 12 weeks. For the evaluation of the treatment, adequate relief (AR) of IBS symptoms, bowel symptom score (BSS), and IBSQOL parameters were evaluated. The BSS scores in all of diarrhea, constipation, and mixed IBS groups were lower in *H. perforatum* treatment group compared with the placebo group at 12 weeks ($p = 0.03$). When the AR scores were evaluated, it was observed that the scores of the placebo group were higher than the treatment group ($p = 0.02$), and no differences were observed between IBSQOL scores. Therefore, *H. perforatum* was not found more effective against IBS than the placebo.[53]

12.4.7   *Mentha piperita L.*

Peppermint oil obtained by steam distillation from dried or fresh aerial parts of *M. piperita* contains menthol (about 50–60%), number of esters (about 5–10%), menthone (5–30%), cineole and other terpenes. *Mentha* species are used traditionally for gastrointestinal disorders. Except the antispasmodic effect, *M. piperita* can also treat gastric ulcer.[20,63]

In a double-blind clinical trial, the activity of *M. piperita* essential oil that was entrapped with site-specific targeting technology (sustained-release) on diarrhea-predominant or mixed-type IBS patients based on Rome III criteria, was evaluated. The 72 patients were divided into two groups. Before the study, the patients were allowed for medical washout for 3 weeks. The first group (*n* = 37) was given placebo capsules that contained 100% fiber and the latter group (*n* = 35) was given capsules that contained 60% fiber and entrapped 180 mg *M. piperita* essential oil 3 times daily for 4 weeks. The total IBS symptom score (TISS) was evaluated at the beginning, 24 h and 28 days after the first dose. As a result, the disquieting gastrointestinal symptoms were reduced significantly in *M. piperita* oil group patients compared with the placebo group patients.[12]

The activity of enteric-coated peppermint oil (Colpermin®) that contained 187 mg peppermint oil was tested on 42 children with IBS by Manning or Rome criteria. The study was conducted for 14 days in a randomized, double-blind control trial.[30] To the upper 45 kg, children were given two capsules three times a day, and the 30–45 kg children were given one capsule three times a day. As a result, in patients receiving peppermint oil, the abdominal pain was diminished by 75%. However, there did not show significant differences in other symptoms.

Antispasmodic effect of peppermint oil on gastric spasm that was induced during the endoscopy applied without anesthesia was investigated in a double-dummy, double-blind controlled study on 100 patients.[23] In this study, the peppermint oil was applied intraluminally and the effect on gastric antral contractions was compared with Hyoscine-*N*-butylbromide that was applied intramuscularly. The opening of the pyloric ring before and after the administration and contraction of the pyloric ring was evaluated. The opening ratio was higher, and the contraction ratio of the pyloric ring was lower in the peppermint oil-treated group when compared with Hyoscine-*N*-butylbromide. Also, while the Hyoscine-*N*-butylbromide caused side effects, the peppermint oil did not cause any side effects. The administration of peppermint oil was preferred intraluminally in the study because it was known that when the essential oil administered orally the main compound of the essential oil, menthol, is absorbed from proximal gut quickly, metabolized to menthol-glucuronide, and excreted with urine. For the extended peak amount of menthol, enteric-coated capsules were studied in a pharmacokinetic study, and it was shown that when compared with soft gelatin capsules, the metabolize of menthol was delayed in the enteric-coated capsules (Colpermine®).[56] The peppermint oil showed antispasmodic activity on gastrointestinal smooth muscle via mobilization of calcium ions.[57] Due to its antispasmodic effect, peppermint oil may relief the IBS symptoms.

An aqueous extract of *M. piperita* leaf was studied against gastric ulcer with 250 and 500 mg/kg dose orally on Wistar albino rats. As a result, the extract showed a gastric mucosa protective effect against indomethacin-induced damage. Also, the extract reduced gastric ulceration induced by ethanol and alkali solutions. Also it is shown in the histopathological examination, the extract diminished inflammation, edema, and necrosis of the lesions at 500 mg/kg.[49]

Effect of enteric-coated peppermint oil capsules in a double-blind, placebo-controlled clinical trial on 50 patients with a diagnosis of IBS according to the Rome II criteria was assessed. Changes in IBS symptoms (such as constipation, diarrhea, sense of lacking evacuation, the urgency of intestinal movement, abdominal pain and bloating, discomfort at evacuation, and passage of gas or mucus) were recorded periodically (baseline, at 4th week after the end of therapy). Treatment group patients ($n = 24$) received peppermint oil capsules (225 mg Mintoil®) capsules twice daily for 4 weeks. Whereas placebo group patients received a mint-flavored enteric-coated capsule during the same time. The results showed that treatment with enteric-coated peppermint oil capsules produced significant improvements in IBS symptoms compared with those of placebo group. In this report, both antibacterial effect of peppermint oil on enteric bacteria and its relaxant effect on smooth muscle tissue were held responsible for its useful effects on IBS symptoms.[11]

Weerts et al.[61] conducted a double-blind clinical study with 178 IBS patients (Rome IV criteria). Peppermint oil formulations with different release properties were tested in patients for 8 weeks. For this reason, one group of patients used 0.182 g of small-intestinal-release peppermint oil (Tempocol®) and the other group used 0.182 g of ileocolonic-release peppermint Q14 essential oil (Tempocol®, coated with a ColoPulse coating layer, core capsules). Thirty minutes before each meal, microcrystalline cellulose was given orally to placebo group patients. Previous clinical studies have shown that the 8-week period is appropriate for predicting the effect. Therefore, the application period was chosen as 8 weeks. The efficacy of treatment was evaluated according to the IBS-SSS, the generalized anxiety disorder-7, IBSQOL, the EuroQoL-5D, and the patient health survey (patient follow-up was scheduled at 1st, 2nd, 4th, 6th, and 8th weeks and at 3rd and 6th months of after the treatment period). Additionally, changes in IBS symptoms (such as stool evacuation frequency and consistency, abdominal bloating and cramping, abdominal pain and discomfort, belching, and nausea) have been reported. The results of the study showed no statistically changes in abdominal pain response or whole symptom relief in both treatment groups. The peppermint oil formulation released in the small intestine prominently reduced abdominal discomfort, abdominal pain and IBS intensity.

The effect of the product named Menthacarin®, a combination of caraway and peppermint oil, used in the cure of functional dyspepsia was assessed in IBS patients in randomized controlled and double-blind clinical trials.[22,36,37,41] For this purpose, the effects of Menthacarin® on symptoms were investigated in 111 patients with IBS in three different clinical trials. Details and results of the three clinical trials are presented in Table 12.2.

TABLE 12.2   Clinical Trials with Menthacarin® (Enteric-Coated Capsule) in Patients with IBS.

Treatment procedure	Study 1	Study 2	Study 3
	Thrice a day (270 mg peppermint oil and 150 mg caraway oil per day) or placebo for 4 weeks	Thrice a day (150 mg caraway oil and 270 mg peppermint oil per day) or enteric soluble capsule for 4 weeks (60 mg caraway oil and 108 mg peppermint oil per day)	Twice a day (180 mg peppermint oil and 100 mg caraway oil per day) or 3 × 10 mg cisapride for 4 weeks
Patients with IBS (No.)	21	82	8
Selection criteria	Outpatients with functional dyspepsia, with or without accompanying IBS symptoms, presence of at least two bowel or/and dyspeptic-related symptoms for more than 14 days		
Primary outcome	CGI item 2, pain intensity	pain intensity	pain intensity
Secondary outcome	Diarrhea, flatulence, feelings of fullness, CGI items 1 + 3.	Flatulence, feelings of fullness, diarrhea, CGI items 1–3.	

The findings indicated that mean pain reduction values ranged from 50 to 75%. The reduction in IBS-associated symptoms in patients with functional dyspepsia has shown that Menthacarin® can also be an option for IBS treatment.

The effect of Colpermin® (peppermint oil 0.2 mL) was investigated in a randomized, double-blind clinical, placebo-controlled trial in 90 outpatients diagnosed with the Rome II criteria. Colpermin® is an enteric-coated, delayed-release peppermint oil formulation. During 8 weeks, patients received one enteric-coated capsule or placebo thrice a day 30 min before the meals. The patients were visited in the Ist, 4th, and 8th weeks after the beginning of the treatment to observe the improvements in their symptoms and quality of life. There was a significant decrease in abdominal pain in the Colpermin® group compared to placebo. These results showed that Colpermin® is a confident and efficacious medication for IBS patients.[42]

Khanna et al.[29] conducted a meta-analysis on nine double-blind clinical trials with peppermint oil preparations. In these studies, the number of patients was between 47 and 178 and the duration of treatment was between 2 and 12 weeks. Patients generally took three to six capsules (Mintoil®: microencapsulated peppermint oil, Colpermin®: 0.1, or 0.2 mL peppermint oil/capsule) per day. A total of 726 patients with IBS were evaluated. Significant improvements in IBS symptoms and abdominal pain were observed in the treatment group compared to the placebo groups. In this meta-analysis, short-term use of peppermint oil was found to be effective and reliable in improving abdominal pain and IBS symptoms.

As a result of PubMed literature research, Chumpitazi et al.[15] evaluated more than 2800 cited references related to the use of peppermint and peppermint oil in gastrointestinal disorders. When only randomized clinical studies were examined, it was reported that peppermint oil was effective in the gastrointestinal tract by various mechanisms:

- Anti-inflammatory activity
- Antimicrobial activity
- Modulation of psychosocial distress
- Modulation of visceral sensitivity (via transient receptor potential cation channels)
- Relaxation of smooth muscle (via affect enteric nervous system or calcium channel blockade).

This report[15] concluded that peppermint oil has physiological effects in the gastrointestinal system and it is safe to use.

The mixture of *Cyperus rotundus* L., *M. longifolia*, and *Zingiber officinale* was studied on 40 IBS patients (based on Rome III criteria) for 8 weeks. The plants were chosen for their traditional consumption for the treatment of gastrointestinal disorders. The mixture was prepared with mixing powders of 150 mg *C. rotundus* tuber, 150 mg *M. longifolia* leaf, and 150 mg *Z. officinale* tuber. The combination was used three times daily 1 h after the meal. The 135 mg mebeverine (positive control) was given to the first group; and the capsule, which contained the plants, was given to the second group. Consequently, the combined plant treatment reduced IBS symptoms and the result was shown comparable with mebeverine.[52]

12.4.8   Panax ginseng C.A. Mey

The roots of ginseng are used as tonic and adaptogen in Traditional Chinese Medicine. This medicinal plant contains a wide variety of secondary metabolites, such as ginsenosides or triterpenoid saponins, volatile oils, amino acids, vitamins, and fatty acids. To date, many scientific studies have been carried out on the biological activities (such as anti-inflammatory, hypotensive, hypoglycemic, sexual dysfunctions, antineoplastic agents, improve vitality, anti-stress, and promote healing process) of *P. ginseng*.[46]

The effect of standardized dry *P. ginseng* leaf and stem extract (containing 26.66% of total ginsenosides) on abdominal pain in IBS patients was assessed by a double-blind, prospective, and randomized clinical experimental study.[51] The patients ($n = 24$) were chosen based on Rome III criteria and were divided into two groups each with 12 patients. The *P. ginseng* was given to the first group at 300 mg/day dose daily. To the latter group, trimebutine (600 mg/day) was given. The condition of the patients was evaluated at baseline, after 1 week, 30 and 60 days. For the determination of the severity of the pain, the Likert scale was used: (1) the scale at −7 that indicated the enormous pain and (2) the scale at (+7) that indicated painless symptoms. After 8 weeks of the treatment, it is shown that the pain scores in all patients in both groups become positive and indicated significant differences when compared to the baseline ($p < 0.05$). Furthermore, no significant differences were shown between *P. ginseng* and trimebutine (positive control) groups. In the group that used

P. ginseng, two patients (16.66%) experienced a headache as a side effect. In the study, the positive effect of *P. ginseng* on IBS patients was attributed to the body tonic and antinociceptive activity of the plant.

12.4.9   Plantago major L.

In general, *Plantago* species are used due to their anesthetic, antiviral, anti-inflammatory, antihelminthic analgesic, analeptic, antirheumatic, antitumor, antiulcer, diuretic, expectorant effects. In traditional medicine, *P. major* has been utilized for the treatment of viral diseases (cold, influenza, etc.) and to protect against snake bites. The leaves of the plant contain flavonoids, organic acids, terpenoids, fatty acids, carotenes, and phenolic acids.[45]

In a double-blinded clinical trial conducted, the effect of *P. major* versus Colofac® was investigated on 51 patients with IBS based on Rome II criteria. Colofac® is a musculotropic antispasmodic containing mebeverine hydrochloride. Powdered *P. major* (4.5 g) in capsule form was given to patients twice daily before meal for 3 months. Other group patients received Colofac capsule (200 mg) at the same time. During treatment, diarrhea, constipation, and defecation number were used as the evaluation criteria. In fact, no difference was observed between the two groups in terms of efficacy. However, *P. major* capsules were found to be more effective than Colofac® in reducing the number of defecations.[44]

12.5   SUMMARY

A diet program, medication (conventional drug and phytotherapeutics) and psychotherapy program should be designed for the patients with IBS symptoms. Clinical studies of *Aloe vera, Cynara scolymus, Hypericum perforatum, Panax ginseng, Carum carvi,* and *Cuminum cyminum* were found to be extremely inadequate and few. Clinical studies on *Curcuma* species and *M. piperita* essential oil (peppermint oil) have provided more promising data for the relief of IBS symptoms. Results of many randomized, double-blind, placebo-controlled clinical trials with some formulations containing peppermint oil have shown that the use of this essential oil for at least 8 weeks is the most promising natural product in alleviating abdominal pain and improving quality of life in IBS patients. It was also concluded that the side effect profiles of peppermint oil were extremely low and safe.

KEYWORDS

- *Aloe vera*
- *Carum carvi*
- *Cuminum cymnium*
- *Curcuma* sp.
- *Cynara scolymus*
- *Hypericum perforatum*
- irritable bowel syndrome
- *Mentha piperita*
- *Panax ginseng*

REFERENCES

1. Agah, S.; Taleb, A. M.; Moeini, R.; Gorji, N.; Nikbakht, H. Cumin Extract for Symptom Control in Patients with Irritable Bowel Syndrome: A Case Study in Iran. *Middle East J. Digest. Dis.*, **2013,** *5* (4), 217–222.
2. Akalın, Ç. Correlation of Irritable Bowel Syndrome Subtype Based on the Rome IV Criteria with Body Mass Index. *Ankara Eğitim ve Araştırma Hastanesi Dergisi (J. Ankara Train. Res. Hosp.)* **2019,** *52* (2), 149–152.
3. Amira, S.; El Senousy Farag, M. A. Developmental Changes in Leaf Phenolics Composition from Artichoke (*Cynara scolymus*) as Determined via UHPLC–MS and Chemometrics. *Phytochemistry* **2014,** *108*, 67–76.
4. Behnke, K.; Jensen, G. S.; Graubaum, H. J.; Gruenwald, J. *Hypericum Perforatum* versus Fluoxetine in the Treatment of Mild to Moderate Depression. *Adv. Therap.* **2002,** *19* (1), 43–52.
5. Ben-Eliezer, D.; Yechiam, E. *Hypericum perforatum* as a Cognitive Enhancer in Rodents: A Meta-analysis. *Sci. Rep.* **2016,** *6*, article ID: 35700.
6. Brinkhaus, B.; Hentschel, C.; Von Keudell, C. Herbal Medicine with Curcuma and Fumitory in the Treatment of Irritable Bowel Syndrome: A Randomized, Placebo-controlled, Double-blind Clinical Trial. *Scand. J. Gastroenterol.* **2005,** *40*, 936–943.

7. Bundy, R.; Walker, A. F.; Middleton, R. W.; Marakis, G.; Booth, J. C. Artichoke leaf Extract Reduces Symptoms of Irritable Bowel Syndrome and Improves Quality of Life in Otherwise Healthy Volunteers Suffering from Concomitant Dyspepsia: A Subset Analysis. *J. Altern. Complem. Med.* **2004,** *10* (4), 667–669.

8. Bundy, R.; Walker, A. F.; Middleton, R. W.; Booth, J. Turmeric Extract May Improve Irritable Bowel Syndrome. *J. Altern. Complem. Med.* **2004,** *10* (6), 1015–1018.

9. Can, G.; Yılmaz, B. Approaches in the Diagnosis and Treatment of Irritable Bowel Syndrome. *Curr. Gastroenterol.* **2015,** *19* (3), 171–181.

10. Canavan, C.; West, J.; Card, T. The Epidemiology of Irritable Bowel Syndrome. *Clin. Epidemiol.* **2014,** *6,* 71–80.

11. Cappello, G.; Spezzaferro, M.; Grossi, L.; Manzoli, L.; Marzio, L. Peppermint Oil (Mintoil[r]) in the Treatment of Irritable Bowel Syndrome: A Prospective Double blind Placebo-controlled Randomized trial. *Digest. Liver Dis.* **2007,** *39* (6), 530–536.

12. Cash, B. D.; Epstein, M. S.; Shah, S. M. Novel Delivery System of Peppermint Oil is an Effective Therapy for Irritable Bowel Syndrome Symptoms. *Digest. Dis. Sci.* **2015,** *61* (2), 560–571.

13. Charapata, C.; Mertz, H. Physician Knowledge of Rome symptom Criteria for Irritable Bowel Syndrome is Poor Among Non-gastroenterologists. *Neurogastroenterol. Motility* **2006,** *18,* 211–216.

14. Cho, H. S.; Park, J. M.; Lim, C. H. Anxiety, Depression and Quality of Life in Patients with Irritable Bowel Syndrome. *Gut Liver* **2011,** *5* (1), 29–36.

15. Chumpitazi, B. P.; Kearns, G. L.; Shulman, R. J. The Physiological Effects and Safety of Peppermint Oil and Its Efficacy in Irritable Bowel Syndrome and other Functional Disorders. *Aliment. Pharmacol. Therap.* **2018,** 47, 738–752.

16. Committee on Herbal Medicinal Products (HMPC). *Assessment Report on Curcuma longa L., rhizome.* EMA/HMPC/329745/2017, 2017; pp 1–34; https://www.ema.europa.eu/en/documents/herbal-report/final-assessment-report-curcuma- longa-l-rhizoma-revi-sion-1_en.pdf; Accessed on November 22, 2020.

17. Çöteli, E.; Karataş, F. Determination of Amounts of Antioxidant Vitamins and Glutathione with Total Antioxidant Capacity in *Curcuma longa* L. *Erciyes Univ. J. Nat. Appl. Sci.* **2017,** *33* (2), 91–101.

18. Davis, K.; Philpott, S.; Kumar, D.; Mendall, M. Randomised Double-blind Placebo-controlled Trial of *Aloe vera* for Irritable Bowel Syndrome. *Int. J. Clin. Pract.* **2006,** *60* (9), 1080–1086.

19. Di Ciaula, A.; Portincasa, P.; Maes, N.; Albert, A. Efficacy of Bio-optimized Extracts of Turmeric and Essential Fennel Oil on the Quality of Life in Patients with Irritable Bowel Syndrome. *Ann. Gastroenterol.* **2018,** *31,* 1–7.

20. Emendorfer, F.; Emendorfer, F.; Bellato, F. Antispasmodic Activity of Fractions and Cynaropicrin from *Cynara scolymus* on Guinea- pig ileum. *Biol. Pharmacol. Bull.* **2005,** *28* (5), 902–904.

21. Ford, A. C.; Lacy, B. E.; Talley, N. J. Irritable Bowel Syndrome. *New Engl. J. Med.* **2017,** *376* (26), 2566–2578.

22. Freise, J.; Köhler, S. *Pfefferminzöl/ Kümmelöl-Fixkombination bei nicht-säurebed-ingter Dyspepsie-Vergleich der Wirksamkeit und Verträglichkeit zweier galenischer Zubereitungen* (Peppermint Oil/Caraway Oil Fixed Combination for Non-Acidic

Dyspepsia Comparison of the Effectiveness and Tolerability of Two Pharmaceutical Preparations). *Pharmazie (Pharmacy)* **1999,** *54,* 210–215.

23. Hiki, N.; Kurosaka, H.; Tatsutomi, Y. Peppermint Oil Reduces Gastric Spasm During Upper Endoscopy: A Randomized, Double-blind, Double-dummy Controlled Trial. *Gastrointest. Endoscop.* **2003,** *5* 7(4), 475–482.

24. Holtmann, G.; Adam, B.; Haag, S.; Collet, W.; Grunewald, E.; Windeck, T. Efficacy of Artichoke Leaf Extract in the Treatment of Patients with Functional Dyspepsia: A Six-week Placebo-controlled, Double-blind, Multicentre Trial. *Aliment. Pharmacol. Therap.* **2003,** *18* (11–12), 1099–1105.

25. Hutchings, H. A.; Wareham, K. Randomised, Cross-over, Placebo-controlled Study of *Aloe vera* in Patients with Irritable Bowel Syndrome: Effects on Patient Quality of Life. *Int. Scholar. Res. Netw. ISRN Gastroenterol.* **2011,** *2011,* article ID 206103; p 8.

26. Hypericum Depression Trial Study Group. Effect of *Hypericum perforatum* (St John's wort) in Major Depressive Disorder: Randomized Controlled Trial. *JAMA* **2002,** *287* (14), 1807–1814.

27. Johri, R. K. *Cuminum Cyminum* and *Carum carvi*: An Update. *Pharmacognosy Rev.* **2011,** *5* (9), 63–72.

28. Kaya, M.; Kaçmaz, H. *Rome IV kriterlerine göre fonksiyonel bağırsak hastalıklarının yeniden değerlendirilmesi* (Re-evaluation of Functional Bowel Disease According to Rome IV Criteria). *Güncel Gastroenteroloji (Curr. Gastroenterol.)* **2016,** *20* (4), 393–407.

29. Khanna, R.; MacDonald, J. K.; Levesque, B. G. Peppermint Oil for the Treatment of Irritable Bowel Syndrome A Systematic Review and Meta-analysis. *J. Clin. Gastroenterol.* **2014,** *48* (6), 505–512.

30. Kline, R. M.; Kline, J. J.; Di Palma, J.; Barbero, G. J., Enteric-coated, pH-dependent Peppermint Oil Capsules for the Treatment of Irritable Bowel Syndrome in Children. *J. Pediatr.* **2001,** *138* (1), 125–128.

31. Kumar, V., Khanna, K.; Seth, K. Brain Neurotransmitter Receptor Binding and Nootropic Studies on Indian *Hypericum perforatum* Linn. *Phytotherap. Res.* **2002,** *16,* 210–216.

32. Lacy, B. E.; Patel, N. K. Rome Criteria and a Diagnostic Approach to Irritable Bowel Syndrome. *J. Clin. Med.* **2017,** *6,* 99–102.

33. Lauche, R.; Janzen, A.; Lüdtke, R.; Cramer, H.; Dobos, G.; Langhorst, J. Efficacy of Caraway Oil Poultices in Treating Irritable Bowel Syndrome: Randomized Controlled Cross-over Trial. *Digestion* **2015,** *92,* 22–31.

34. Lea, R.; Hopkins, V.; Hastleton, J.; Houghton, L. A.; Whorwell, P. J. Diagnostic Criteria for Irritable Bowel Syndrome: Utility and Applicability in Clinical Practice. *Digestion* **2004,** *70* (4), 210–213.

35. Lior, O.; Sklerovsy-Benjaminov, F.; Lish, I. Treatment of Irritable Bowel Syndrome with a combination of Curcumin, Green Tea and Selenomethionine has a Positive Effect on Satisfaction with Bowel Habits. *J. Biosci. Med.* **2019,** *7,* 170–179.

36. Madisch, A.; Heydenreich, C. J.; Wieland, V.; Hufnagel, R.; Hotz, J. Treatment of Functional Dyspepsia with a Fixed Peppermint Oil and Caraway Oil Combination Preparation as Compared to Cisapride. A Multicenter, Reference-controlled Double-blind Equivalence Study. *Arzneimittelforschung (Drug Res.)* **1999,** *49,* 925–932.

37. Madisch, A.; Miehlke, S.; Labenz, J.; Stracke, B.; Köhler, S. Effectiveness of Menthacarin on Symptoms of Irritable Bowel Syndrome. *Wiener Medizinische Wochenschrift (Vienna Medical Weekly)*, **2019**, *169*, 149–155.

38. Manning, A. P.; Thompson, W. G.; Heaton, K. W.; Morris, A. F. Towards Positive Diagnosis of the Irritable Bowel. *Br. Med. J.* **1978**, *2*, 653–654.

39. Masand, P. S.; Kaplan, D. S.; Gupta, S. Major Depression and Irritable Bowel Syndrome: Is there a Relationship? *J. Clin. Psych.*, **1995**, *56* (8), 363–367.

40. Maxwell, P. R.; Mendall, M. A.; Kumar, D. Irritable Bowel Syndrome. *Lancet* **1997**, *350* (9092), 1691–1695.

41. May, B.; Kuntz, H. D.; Kieser, M.; Köhler, S. Efficacy of a Fixed Peppermint oil/caraway Oil Combination in Non-ulcer Dyspepsia. *Arzneimittelforschung (Drug Res.)* **1996**, *46*, 1149–1153.

42. Merat, S.; Khalili, S.; Mostajabi, P.; Ghorbani, A.; Ansari, R.; Malekzadeh, R. The Effect of Enteric-coated, Delayed-release Peppermint Oil on Irritable Bowel Syndrome. *Digest. Dis. Sci.* **2010**, *55*, 1385–1390.

43. Monsbakken, K. W.; Vandvik, P. O.; Farup, P. G. Perceived Food Intolerance in Subjects with Irritable Bowel Syndrome-Etiology, Prevalence and Consequences. *Eur. J. Clin. Nutr.* **2006**, *60* (5), 667–672.

44. Nagafabadi, M.; Yousefi, A. S.; Kamalinejad, S. Comparison of the Plant *Plantago major* and the Drug Colofac on Clinical Symptoms in IBS Patients. *Int. J. Life Sci.* **2015**, *9* (5), 108–112.

45. Nazarizadeh, A.; Mikaili, P.; Moloudizargari, M. Therapeutic Uses and Pharmacological Properties of *Plantago major* L. and Its Active Constituents. *J. Basic Appl. Sci. Res.* **2013**, *3* (9), 212–221.

46. Nuri, T. H. M.; Yee, J. C. W.; Gupta, M.; Khan, M. A. N. Review of *Panax Ginseng* as an Herbal Medicine. *Arch. Pharm. Pract.* **2016**, *7*, 61–65.

47. Portincasa, P.; Bonfrate, L.; Scribano, M. L. Curcumin and Fennel Essential Oil Improve Symptoms and Quality of Life in Patients with Irritable Bowel Syndrome. *J. Gastrointest. Liver Dis.* **2016**, *25* (2), 151–157.

48. Prakash, S.M.; Gupta, S.; Schwartz, T.L.; Virk, S.; Hameed, A.; Kaplan, D.S. Open-label Treatment with Citalopram in Patients with Irritable Bowel Syndrome: A Pilot Study. *Prim. Care Compan. J. Clin. Psych.* **2005**, *7* (4), 162–166.

49. Rafatullah, S.; Al-Mofleh, I.; Alhaider, A. Antisecretagogue, Antiulcer and Cytoprotective Effects of' Peppermint' *Mentha piperita* L. in Laboratory Animals. *J. Med. Sci. (Faisalabad, Pakistan)* **2006**, *6* (6), 930–936.

50. Rao, G. V.; Annamalai, T.; Sharlene, C. Secondary Metabolites and Biological Studies of Seeds of *Carum carvi* Linn. *J. Pharm. Res.* **2011**, *4* (7), 2126–2128.

51. Rocha, H. A. C.; Rocha, T. V. Randomized Controlled Trial of *Panax ginseng* in Patients with Irritable Bowel Syndrome. *Braz. J. Pharmacognosy* **2018**, *28* (2), 218–222.

52. Sahib, A.S. Treatment of Irritable Bowel Syndrome Using a Selected Herbal Combination of Iraqi Folk Medicines. *J. Ethnopharmacol.* **2013**, *148* (3), 1008–1012.

53. Saito, Y. A.; Rey, E.; Almazar-Elder, A. E. Randomized, Double-blind, Placebo-controlled Trial of St John's Wort for Treating Irritable Bowel Syndrome. *Am. J. Gastroenterol.* **2010**, *105* (1), 170–177.

54. Schmulson, M. J.; Drossman, D. A. What Is New in Rome IV. *J. Neurogastroenterol. Motility* **2017**, *23* (2), 151–163.

55. Shih, D. Q.; Kwan, L. Y. All Roads Lead to Rome: Update on Rome III Criteria and New Treatment Options. *Gastroenterology Report*, **2007,** *1* (2), 56–65.
56. Somerville, K. W.; Richmond, C. R.; Bell, G. D. Delayed Release Peppermint Oil Capsules (Colpermin) for the Spastic Colon Syndrome: Pharmacokinetic Study. *Br. J. Clin. Pharmacol.* **1984,** *18* (4), 638–640.
57. Taylor, B. D.; Luscombe, D. K.; Duthie, H. L. Inhibitory Effect of Peppermint Oil on a Gastrointestinal Smooth Muscle. *Gut* **1983,** *24* (10), A992.
58. Tomasello, G.; Palumbo, V. D.; Sinagra, E. Mixture of Vegetable Extracts (Chamomile, Passionflower, Caraway, Fennel) and Enzymes (Beta-galactosidase) for Irritable Bowel Syndrome (IBS): An Observational Study. *Progr. Nutr.* **2018,** *20* (3), 526–531.
59. Vahedi, H.; Ansari, R.; Mir-Nasseri, M.; Jafari, E. Irritable Bowel Syndrome: A Review Article. *Middle East J. Digest. Dis.* **2010,** *2* (2), 66–77.
60. Walker, A. F.; Middleton, R. W.; Petrowicz, O. Artichoke Leaf Extract Reduces Symptoms of Irritable Bowel Syndrome in a Post-marketing Surveillance Study. *Phytotherap. Res.* **2001,** *15* (1), 58–61.
61. Weerts, Z. R. M.; Masclee, A. A. M. Efficacy and Safety of Peppermint Q3 Oil in a Randomized, Double-blind Trial of Patients with Irritable Bowel Syndrome. *Gastroenterology* **2020,** *158* (1), 123–136; doi: 10.1053/j.gastro.2019.08.026.
62. Whitehead, W. E.; Engel, B. T.; Schuster, M. M. Irritable Bowel Syndrome: Physiological and Psychological Differences between Diarrhea-predominant and Constipation-predominant Patients. *Digest. Dis. Sci.* **1980,** *25* (6), 404–413.
63. Yeşilada, E.; Honda, G.; Sezik, E.; Tabata, M.; Goto, K.; Ikeshiro, Y. Traditional Medicine in Turkey, Part IV: Folk Medicine in the Mediterranean Subdivision. *J. Ethnopharmacol.* **1993,** *39* (1), 31–38.

CHAPTER 13

Role of Plant-Based Medicines for Gallstones

VIVEK KUMAR, ANJU DHIMAN, POOJA CHAWLA, and
VINEY CHAWLA

ABSTRACT

Phytomedicines play an important role in the prevention and treatment of various diseases as they are a rich source of active constituents. Cholecystectomy (gallbladder removal) is the surgical and most frequently used conventional solution to get rid of gallstones. However, the nonsurgical management and treatment of gallstone has become desirable using medicinal plants (such as *Gomphrena globosa, Kalanchoe pinnata, Portulaca oleracea,* and *Solanum melongena*) and bile salts (such as ursodeoxycholic acid (UDCA) and chenodeoxycholic acid (CDCA)). This chapter provides an overview about the pathways for management and treatment of gallstone diseases.

13.1 INTRODUCTION

Lithiasis (Greek, *Lithos* (stone)) is the process of formation of calculus (*plural calculi*) in which the concretion of mineral salts occur in gallbladder. Calculi may occur in urinary system (urinary calculi, urolithiasis, nephrolithiasis, and renal calculi), bladder (vesical calculi or cystoliths), gallbladder and bile ducts (gallstones), nasal passages (rhinoliths), gastrointestinal tract (entroliths), stomach (gastroliths), salivary glands (sialoliths), tonsils (tonsilloliths), veins (venous calculi, phleboliths), and skin (such as sweat glands). Out of these, kidney stones and gallstones are most common. The main issue is the removal of gallstones due to the position and shape of the gallbladder.[7]

In this chapter, authors have discussed the pathogenesis, factors affecting gallstone formation, and the role of complementary and alternative medicine (CAM) in the treatment of gallstones.

Almost 75% of the gallstones are composed of cholesterol and rest of these are of black and brown pigments. The brown pigmented (5%) stones are composed of calcium bilirubinate, mucin glycoproteins and calcium soaps (such as calcium palmitate and calcium stearate). Soft and greasy type gallstones generally occur in bile ducts due to infections, such as biliary obstruction and biliary tract infestation (such as *Ascaris, Opisthorchis viverrini and Clinor chussinesis*).[31,32] The black pigmented (20%) stones are composed of bilirubin pigment mixed with calcium carbonate, phosphate, and cholesterol.

Bile is composed of bile salts, cholesterol, and phospholipids, which are present in major proportions and bile pigments are present in minor proportions. In addition to these compounds, lipids, proteins (such as albumin, insulin, haptaglobin, cholecyskinin, lysosomal hydrolase, and amylase) and elements (such as strontium, zinc, sodium, potassium, phosphorus, copper, calcium, manganese, iron, magnesium, molybdenum, and sodium) are also found in the bile. These proteins and elements bind to cholesterol and bile salts, and can affect the crystallization or precipitation of cholesterol in bile.[12] This disturbance in physiochemical balance of cholesterol solubility in bile results in cholelithiasis.[42]

13.2   MECHANISM OF GALLSTONE FORMATION

The cholelithiasis results from the disturbance in cholesterol metabolism. Cholesterol is virtually water insoluble and forms a micellar solution with bile acids, phospholipids by the action of bile acids.[28] Phospholipids and bile salts are key members that are responsible for the dissolution of cholesterol in bile.[12] It involves metabolic disturbance that causes an increase in the amount of cholesterol with respect to bile acids and phospholipids and form unsteady vesicles of cholesterol, which in turn join to form large multilayered vesicles leading to crystals of cholesterol precipitation.[28] Mainly three types of disturbances are considered to be responsible for cholelithiasis occurrence: The first disturbance includes the supersaturation of bile with cholesterol. It is the main and essential requirement for cholelithiasis and might be helped by two additional metabolic disturbances, such as reduction of the bile acid pool, and enhancement in the conversion of cholic acid to deoxycholic acid. Bile acid pool reduction is caused by snappy depletion of bile acid from the small intestinal tract into the colon. The enhancement in deoxycholic acid results due to the dehydroxylation of cholic acid and expanded absorption of recently made deoxycholic acid. The cholesterol hypersecretion is caused by the updated level of deoxycholate and hence causing the supersaturation of bile with cholesterol.

The second mechanism includes nucleation of cholesterol crystals. It may be due to either increase in pronucleating factors or lack of anti-nucleating factors. The pronucleating factors promote the cholesterol crystallization and antinucleating agents inhibit the cholesterol crystallization. The imbalance between these promoters and inhibitors stimulates the cholesterol crystallization in bile.[12,28,37,44] Mucin (pronucleating agent) and many other glycoproteins are known to act as a matrix to keep cholesterol crystals aggregated to form a stone. The glycoproteins (such as aminopeptidase N, immunoglobulins, alpha 1-acid glycoproteins, phospholipase C, haptoglobin, and fibronectin) promote the cholesterol crystallization. The calcium-binding proteins, albumin–lipid complexes and group II phospholipase A_2 are also promoters. The nonprotein components of bile (such as calcium and low-density particles of lipids) are also responsible for the crystallization of cholesterol. Antinucleating agents include apolipoproteins AI and AII and secretory immunoglobulin A and its heavy and light chains. These prolong and inhibit cholesterol nucleation.

The third mechanism includes in cholelithiasis is gallbladder hypomotility. The hypomotility cause delay in gallbladder emptying and lead to an increase in bile storage time. Good motility leads to complete emptying of supersaturated bile and stone would not grow further.[12,28,37,44]

13.3 FACTORS AFFECTING GALLSTONE FORMATION

The formation of gallstone is a complex and multifactor influenced process. There are number of factors, which are responsible for the gallstone formation and include both biological and acquired factors as follows:

- **Biological risk factors:** Gender,[13,14] age,[13] genetic factor.[1,37]
- **Acquired risk factors:** Body mass index,[24,30] rapid weight loss,[9,13,31,37] diet,[6,9,13,24,30,31,33,34,36,37,41] pregnancy,[38,39] drugs,[31] and intestinal motility.[12]

These factors affect the metabolic process and create a disturbance, which leads to the supersaturation of bile with cholesterol, promote nucleation, gallbladder motility, and finally leads to the formation of a gallstone.

13.4 COMPLEMENTARY AND ALTERNATIVE MEDICINE IN CHOLELITHIASIS

Ursodeoxycholic acid and chenodeoxycholic acid, extracorporeal shock wave lithotripsy (ESWL), contact dissolution therapy (injection of methyl tertiary-butyl ether (MTBE) into the gallbladder to break down the gallstones), percutaneous cholecystectomy are successful nonsurgical treatments. Clearly, there is a critical need of assistance from alternative treatment to counter these troubles.[4,5,10,11,15,20,21,35]

According to the National Centre for Complementary and Integrative Health (NCCIH), "Complementary medicines are used along with the conventional medicine and Alternative medicines are used in place of conventional medicine." CAM is expansively characterized as framework of drug that falls outside of standard consideration. In this definition, both complementary and alternative medicines are utilized conversely.[17]

The limits among CAM and conventional medication are not supreme, and CAM rehearses may become broadly acknowledged. To confound the matter further, certain treatments that are considered as CAM in the West are piece of regular drug in the East. For instance, needle therapy (acupuncture) and Chinese homegrown medication are conventional medicinal frameworks in China. The National Centre for CAM has classified CAM therapies into five major categories[26]:

- Alternative medical systems, such as traditional Chinese medicine or Ayurveda.
- Biologically based therapies (Herbs, dietary supplement, and vitamins).
- Energy therapies (bioelectromagnetic-based therapies, such as magnetic fields).
- Manipulation and body-based methods (massage, chiropractic, and osteopathy).
- Mind–body interventions, such as meditation and prayer

13.5 ROLE OF HERBS IN MANAGEMENT OF GALLSTONES

Phytomedicines play a vital part in the avoidance and treatment of several diseases as they are a rich source of naturally active constituents. These active constituents strengthen and tone up the systems of the body and also help to treat and manage diseases. The herbal constituents can be used as tinctures (alcoholic extracts), galenicals, glycerites (glycerine extracts) or as dried extracts (in the form of powder, capsules, or tablets). There are many herbs that are used to manage the gallstone conditions, some of which are listed in Table 13.1. Some important bioactive compounds from medicinal plants acting against gallstones are:

- Afzelin
- Ascorbic acid
- Campesterol
- Carvone
- Coumaric acid
- Ferulic acid
- Gallic acid
- Limonene
- Linoleic acid
- Protocatechuic acid
- Syingic acid

13.6 ACUPUNCTURE

This therapy might be particularly useful to relieve from discomfort, lessening fit, facilitating bile stream, and restoring proper liver and gallbladder functions. Needle therapy (acupuncture) encourages the removal of gallstones in 70% of patients. Stagnation of liver-Qi is treated with needle therapy at the GB-34 and LIV-14. Moist warmth in gallbladder and liver is treated by needle therapy at focuses SP-9, GB-34, GB-24, and GV-9.

In the hamster model of cholelithiasis, needle therapy at GB-34, GB-24, and LIV-14 decreased the development of cholelithiasis, diminished the biliary and plasma cholesterol, and altogether expanded the degrees of cholic acid in bile. Synergistic effect of decreased biliary cholesterol and expanded cholic acid in bile would lower the lithogenicity. These outcomes recommend that needle therapy beneficially affects the bile organization.

TABLE 13.1 Herbal Medicines in the Treatment of Gallstones.[2,3,8,14,16,18,20,22,23,25,29,43]

Botanical name	Common name	Parts used	Bioactive constituent
Apium graveolens (Apiaceae)	Celery	Seeds	Limonene, caryophyllene, linalool, isovalaric acid, carvone, and vitamin B
Bauhinia cumanensis (Fabaceae)	Crown vine, Wreath vine	Stem	Nonadecyl, p-coumarate, Arachidyl p-coumarate, Heneicosyl p-coumarate, 1,2-benzopyrone, and p-Coumaric acid
Capraria biflora (Scrophulariaceae)	Goat weed, Stow weed	Leaves, stem, roots	β-sitosterol, naphthoquinone biflorin, myopochlorin, and caprarioside
Chamaesyce hirta (Euphorbiaceae)	Asthma plant, Cat's hair	Leaves, stem, flower	Afzelin, quercitrin, myricitrin, rutin, and gallic acid
Cissus verticillata (Vitaceae)	Princess vine	Leaves, stem	Coumarins, flavonoids, anthocyanins, steroids, and tannins
Cocos nucifera (Arecacae)	Coconut	Shell fiber, root, solid albumen, coconut water, leaves	Vitamin C, lauric acid, L-arginine, catechin, skinmiwallin, and saponin
Eleusine indica (Poaceae)	Indian crowfoot grass, Goose grass	Whole plant	Cyan genetic glycoside, albuminoids, starch, fatty oils, and flavonoids
Ficus carica (Moraceae)	Anjeer, Fig	Fruits, root, leaves	Ferulic acid, psoralen, bergapten, fumaric acid, bauerenol, and methyl maslinate
Gomphrena globosa (Amaranthaceae)	Globe amaranth, Makhmali	Stem, leaves, flowers	Kaempferol-3-o-rutinoside, campesterol, betanin, gomphrenin, amaranthin, and bougainvillein
Kalanchoe pinnata	Air plant, Cathedral bells, Miracle leaf, life plant	Leaves	Bufadienolides, syringic acid, caffeic acid, bryophollenone, bryophollone, and palmitic acid
Portulaca oleracea (Portulacaceae)	Purslane	Leaves, stem, seeds	Kaempferol, apigenin, thymine, uracil, portulene, lupeol, linoleic acid, and stearic acid
Solanum melongena (Solanaceae)	Eggplant	Fruits, leaves, seeds, root	Arginine, aspartic acid, histidine, chlorogenic, hydro-caffeic, protocatechuric acids, tropane, and pyrrolidine

13.7   PHYSICAL ACTIVITY

Physical movement may play a significant role in the treatment of cholelithiasis. The danger of gallstone development is fundamentally expanded in individuals with an inactive way of life. Reduction in muscle mass is related to tocholelithiasis in humans. A little time for exercise per week diminished the danger of cholelithiasis in ladies by 20%. It might be due to the digestion of glucose that is affected by regular physical exertion. Insulin level in plasma during fasting is fundamentally diminished after an activity program. In individuals other than diabetics, plasma levels of insulin during an oral glucose resilience test are lower in persons with the most noteworthy physical movement.[19,40]

13.8   FUTURE PROSPECTS

In any event, four imperfections must happen for nucleation and crystallization of cholesterol monohydrate stones in bile. These are un-physiological supersaturation with cholesterol, quickened cholesterol nucleation/crystallization, gallbladder hypomotility, and expanded measures of cholesterol from the digestive tract. Development of stones to shape into gallstones is a result of both gallbladder mucin hypersecretion and gel arrangement with deficient clearing by the gallbladder. Proof for varieties in frequency rates of gallstones among topographically and ethnic populations just as family and twin investigations emphatically bolster hereditary helplessness to the development of cholesterol gallstones. In future, CAM therapy is becoming an alternate choice to treat and manage the gallstones. This therapy works on the root cause of gallstone formation and stimulates the inhibiting factors to stop gallstone formation. Hence, it avoids any unwanted side effects in the body. It is also an alternate for the surgical treatment for gallstone.

13.9   SUMMARY

Literature survey reveals that there are lot of surgical and nonsurgical treatments available for the cholelithiasis management, but none of them is precise and satisfactory treatment. Therefore, CAM is an alternative as it includes the traditional Chinese system and Ayurveda, and use of herbs to treat the cholelithiasis.

KEYWORDS

- cholecystectomy
- gallstones
- herbal treatment
- phytomedicine
- ursodeoxycholic acid

REFERENCES

1. Acalovschi, M. Cholesterol Gallstones: from Epidemiology to Prevention. *Postgrad. Med. J.* **2001,** *77* (906), 221–229.
2. Al-Snafi, A. E. Pharmacology and Therapeutic Potential of *Euphorbia hirta* (Syn: *Euphorbia pilulifera*)—A Review. *IOSR J. Pharm.* **2017,** *7* (3), 7–20.
3. Allen, M. J.; Borody, T. J.; Thistle, J. L. *In Vitro* Dissolution of Cholesterol Gallstones. *Gastroenterology* **1985,** *89* (5), 1097–1103.
4. Bari, O. D.; Wang, T. Y.; Liu, M.; Paik, C. N.; Porticasa, P. Cholesterol Cholelithiasis in Pregnant Women: Pathogenesis, Prevention and Treatment. *Ann. Hepatol.* **2014,** *13* (6), 728–745.
5. Beserra, F. P.; Santos, R. C.; Perico, L. L. *Cissus sicyoides*: Pharmacological Mechanisms Involved in the Anti-Inflammatory and Anti-diarrheal Activities. *Int. J. Mol. Sci.* **2016,** *17* (2), 149–153.
6. Brauwald, E.; Fauci, A. S.; Kasper, D. L. *Harrison's Principles of Internal Medicine*, 15th ed.; McGraw Hill: New York, 2001; p 1707.
7. Brewer, N. D. The Role of Complementary and Alternative Medicine for the Management of Fibroids and Associated Symptomatology. *Curr. Obstetr. Gynecol. Rep.* **2016,** *5* (2), 110–118.
8. Campos, R.; Lima, C. P.; Duarte, A. F. S. Coumaric Derivates Identified from the Extract of the Stems of *Bauhinia glabra*. *Latin Am. J. Pharm.* **2016,** *35* (4), 712–715.
9. Chandana, E.; Kumar, P. Review on Different Pharmacological Activities of *Gomphrena globosa* L. *World J. Pharm. Pharma. Sci.* **2018,** *7* (8), 386–394.
10. Choong, M. K.; Phillips, G. W. L. Gallstone Dissolution by Methyl-Tert-Butyl Ether (MTBE) via Percutaneous Transhepatic Cholecystostomy. *Aust. Radiol.* **1990,** *34* (4), 339–342.
11. Ciaula, A. D.; Portincasa, P. Recent Advances in Understanding and Managing Cholesterol Gallstone. *F1000-Research,* **2018,** *2018,* 7-11.
12. Ciaula, A. D.; Wang, D. Q. H. Targets for Current Pharmacologic Therapy in Cholesterol Gallstone Disease. *Gastroenterol. Clin.* **2010,** *39* (2), 245–264.
13. Cuevas, A.; Miquel, J. F.; Reyes, M. S. Diet as a Risk Factor for Cholesterol Gallstone Disease. *J. Am. Coll. Nutr.* **2004,** *23* (3), 187–196.

14. Dayan, Y. B.; Vilkin, A.; Niv, Y. Gallbladder Mucin Plays a Role in Gallstone Formation. *Eur. J. Intern. Med.* **2004,** *15* (7), 411–414.

15. Desai, A. V.; Patil, V. M. Phytochemical Investigation of *Eleusine indica* for *in-vivo* Anti-Hypertensive Activity. *Int. J. Innov. Sci. Res. Technol,* **2017,** *2* (6), 405–416.

16. Eidsvoll, B. E.; Aadland, E.; Stiris, M.; Lunde, O. C. Dissolution of Cholesterol Gallbladder Stones with Methyl Tert-Butyl Ether in Patients with Increased Surgical Risk. *Scandavian J. Gastroenterol.* **1993,** *28* (8), 744–748.

17. Fazal, S. S.; Singla, R. K. Review on the Pharmacognostical and Pharmacological Characterization of *Apium Graveolens* Linn. *Indo Global J. Pharma. Sci.* **2012,** *2* (1), 36–42.

18. Fromm, H. Gallstone Dissolution Therapy. *Gastroenterology* **1986,** *91* (6), 560–567.

19. Gaby, A. R. Nutritional Approaches to Prevention and Treatment of Gallstones. *Altern. Med. Rev.* **2009,** *14* (3), 258–267.

20. Hayes, K. C.; Livingston, A. Dietary Impact on Biliary Lipids and Gallstones. *Annu. Rev. Nutr.* **1992,** *12* (1), 299–326.

21. https://en.wikipedia.org/wiki/Calculus_(medicine); Accessed on 07 August, 2020. 6.

22. Kaur, K.; Singh, B.; Kaur, G. Complementary and Alternative Medicine Usage in Patients for Different Ailments in Rural Region of Malwa Area of Punjab: A Cross-Sectional Study. *Natl. J. Physiol. Pharm. Pharmacol.* **2016,** *6* (5), 394–398.

23. Lemus, C.; Grougnet, R.; Ellong, E. N. Phytochemical Study of *Capraria biflora* L. Aerial Parts from Martinique Island (French West Indies). *Phytochem. Lett.,* **2015,** *13*, 194–199.

24. Lima, E. B. C.; Sousa, C. N. S.; Meneses, L. N. *Cocos nucifera*: Phytochemical and Pharmacological Review. *Braz. J. Med. Biol. Res.* **2015,** *48* (11), 953–964.

25. Mava, S.; Husain, K.; Jantan, I. *Ficus carica*: Phytochemistry, Traditional Uses and Biological Activities. *Complemen. Altern. Med.* **2013,** *2013*, Article ID 974256; 8 p.

26. Moga, M. M. Alternative Treatment of Gallbladder Disease. *Med. Hypotheses* **2003,** *60* (1), 143–147.

27. Pattewar, S. V. *Kalanchoe pinnata*: Phytochemical and Pharmacological Profile. *Int. J. Phytopharm.* **2012,** *2* (1), 1–8.

28. Raj, A.; MP, G.; Joshi, H.; Shastry, C. S. *Kalanchoe pinnatum* in Treatment of Gallstones: Ethnopharmacological Review. *Int. J. Pharm Tech Res.* **2014,** *6* (1), 252–261.

29. Reshetnyak, V. I. Concept of the Pathogenesis and Treatment of Cholelithiasis. *World J. Hepatol.* **2012,** *4* (2), 18–34.

30. Saleh, G. S. Chemical Detection of some Active Compounds in Egg Plant (*Solanum melongena*) Callus as Compared with Fruit and Root Contents. *Int. J. Curr. Microbiol. Appl. Sci.* **2015,** *4* (5), 160–165.

31. Sanchez, N. M.; Chaves-Tapia, N. C. Pregnancy and Gallbladder Disease. *Ann. Hepatol.* **2006,** *5* (3), 227–230.

32. Sanchez, N. M.; Valdes, D. Z. Role of Diet in Cholesterol Gallstone Formation. *Clin. Chim. Acta* **2007,** *376* (1–2), 1–8.

33. Shaffer, E. A. Epidemiology of Gallbladder Stone Disease. *Best Pract. Clin. Res. Clin. Gastroenterol.* **2006,** *20* (6), 981–996.

34. Shankar, A. Cholelithiasis and Ayurveda. *Int. J. Complemen. Altern, Med.* **2017,** *7* (5), 239–245.

35. Sharma, R. K.; Shah, H. S.; Gohel, J. K. Non Surgical Management of Cholelithiasis: A Case Study. *Asian J. Pharma. Res. Dev.* **2019,** *7* (1), 34–37.

36. Stinton, L. M.; Shaffer, E. A. Epidemiology of Gallbladder Disease: Cholelithiasis and Cancer. *Gut Liver* **2012,** *6* (2), 172–187.

37. Stokes, C. S.; Krawczyk, M.; Lammert, F. Gallstones: Environment, Lifestyle and Genes. *Digest. Dis.* **2011,** *29* (2), 191–201.

38. Thistle, J. L.; May, G. R.; Bender, C. E. Dissolution of Cholesterol Gallbladder Stone Methyl Tert-Butyl Ether Administered by Percutaneuos Transhepatic Catheter. *New Engl. J. Med.* **1989,** *320* (10), 633–639.

39. Tseng, M.; Everhart, J. E.; Sandler, R. S. Dietary Intake and Gallbladder Disease: A Review. *Public Health Nutrition,* **1999,** 2 (2), 161-172.

40. Wang, H. H.; Portincasa, P.; Bari, O. D. Prevention of Cholesterol Gallstones by Inhibiting Hepatic Biosynthesis and Intestinal Absorption of Cholesterol. *Eur. J. Clin. Invest.* **2013,** *43* (4), 413–426.

41. Wang, H. H.; Portincasa, P. Effect of Ezetimibe on the Prevention and Dissolution of Cholesterol Gallstones. *Gastroenterology* **2008,** *134* (7), 2101–2110.

42. Wang, H. H.; Portincasa, P. Molecular Pathophysiology and Physical Chemistry of Cholesterol Gallstones. *Front. Biosci.* **2008,** *13* (4), 401–423.

43. Yoo, E. H.; Lee, S. Y. The Prevalence and Risk Factors for Gallstone Disease. *Clin. Chem. Lab. Med.* **2009,** *47* (7), 795–807.

44. Zhou, Y. X.; Xin, H. L.; Rahman, K. *Portulaca oleracea*: Review of Phytochemistry and Pharmacological Effects. *BioMed Res. Int.,* **2015,** *2015,* Article ID 925631; p 11.

CHAPTER 14

Potential of Pseudocereals in Celiac Disease

CATERINA ANANIA and FRANCESCA OLIVERO

ABSTRACT

Although gluten-free diet (GFD) is currently the efficacious therapy for celiac disease (CD), yet GFD has been shown to be responsible: for deficiencies in macro- and micronutrients. Pseudocereals are naturally gluten-free crops, which may be healthier alternative for GFD. The authors of this chapter have described the nutritional characteristics of pseudocereals and their use in the treatment of CD. The aim of this chapter is to highlight the properties of GFD to support its use as a potential healthier strategy in CD management.

14.1 INTRODUCTION

Attentive gluten-free diet (GFD) adherence results in the normalization of serological markers, complete clinical and histological relief and it prevents long-term complications in patientswith CD.[20,28] However, available gluten-free products are of low quality and poor nutritional value. For example, some articles have shown that GFD may result in macro- and micronutrient deficiencies. Specifically, the dietary intake of patients following GFD is characterized by the low amount of fiber, vitamin B, folate, vitamin D, calcium, iron, zinc, and magnesium.[5,61,64]

Also, gluten-free products (GFD) contain high amounts of lipids, sugar, and salt to enhance food taste and consistency.[3,42] As a result, CD subjects often reveal an exaggerated utilization of hypercaloric and hyperlipidic foods to balance for the limitations that result from a typical GFD. Therefore, GFD may have a negative effect on cardiometabolic factors (obesity, serum lipid levels, insulin resistance, metabolic syndrome, etc.), and atherosclerosis. The ideal GFD diet should contain both macro and micronutrients to a high degree, be affordable, and readily available and obviously gluten-free.

The pseudocereals (quinoa, amaranth, buckwheat, etc.) are naturally gluten-free and provide a wide range of nutrients, in addition to being an excellent source of vitamins and minerals.

The focus of this chapter is on: (1) the nutritional characteristics of gluten-free pseudocereals and (2) their use in the prevention of cardio-metabolic risk factors and nutritional deficiencies in celiac patients.

14.2   PSEUDOCEREALS

The pseudocereals refer to non-grass species of dicotyledonous plants that are cultivated for their starchy grains for human consumption. They have been significant contributors to the diet of Latin American habitants and could be developed again as important new crops in other areas. These have shown a strong tolerance to various stress factors (such as water shortage and heat) and as a result, these represent an alternative crop source to meet the increasing food demand in the world.[2] Recently, pseudocereals have received particular attention due to their nutritional characteristics, such as being rich in important nutrients, including proteins, carbohydrates, lipids (especially unsaturated fatty acids), fiber, vitamins, minerals, and phytochemicals.[38,51]

It should also be noted that pseudocereals are naturally gluten-free and represent a healthy alternative to grain products for improving the nutrition quality of GFD. Collectively, these positive features make pseudocereals of particular interest and justify the title, "cereals of the 21st century".[35] There are number of diverse pseudocereals available, and at present, the most widely known and used are quinoa, amaranth, and buckwheat. Table 14.1 depicts the nutritional properties of quinoa, amaranth, and buckwheat.

14.2.1   Quinoa

Quinoa plant (*Chenopodium quinoa*) is a pseudocereal. They are principally cultivated in Bolivia, Ecuador, Peru, Argentina, Chile, and Colombia. Though in recent years, they have also been introduced into Europe, North America, and Africa.[1] Quinoa is capable of producing grains even at altitudes of 4500 m above m.s.l. (mean sea level) and has a higher nutritional value than the traditional cereals.[65] The comparison between the nutritional properties of quinoa to common grains (rice, wheat, rye, barley, corn, and sorghum) clearly shows the superiority of quinoa with respect to its protein, lipid, micronutrient, and fiber content.[66] Because of high nutritional value, this quinoa has been given the name "golden grain" by various ancient populations.[30]

TABLE 14.1 Chemical Composition of Pseudocereals Seeds and their Comparison with Wheat.

Chemical	Quinoa	Amaranth	Buckwheat	Wheat
		g/100 g edible material		
Carbohydrate	69[*]	70.3[@]	67–70[**]	63.7[@]
Fat	5.5–7.4[*]	5.7 (5.7–10.9)	2.1[@]	1.7[@]
Fiber	7.0–9.7[***]	7.1–16.4[@]	27.4[@]	12.2[@]
Protein	15[*]	16.5[@]	11.7[@]	12[@]
Starch	52–69[***]	48–69[@]	29.5[@]	–

Notes: [*]Koziol 1992[36]; [**]Steadman 2001[59]; [***]Abugoch 2009[1]; [@]Alvarez-Joubete 2010[2].

The average protein content of quinoa seeds (expressed as g/100 g edible matter) is 15%.[36] The major quinoa storage proteins are composed of albumin (35%) and globulins (37%), which are in higher concentrations than the normal values in major cereals,[66] and prolamins are present in low concentrations[1] rendering the plant useful in GFD. Nutrition quality is also very high in quinoa as a result of its proportion of essential amino acids, all of which are contained in values which closely approximate those suggested by the Food and Agriculture Organization (FAO).

Essential amino acids in quinoa include high content of lysine (2.4–7.8/100 g protein), methionine (0.3–9.1/100 g protein), and threonine (2.1–8.9/100 g protein), which represent the limiting amino acids in traditional cereals, such as, wheat and maize.[13,14] It should also be noted that the protein bioavailability of amino acids in quinoa differs consistently with the type and treatment of the grain and increases significantly as a result of cooking.[36]

In terms of carbohydrate content, quinoa is analogous to wheat and rice. The main carbohydrate component of quinoa is starch constituting 52%–69% of the dry matter[1] of which, 11% is amylose.[55] Similarly, the total dietary fiber in quinoa is comparable to that in wheat (7–9.7 g/100). The content of soluble fiber, on the other hand, ranges from 1.3 to 6.1/100 g.[1] The simple sugar content of quinoa seeds is approximately 3% consisting primarily of D-galactose and D-ribose, and an elevated percentage of D-xylose and maltose and a low percentage of fructose and glucose.[1]

The overall content of maltose, D-galactose, and D-ribose would result in low glycemic index (GI). The fat content in quinoa seeds ranges from 1.8% to 9.5%,[36] which is higher than wheat (1.7%), corn (4.7%), and rice (0.7%), but lower than that of soybeans (19.0%).[46] However, poly-unsaturated fatty acids are found plentifully in quinoa seeds, and among these, linoleic acid is the primary contributor (49.0–54.6%), followed by oleic acid (24.5–26.7%) and palmitic acid (11%).[46] Also, quinoa contains large amount of vitamins and minerals, including folic acid, pyridoxine (B6), riboflavin (B2), and vitamin E, and quinoa is notably superior to wheat, barley, rice, and corn.[66]

Moreover, the levels of pyridoxine and folic acid in 100 g of quinoa have been shown to meet the adult daily requirement, whereas 80% of childhood and 40% of adult requirements for riboflavin are further provided.[1] Quinoa contains a considerable amount of vitamin C, which ranges from 4.0 to 16.4 mg/100 g of dry matter.[66] The vitamin E content of quinoa (8.7 mg/100) is excellent and acts as an antioxidant in protecting the cell membranes against damage resulting from free radicals.[1,55] On the other hand, thiamine (B1) content in quinoa is less than that of oats or barley.[46]

Quinoa also has large mineral content. Calcium (87 mg/100 g dry matter) and iron (9.47 mg/100 g dry matter) are reported to be higher than that found in common grain.[49] Furthermore, quinoa contains 0.26% magnesium, which is higher against wheat (0.16%) and corn (0.14%).[46] The mineral content in quinoa is adequate for a well-balanced diet as a consequence of its bioavailable form.[35,46,55,65] Quinoa contains high amount of bioactive compounds (such as flavonoids), which have demonstrated positive health effects. The flavonoid content in quinoa is about 58/100 g compared with many common cereals. The most important of these are flavonols, quercetin, and kaempferol.[49] With their antioxidant properties, quinoa biocomponents have been reported to exert inhibitory activity on glucosidase and pancreatic lipase.[60]

The antinutritional substances in quinoa include saponins, phytic acid, and protease inhibitors[21,29] in significant amounts. Saponins are toxic substances, which interfere with palatability and digestibility resulting in the need for their removal before seed consumption[23]. Nevertheless, they do also contain a variety of important biological properties, such as anti-inflammatory, diuretic, antithrombotic, hypoglycemic, hypocholesterolemic, anticarcinogenic, fungicidal, and antiviral properties.[23] The protease inhibitor contents in quinoa, which are known to bind in very stable complexes involving proteolytic enzymes, are lower than that in common grains. Phytic acid content of quinoa ranges from 10.5 to 13.5 mg/g.[36]

Phytic acid is important in binding minerals resulting in their unavailability for metabolism.[6,33] Therefore, few clinical studies have been conducted to explore the overall repercussions on the quinoa consumption on human health. A childhood nutrition study was carried out on 50–65 months-old children from low-income families in Ecuador. The findings showed that the 100 g utilization of quinoa supplemented to infant food products twice a day for 15 days considerably enhanced plasma insulin-like growth factor-1 levels in children in comparison to the control group. This study demonstrated that adequate levels of protein and other necessary nutritional factors were provided by quinoa, all of which having a fundamental function in preventing malnourishment in infants.[56]

Zevallos et al.[70] evaluated the diet, serology, and gastroenterology parameters in 19 celiac patients following a 6-week consumption of 50 g of quinoa daily for 6 weeks as constituent of their usual GFD and they noted an improvement in gastrointestinal parameters as well as a small decrease in the levels of total cholesterol, low-density cholesterol (LDL), high-density cholesterol (HDL), and triglyceride levels. Further studies have demonstrated that a diet containing quinoa helps to prevent cardiovascular disease in healthy subjects[19] and also modulates metabolic parameters in postmenopausal overweight women.[12]

14.2.2 Amaranth

The genus *Amaranthus* belongs to the *Amaranthaceae* family which consists of over 60 species of which *Amaranthus hypochondriacus, A. cruentus*, and *A. caudatus* are essential grain species.[31] The cultivation of amaranth as a food crop began in ancient Mayan civilization. Throughout Central and South America, and in some parts of Africa and Asia, the amaranth plant has been cultivated as a minor crop for centuries. These crops are relatively fast-growing and are well-regarded for their resistance to hostile conditions resulting from moisture or low temperatures.[35]

The nutritional value of amaranth grains primarily results from the protein and lipid contents, which are of very high quality. Amaranth protein content ranges from 14.5% to 16%, which is superior to that found in conventional cereals.[2] Due to its amino acid balance, the unique protein characteristics of amaranth have been shown to closely approximate the optimal balance suggested for human nutrition.[15] As with quinoa and buckwheat, amaranth protein is primarily composed of globulins and albumins with very few or no prolamin storage proteins. Prolamin storage proteins act as the principal proteins found in common cereals as well as the toxic proteins involved in CD.[16]

It has been shown that globulins and albumins have lower level of glutamic acid and proline than prolamins along with a greater number of essential amino acids, including arginine, tryptophan, and lysine. Indeed, lysine content in amaranth is considerably high[22] in comparison to conventional cereals, and as an added advantage can supplement those amino acids found in other cereals including wheat.[17]

It has also been demonstrated in several studies that protein bioavailability in amaranth is of a high level and is significantly greater than that found in common cereals.[2] In both amaranth, lipid content is between 2 and 3 times higher than that found in wheat.[2] Fat content in amaranth rangrs from 5.7% to 10.9%[56] and contains a high level of unsaturated fatty acids (75%–77.1%). Of these, the most common fatty acids are linoleic acid (50% of total), oleic acid (25%), and palmitic acid (20%).[2] In addition, amaranth is an excellent source of 6% squalene, which is significantly higher than that commonly found in oils from other cereal grains.[2] Squalene is a terpenoid compound, which is common in the unsaponifiable elements of cereal grains often used in the cosmetic industry and in skincare products. As a food constituent, squalene is important as a result of its cholesterol-lowering abilities that result from the inhibition of cholesterol synthesis in the liver.[18]

Amaranth is also rich in starch and is an excellent source of fiber, vitamins (A, K, B2, B6, C, E, etc.) and minerals (such as calcium, iron, magnesium, and zinc).[2] It has also been shown that the levels of phosphorus, calcium, potassium, and magnesium found in amaranth are in the majority of cases superior to those found in conventional cereals.[36] Amaranth also contains a high level of riboflavin (vitamin B2) and vitamin C than the common cereals, and is an excellent source of vitamin E (5.7 mg/100 g dry weight basis)[11] leading to its antioxidant properties. Moreover, it has been shown that amaranth contains a high concentration of folic acid (102 µg/100 g) compared 40 µg/100 g in wheat. It is an excellent source of dietary fiber depending on the plant species and variety and geographical location.[44]

14.2.3 Buckwheat

Buckwheat belongs to a group of pseudocereals originally found in southwest China and is part of the *Polygonaceae* family. Buckwheat has been cultivated in Europe since the start of the 15th century. Of all the diverse species, those with agricultural importance are common buckwheat (*Fagopyrum esculentum* Moench) and tartary buckwheat (*Fagopyrum tataricum* Gaertn). The latter is cultivated in certain mountainous regions while common buckwheat is widely grown in temperate regions of Europe and Japan.[71] In the last few years, there has been a renewal of interest in the utilization of buckwheat as a food source due to "rediscovery" of its numerous nutritional and health benefits.[39] The same can be said for the fact that buckwheat has been shown to be a candidate for natural, organic production.

The protein content of buckwheat ranges from 7% to 21%, which is highest among all cereals. Buckwheat is of high nutritional and is a well-known dietary source of vitamins, starch, dietary fiber, essential minerals, and trace elements[8,9,57] and source of protein with a beneficial amino acid constitution. Buckwheat has a high content of lysine, which is considered the first limiting amino acid in similar plant proteins, and arginine, histidine, and methionine are other amino acids present in it. Furthermore, the glutamine and prolamine content is considerably less than that found in wheat,[4] which is relevant in terms of their use of this pseudocereal in GFD.

The total lipid content in buckwheat varies from 1.2% to 4.3%. Among these, linoleic acids, oleic acid, and palmitic acid account for 8.8% of the total fatty acids.[59] Total carbohydrate content ranges from 67% to 70%.[58] The vitamin content of buckwheat is comparable to other grains; however, buckwheat contains high levels of niacin (B6) and vitamin K. Buckwheat also contains more nutritionally significant minerals (excluding calcium) than many conventional cereals, being an excellent source of zinc, copper, manganese, magnesium, and selenium.[59] Tartary and common buckwheat both contain similar amount of total dietary fiber (29.5%), which is considerably higher than amaranth and quinoa[2] and common cereals.

As a result of its high fiber content, buckwheat may have a significant role in the prevention and treatment of hypertension and hypercholesterolemia.[27] Due to high level of flavonoids in buckwheat,[72] it has antioxidant activity in comparison to other cereal crops. Tartary buckwheat has also been found to contain even higher flavonoid content than common buckwheat due to chemical constitution. Buckwheat certainly has enormous potential for human health benefits, such as: antioxidation, anti-inflammation, antidiabetic, cholesterol-lowering, antihypertension, and anticancer properties.

Buckwheat also contains high amount of rutin (quercetin-3-rutinoside) and other polyphenols.[41] As a result of their antioxidative properties, rutin, quercetin, and certain other polyphenols in buckwheat may be considered as potent anticarcinogens in the colon and other organs. In addition to this, phenolic compounds may be involved in lowering blood sugar and blood lipid levels as well as contributing to the hypocholesterolemic effect.[62] As a direct result of contributing factors (such as gluten-free content, excellent nutritional value, and therapeutic features), buckwheat has a strong case for representing a valid alternative crop within a gluten-free formulation for celiac patients.

14.3   CELIAC DISEASE

CD is an autoimmune, systemic condition that results from the consumption of gluten and related prolamins in persons who are genetically predisposed. The presence of different clinical signs and symptoms, specific serum autoimmune antibodies, human lymphocyte antigen (HLA) -DQ2 and-DQ8 haplotypes, and slight intestinal enteropathy are typical of this disease.[20,28] Evidence suggests that the prevalence of CD has been increasing in the last few decades.[40] About 1% of the Western population is affected by CD with few regional differences. In Europe, for instance, the prevalence ranges from 0.3% in Germany to 2.4% in Finland[45], in spite of this, regions presenting a similar intake of gluten and frequency of HLA-DQ2 and -DQ8. In recent years, CD has also been found to be increasingly common in developing nations with greatest prevalence in northwestern India.[20,54]

CD is found in subjects with a genetic predisposition and results from environmental components. The presence of HLA-DQ2 and -DQ8 constitute a necessary but not a sufficient explanation for the occurrence of the disorders, and the development of the disease requires gluten ingestion as a further necessary factor. The toxic fractions of gluten are gliadins, which contain large amount of proline and glutamine and are incompletely digested. Certain gliadin peptides manage to cross the intestinal barrier and thereby make their way into the lamina propria of the small intestine via tight junctions of transcellular and paracellular routes.

Glutamine and proline deamidation occurs in the lamina propria through type 2 transglutaminase (TG2). This deamidation increases the affinity for the HLA-DQ2 and -DQ8 on the antigen-presenting cells (APCs).[37] Following these gliadin peptides, attached to DQ2 or DQ8 are submitted to the CD4+T cells, thereby activating an inflammatory response with the release of cytokines. The result of this process is an inflammatory condition of the small intestine leading to mucosal damage disrupting the structure of the mucosa, which results in lymphocytic infiltration into the epithelium plus an increased depth and density to the colon crypts.[24]

14.4   GLUTEN-FREE DIET

GFD consist of a combination of foods, which are naturally lacking in gluten, such as rice, maize, and potatoes along with industrially processed foods with a gluten content <20 ppm. Given the ubiquitous presence of gluten, social limitation and the cross-contamination of foods, it is not always easy to rigidly adhere to the GFD. Compliance with GFD has been shown to be challenging for patients with a negative effect on the quality of life, and further studies have shown similar results in terms of making appropriate nutritional choices.

Even if CD patients manage to strictly follow a GFD, several studies have shown that GFD can be responsible for imbalances and deficiencies in terms of nutrition. As we have seen, the most relevant problems concerning GFD are nutritional deficits and excesses resulting from this diet.

14.4.1   Gluten-Free Diet vs Nutrient Deficiencies

Commercially available gluten-free (GF) are foods, which have been purified of gluten. Gluten removal has a negative influence on nutritional value through the modification of macro and micronutrients, which is an unavoidable result of the elimination process. In recent decades, the nutritional profile of gluten-free food products has been increasingly questioned within the scientific community. Certain available reports have shown that GFD may result in macro and micronutrient deficiencies; For example, it has been shown that low levels of magnesium, zinc, iron, calcium, vitamin D, folate, and vitamin B are typical of patients following GFD.[5,64]

Hallert et al.[25] reported that over 50% of adult subjects with CD adhering to a strict GFD for 10 years had low levels of vitamin B6, B12, and folate. Furthermore, the authors reported an high plasma homocysteine level in CD subjects, which could imply an independent increased risk of cardio-vascular disease (hypertension, hyperlipidemia). However, these authors, in a double-blind placebo-controlled multicenter trial, demonstrated that plasma homocysteine levels returned to normal in CD patients on GFD after they were supplemented for 6 months with folic acid, B12, and pyri-doxine.[26] Also, Martin et al.[43] provided an analysis of the dietary habits of 88 CD patients adhering to GFD in Germany and discovered a suboptimal intake of vitamins B1, B2, B6, and folic acid.[43]

Similarly, Thompson [63] observed that merely 35 out of 368 gluten-free pastas, breads, flours, and cereals were fortified with thiamine, riboflavin, and/or niacin. In an analogous study in 2005, Thompson et al.[64] found that among the 58 gluten-free breads, pastas, and cold cereals, the total enriched with folic acid amounted to only three and not one of the breads or pastas were fortified at all. Two European studies have documented a reduced intake of vitamin D[34,50] among celiac patients. Finally, some studies have also shown that GFD is related to a lower intake of dietary fiber in comparison to a standard, gluten-containing diet.[64,68] It has been suggested that this problem is due to the flour refining process, which removes the outer layer of grain containing most of the fiber.

14.4.2   Impact of Gluten-Free Diet on Cardiometabolic Risk Factors

GFD could also have highly significant reverberations including obesity, which has also been added to the list of possible nutritional reverberations resulting from GFD. This has been in part linked to the hypercaloric content of available commercial gluten-free foods and also clinical evidence indicated a higher caloric intake along with superior consumption of fats, saturated fats, simple carbohydrates, and food with an elevated glycemic index[32,42] in these types of diets.

Gluten-free products contain high amounts of lipids, sugar, and salt to render the available foods more palatable and consistent for CD patients. GFD, may therefore, have negative influence on specific cardiometabolic risk factors, such as obesity, serum lipid concentrations, insulin resistance, metabolic syndrome, and atherosclerosis. Nevertheless, it remains under discussion as to whether the cardiovascular risk profile is influenced by GFD in patients with CD. Indeed, researches have indicated that GFD in adults has a positive influence on cardiovascular profiles as a result of its antiatherosclerotic influence[10,69]; while others have actually demonstrated atherogenic consequences resulting from GFD.[48,67]

In case of children, there are very few studies available on GFD. Long-term dietary guidance, which targets obesity and other factors of metabolic syndrome as well as the careful monitoring of compliance with GFD, may be justified in adolescents with CD.

14.5 SUMMARY

Equilibrated GFD should include a combination of certified, processed, gluten-free products and naturally gluten-free foods. Pseudocereals (quinoa, amaranth, buckwheat, etc.) can be considered a healthier substitute to more commonly used components in GFD and it represents a promising area for further research. Besides being an excellent source of carbohydrates, proteins, dietary fiber, vitamins, and polyunsaturated fatty acids, pseudocereals have an amino acid profile and valuable nutritional characteristics (such as essential amino acid index, biological value, nutritional index, and protein efficiency ratio), which are of far higher value than that found in standard cereals (such as wheat, rice, and maize). In addition to this, numerous health benefits including the prevention and reduction of hypertension, cancer, inflammation, hyperglycemia, and oxidative stress and prevention of cardiovascular complications have resulted from the phenolics in pseudocereals. Further studies into the nutritional and technological properties of pseudocereals as wheat replacements are desirable to not only confirm their role in reducing nutritional deficiencies in CD but also their effects on GFD compliance and economic burden.

KEYWORDS

- amaranth
- buckwheat
- celiac disease
- gluten-free diet
- pseudocereals
- quinova

REFERENCES

1. Abugoch, J. L. E. Quinoa (*Chenopodium Quinoa*): Composition, Chemistry, Nutritional, and Functional Properties. *Adv. Food Nutr. Res.* **2009,** *58*, 1–31.

2. Alvarez-Jubete, L.; Arendt, E. K.; Gallagher, E. Nutritive Value and Chemical Composition of Pseudocereals as Gluten-Free Ingredients. *Int. J. Food Sci. Nutr.* **2009,** *60* (Suppl. 4), 240–257.

3. Alzaben, A. S.; Turner, J.; Shirton, L. Assessing Nutritional Quality and Adherence to the Gluten-Free Diet in Children and Adolescents with Celiac Disease. *Can. J. Diet. Pract. Res.* **2015,** *76* (2), 56–63.

4. Aubrecht, E.; Biacs, P. Á. Characterization of Buckwheat Grain Proteins and its Products. *Acta Aliment.* **2001,** *30* (1), 71–80.

5. Barton, S. H.; Kelly, D. G.; Murray, J. A. Nutritional Deficiencies in Celiac Disease. *Gastroenterol. Clin. North Am.* **2007,** *36* (1), 93–108.

6. Bhargava, A.; Rana, T. S.; Shukla, S.; Ohri, D. Seed Protein Electrophoresis of Some Cultivated and Wild Species of Chenopodium. *Biol. Plant.* **2005,** *49* (4), 505–511.

7. Bonafaccia, G.; Gambelli, L.; Fabjan, N.; Kreft, I. Trace Elements in Flour and Bran from Common and Tartary Buckwheat. *Food Chem.* **2003,** *83* (1), 1–5.

8. Bonafaccia, G.; Kreft, I. Technological and Qualitative Characteristics of Food Products Made with Buckwheat. *Fagopyrum* **1994,** *14*, 35–42.

9. Bonafaccia, G.; Marocchini, M.; Kreft, I. Composition and Technological Properties of the Flour and Bran from Common and Tartary Buckwheat. *Food Chem.* **2003,** *80* (1), 9–15.

10. Brar, P.; Kwon, G. Y.; Holleran, S. Change in Lipid Profile in Celiac Disease: Beneficial Effect of Gluten-Free Diet. *Am. J. Med.* **2006,** *119* (9), 786–790.

11. Bruni, R.; Medici, A.; Guerrini, A.; Scalia, S.; Poli, F. Wild *Amaranthus Caudatus* Seed Oil, a Nutraceutical Resource from Ecuadorian Flora. *J. Agric. Food Chem.* **2001,** *49* (11), 5455–5460.

12. De Carvalho, F. G.; Ovídio, P. P.; Padovan, G. J. Metabolic Parameters of Postmenopausal Women after Quinoa or Corn Flakes Intake: Prospective and Double-Blind Study. *Int. J. Food Sci. Nutr.* **2013,** *65* (3), 380–385.

13. Dini, A.; Rastrelli, L.; Saturnino, P; Schettino, O. A. Compositional Study of *Chenopodium Quinoa* Seeds. *Nahrung* **1992**, *36*, 400–404.

14. Dini, I.; Tenore, G. D.; Dini, A. Nutritional and Antinutritional Composition of Kancolla Seeds: an Interesting and Under-exploited Andine Food Plant. *Food Chem.* **2005**, *92* (1), 125–132.

15. Drzewiecki, J. Similarities and Differences Between Amaranthus Species and Cultivars and Estimation of Out-Crossing Rate on the Basis of Electrophoretic Separations of Urea-Soluble Seed Proteins. *Euphytica* **2001**, *119*, 279–287.

16. Drzewiecki, J.; Delgado-Licon, E. Identification and Differences of Total Proteins and Their Soluble Fractions in Some Pseudocereals Based on Electrophoretic Patterns. *J. Agric. Food Chem.* **2003**, *51* (26), 7798–7804.

17. Duranti, M. Grain Legume Proteins and Nutraceutical Properties. *Fitoterapia* **2006**, *77* (2), 67–82.

18. Escudero, N. L.; Zirulnik, F. Influence of a Protein Concentrate from *Amaranthus Cruentus* Seeds on Lipid Metabolism. *Exp. Biol. Med.* **2006**, *231* (1), 50–59.

19. Farinazzi-Machado, F. M.; Barbalho, S. M. Use of Cereal Bars with Quinoa (*Chenopodium Quinoa*) to Reduce Risk Factors Related to Cardiovascular Diseases. *Food Sci. Technol.* **2012**, *32* (2), 239–244.

20. Fasano, A.; Catassi, C. Clinical Practice: Celiac disease. *New Engl. J. Med.* **2012**, *367*, 2419–2426.

21. Gonzalez, J. A.; Roldan, A.; Gallardo, M.; Escudero, T.; Prado, F. E. Quantitative Determinations of Chemical Compounds with Nutritional Value from Inca Crops: *Chenopodium Quinoa*. *Plant Foods Human Nutr.* **1989**, *39* (4), 331–337.

22. Gorinstein, S.; Pawelzik, E. Characterization of Pseudocereals and Cereal Proteins by Protein and Amino Acid Analyses. *J. Sci. Food Agric.* **2002**, *82*, 886–891.

23. Graf, B. L.; Rojas-Silva, P.; Rojo, L. E. Innovations in Health Value and Functional Food Development of Quinoa (*Chenopodium Quinoa*). *Comprehen. Rev. Food Sci. Food Safe.* **2015**, *14* (4), 431–445.

24. Guandalini, S.; Assiri, A. Celiac Disease. *JAMA Pediatr.* **2014**, *168* (3), 272–278.

25. Hallert, C.; Grant, C.; Grehn, S. Evidence of Poor Vitamin Status in Coeliac Patients on a Gluten-Free Diet for 10 Years. *Aliment. Pharmacol. Therap.* **2002**, *16* (7), 1333–1339.

26. Hallert, C.; Svensson, M.; Tholstrup, J.; Hultber, B. Clinical Trial: Vitamin-B Improve Health in Patients with Coeliac Disease Living on a Gluten-Free Diet. *Aliment. Pharmacol. Therap.* **2009**, *29* (8), 811–816.

27. He, J.; Klag, M. J.; Whelton, P. K.; Mo, J. P.; Chen, J. Y.; Qian, M. C.; He, G. Q. Oats and Buckwheat Intakes and Cardiovascular Disease Risk Factors in an Ethnic Minority of China. *Am. J. Clin. Nutr.* **1995**, *61* (2), 366–372.

28. Husby, S.; Koletzko, S.; Korponay-Szabó, I. R. ESPGHAN Working Group on Coeliac Disease Diagnosis; European Society for Pediatric Gastroenterology, Hepatology, and Nutrition Guidelines for the Diagnosis of Coeliac Disease. *J. Pediatr. Gastroenterol. Nutr.* **2012**, *54* (4),136–160.

29. Improta, F.; Kellens, R. Comparison of Raw, Washed and Polished Quinoa (*Chenopodium Quinoa* Willd.) to Wheat, Sorghum or Maize Based Diets on Growth and Survival of Broiler 17 Chicks. *Livestock Res. Rural Dev.* **2001**, *13* (1), 10–15.

30. Jacobsen, S. E.; Mujica, A.; Ortiz, R. *La Importancia de los Cultivos Andinos* (Importance of Andino Crops). *Fermentum* **2003**, *13*, 14–24.

31. Kaur, S.; Singh, N.; Rana, J. C. *Amaranthus Hypochondriacus* and *Amaranthus Caudatus* Germplasm: Characteristics of Plants, Grain and Flours. *Food Chem.* **2010,** *123* (4), 1227–1234.

32. Kemppainen, T.; Uusitupa, M. Intakes of Nutrients and Nutritional Status in Coeliac Patients. *Scand. J. Gastroenterol.* **1995,** *30* (6), 575–579.

33. Khattak, A. B.; Zeb, A.; Bibi, N.; Khalil, S. A.; Khattak, M. S. Influence of Germination Techniques on Phytic Acid and Polyphenols Content of Chickpea (*Cicer arietinum* L.) Sprouts. *Food Chem.* **2007,** *104* (3), 1074–1079.

34. Kinsey, L.; Burden, S. T.; Bannerman, E. Dietary Survey to Determine if Patients with Coeliac Disease are Meeting Current Healthy Eating Guidelines and how their Diet Compares to that of the British General Population. *Eur. J. Clin. Nutr.* **2007,** *62* (11), 1333–1342.

35. Konishi, Y.; Nojima, H.; Okuno, K.; Asaoka, M.; Fuwa, H. Characterization of Starch Granules from Waxy, Nonwaxy, and Hybrid Seeds of *Amaranthus Hypochondriacus* L. *Agric. Biol. Chem.* **1985,** *49* (7), 1965–1971.

36. Kozioł, M. Chemical Composition and Nutritional Evaluation of Quinoa (*Chenopodium Quinoa* Willd.). *J. Food Compos. Analy.* **1992,** *5* (1), 35–68.

37. Kupfer, S.S; Jabri, B. Pathophysiology of Celiac Disease. *Gastrointest. Endosc. Clin. NA* **2012,** *22* (4), 639–660.

38. Kupper, C. Dietary Guidelines and Implementation for Celiac Disease. *Gastroenterology* **2005,** *128* (4), S121–S127.

39. Li, S.; Zhang, Q. H. Advances in the Development of Functional Foods from Buckwheat. *Crit. Rev. Food Sci. Nutr.* **2001,** *41* (6), 451–464.

40. Ludvigsson, J. F.; Rubio-Tapia, A. Increasing Incidence of Celiac Disease in a North American Population. *Am. J. Gastroenterol.* **2013,** *108* (5), 818–824.

41. Lutar, Z. Polyphenol Classification and Tannin Content of Buckwheat Seeds (*Fagopyrum esculentum* Moench.). *Fagopyrum* **1992,** *12,* 36–42.

42. Mariani, P.; Viti, M. G.; Montouri, M. The Gluten-Free Diet: Nutritional Risk Factor for Adolescents with Celiac Disease? *J. Pediatr. Gastroenterol. Nutr.* **1998,** *27* (5), 519–523.

43. Martin, J.; Geisel, T.; Maresch, C.; Krieger, K.; Stein, J. Inadequate Nutrient Intake in Patients with Celiac Disease: Results from a German Dietary Survey. *Digestion* **2013,** *87,* 240–246.

44. Mir, N. A.; Riar, C. S.; Singh, S. Nutritional Constituents of Pseudo Cereals and their Potential Use in Food Systems: Review. *Trends in Food Science & Technology,* **2018,** *75,* 170–180.

45. Mustalahti, K.; Catassi, C.; Reunanen, A. The Prevalence of Celiac Disease in Europe: Results of Centralized, International Mass Screening Project. *Ann. Med.* **2010,** *42* (8), 587–595.

46. Navruz-Varli, S.; Sanlier, N. Nutritional and Health Benefits of Quinoa (Chenopodium Quinoa Willd.). *J. Cereal Sci.* **2016,** *69,* 371–376.

47. Ng, S.; Anderson, A.; Coker, J.; Ondrus, M. Characterization of Lipid Oxidation Products in Quinoa (*Chenopodium Quinoa*). *Food Chem.,* **2007,** *101* (1), 185–192.

48. Norsa, L. Cardiovascular Disease Risk Factor Profiles in Children with Celiac Disease on Gluten-Free Diets. *World J. Gastroenterol.* **2013,** *19* (34), 5658–5664.

49. Nowak, V.; Du, J.; Charrondière, U. R. Assessment of the Nutritional Composition of Quinoa (*Chenopodium Quinoa* Willd.). *Food Chem.* **2016,** *193,* 47–54.
50. Öhlund, K.; Olsson, C.; Hernell, O.; Öhlund, I. Dietary Shortcomings in Children on a Gluten-Free Diet. *J. Human Nutr. Diet.* **2010,** *23* (3), 294–300.
51. Pagano, A. E. Whole Grains and the Gluten-Free Diet. *Pract. Gastroenterol.* **2006,** *29* (10), 66–78.
52. Penagini, F.; Dilillo, D.; Meneghin, F. Gluten-Free Diet in Children: an Approach to a Nutritionally Adeguate and Balanced Diet. *Nutrients* **2013,** *5,* 4553–4565.
53. Qureshi, A. A.; Lehmann, J. W.; Peterson, D. M. Amaranth and Its Oil Inhibit Cholesterol Biosynthesis in 6-Week-Old Female Chickens. *J. Nutr.* **1996,***126* (8), 1972–1978.
54. Ramakrishna, B.; Makharia, G. K.; Chetri, K. Prevalence of Adult Celiac Disease in India: Regional Variations and Associations. *Am. J. Gastroenterol.* **2016,** *111* (1), 115–123.
55. Repo-Carrasco, R.; Espinoza, C.; Jacobsen, S. Nutritional Value and Use of the Andean Crops Quinoa (*Chenopodium Quinoa*) and Kañiwa (*Chenopodium Pallidicaule*). *Food Rev. Int.* **2003,** *19* (1–2), 179–189.
56. Ruales, J.; Grijalva, Y. D.; Lopez-Jaramillo, P.; Nair, B. M. The Nutritional Quality of an Infant Food from Quinoa and its Effect on the Plasma Level of Insulin-Like Growth Factor-1 (IGF-1) in Undernourished Children. *Int. J. Food Sci. Nutr.* **2002,** *53* (2), 143–154.
57. Skrabanja, V.; Kreft, I.; Golob, T.; Modic, M. Nutrient Content in Buckwheat Milling Fractions. *Cereal Chem. J.* **2004,** *81* (2), 172–176.
58. Steadman, K.; Burgoon, M.; Lewis, B.; Edwardson, S.; Obendorf, R. Buckwheat Seed Milling Fractions: Description, Macronutrient Composition and Dietary Fiber. *J. Cereal Sci.* **2001,** *33* (3), 271–278.
59. Steadman, K. J.; Burgoon, M. S. Minerals, Phytic Acid, Tannin and Rutin in Buckwheat Seed Milling Fractions. *J. Sci. Food Agric.* **2001,** *81* (11), 1094–1100.
60. Tang, Y.; Zhang, B.; Li, X.; Chen, P. X.; Zhang, H.; Liu, R.; Tsao, R. Bound Phenolics of Quinoa Seeds Released by Acid, Alkaline, and Enzymatic Treatments and their Antioxidant and α-Glucosidase and Pancreatic Lipase Inhibitory Effects. *J. Agric. Food Chem.* **2016,** *64* (8), 1712–1719.
61. Thompson, T. Folate, Iron, and Dietary Fiber Contents of the Gluten-Free Diet. *J. Am. Diet. Assoc.* **2000,** *100* (11), 1389–1396.
62. Thompson, L. U. Potential Health Benefits and Problems Associated with Antinutrients in Foods. *Food Research International,* **1993,** *26* (2), 131–149.
63. Thompson, T. Thiamin, Riboflavin, and Niacin Contents of the Gluten-Free Diet. *J. Am. Diet. Assoc.* **1999,** *99* (7), 858–862.
64. Thompson, T.; Dennis, M.; Higgins, L. A.; Lee, A. R.; Sharrett, M. K. Gluten-Free Diet Survey: Are Americans with Coeliac Disease Consuming Recommended Amounts of Fiber, Iron, Calcium and Grain Foods? *J. Human Nutr. Diet.* **2005,** *18* (3), 163–169.
65. Vega-Gálvez, A.; Miranda, M.; Vergara, J. Nutrition Facts and Functional Potential of Quinoa (*Chenopodium Quinoa* Willd.), an Ancient Andean Grain: A Review. *J. Sci. Food Agric.* **2010,** *90* (15), 2541–2547.

66. Vilcacundo, R.; Hernandez-Ledesma, B. Nutritional and Biological Value of Quinoa (*Chenopodium Quinoa*). *Curr. Opin. Food Sci.* **2017,** *14*, 1–6.

67. Wei, L.; Spiers, E.; Reynolds, N.; Walsh, S.; Fahey, T.; MacDonald, T. M. The Association Between Coeliac Disease and Cardiovascular Disease. *Aliment. Pharmacol. Therap.* **2007,** *27* (6), 514–519.

68. Wild, D.; Robins, G. G.; Burley, V. J.; Howdle, P. D. Evidence of High Sugar Intake, and Low Fiber and Mineral Intake, in the Gluten-Free Diet. *Aliment. Pharmacol. Therap.* **2010,** *32* (4), 573–581.

69. Zanini, B.; Mazzoncini, E.; Lanzarotto, F. Impact of Gluten-Free Diet on Cardiovascular Risk Factors: Retrospective Analysis in a Large Cohort of Coeliac Patients. *Digest. Liver Dis.* **2013,** *45* (10), 810–815.

70. Zevallos, V. F.; Herencia, I. Gastrointestinal Effects of Eating Quinoa (*Chenopodium Quinoa*) in Celiac Patients. *Am. J. Gastroenterol.* **2014,** *109* (2), 270–278.

71. Zhang, Z.; Zhou, M.; Tang, Y.; Li, F.; Tang, Y.; Shao, J.; Wu, Y. Bioactive Compounds in Functional Buckwheat Food. *Food Res. Int.* **2012,** *49* (1), 389–395.

72. Zielińska, D.; Turemko, M.; Kwiatkowski, J.; Zieliński, H. Evaluation of Flavonoid Contents and Antioxidant Capacity of the Aerial Parts of Common and Tartary Buckwheat Plants. *Molecules* **2012,** *17*, 9668–9682.

CHAPTER 15

Role of Amla (*Emblica officinalis*) in Peptic Ulcer

DILIPKUMAR PAL and SOUVIK MUKHERJEE

ABSTRACT

Emblica officinalis (EO: Indian gooseberry or Amla) has extended appraisal in an old and wise system of medicinal system. The plant has significant amounts of polyphenols, such as: gallic acid, ellagic acid and terpenoids, which act as therapeutic agents in different chronic peptic ulcer (PU). The fruit extract of amla is an anti-ulcer agent and pain reducing therapy. This book chapter covers its ethnopharmacology, chemistry, clinical and preclinical studies focusing on the use of the plant in PU. This chapter provides information on ethnopharmacology, chemistry, clinical and preclinical studies of Amla in Peptic ulcer disease.

15.1 INTRODUCTION

Ulcers are an open broken of the skin or mucous membrane. It is represented by the sloughing of rubbed red dead tissue. These diseases are most common on the skin of the lower portion and in the GI tract.[5] Many types of ulcers (such as: mouth ulcer (MU), throat ulcer (TU), peptic ulcer (PU) and Gastric ulcer (GU)) are mostly seen in patients. Amongst these, PU are very common. The PU are rubbing away from the lining of the stomach or the duodenum.

There are two common types of PU, such as, GU and duodenal ulcer (DU).[2] Ulcers generally occur in older persons. There are various symptoms, such as, nausea, vomiting, and weight loss in ulcer patients.[1] DU occurs at the orifice of the small intestine with the burning sensation in the upper abdomen. Generally, pain takes place, when the stomach is empty and comforts after taking the food.[4] The DU is more common in younger male persons. In the duodenum, ulcers may come into view on both the anterior and posterior walls. In some cases, PUs may be the living suggestions of violent behavior with symptoms, such as, bloody stool, serious abdominal pain and cramps with vomiting blood.[18]

The pathophysiology of PU disease deals with the imbalance between disgusting agents (such as: acid, pepsin, *H. pylori*) and attack-stopping factors (such as: mucin, PG, bicarbonate, nitric oxide) and growth factors.[9] PU are believed to be caused by strong taste foods.[34] The PU is one of the important GI diseases. About 19 out of 20 cases are found to have DU.[11] In the Indian pharmaceutical industry, antacids and antiulcer drugs take a major role in the market. However, the ready treatment plans of PU are related to anti-histamine medicines, sometimes used for amusement, but each of them has its own unwanted, unhealthy side-effects. Scientists are in search for the new compounds based on indigenous plants to treat PU.

Plants having potential medical values are commenced as a mixture in herbal constitution containing Indian old, conventional Ayurveda.[17] Amla (or Ama) is the very familiar medicinal plant used in Ayurveda system.[13] It has been used as a good medicine fruit and good tonic, because of the presence of amino acid (AA) and vitamin (VM).

While every part of Amla plant is used for medical usage, yet the fruits are more widely used either alone or in a mixture with other herbs for the treatment of numerous contagious and non-contagious diseases.[20] In India, fruits of Amla are extensively consumed to treat the swelling of the gastrointestinal system and chronic PU disease. It also has antipyretic activity in addition to its familiar utilization as a livener.[19,29]

This book chapter deals with ethnopharmacology, chemistry, clinical and preclinical studies focusing on the use of Amla in PU disease.

15.2   DESCRIPTION OF *EMBLICA OFFICINALIS*

Amla is a primitive tree that is extensively scattered in tropical and subtropical continents of China, India, Indonesia, and Southeast Asia.[30–32] This plant has been exploited for controlling various ailments and different lifestyle sickness.[13,14]

The plant is medium-sized tree with 8–18 m in height having a twisting stalk.[24] The leaves are too much abbreviated having size up to 7–10 cm long, sub-sessile and closely fixed in conjunction with wings. The ripe fruits (Fig. 15.1) with greenish-yellow color are ball-shaped with six vertical bands have an astringent sour and acidic taste.[3]

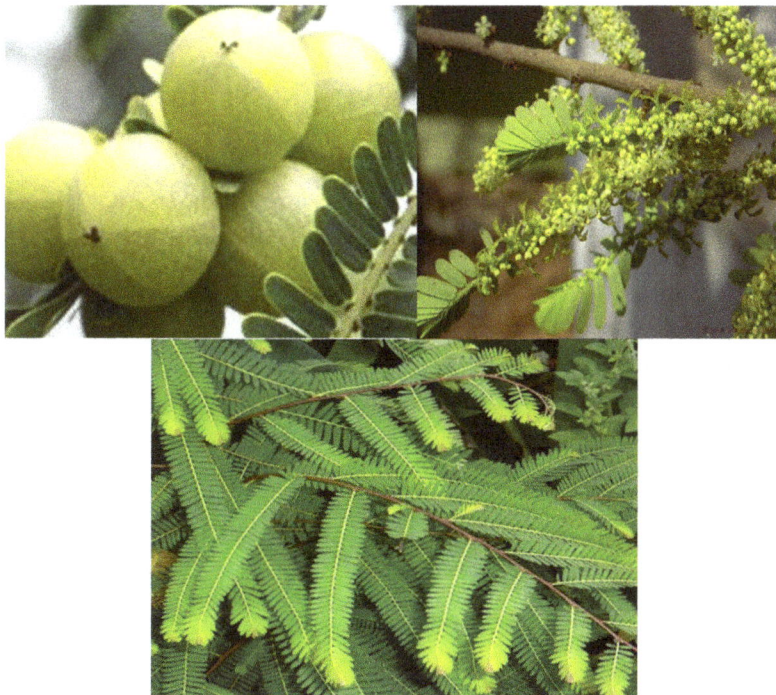

FIGURE 15.1   *Emblica officinalis* flowers, leaves and round fruits.

15.3   PHYTOCHEMICAL CONSTITUENTS

Amla plant contains a variety of following biochemical constituents[6–8,11,12,26,27]:

- 1-O-galloyl-beta-D-glucose
- 1,6-di-O-galloyl-beta-D-glucose
- 2,3,7,8-tetrahydroxy-chromene
- 3,6-di-O-galloyl-D-glucose
- alkaloids

- amino acids
- apigenin
- chebulagic acid
- chebulinic acid
- corilagin
- ellagic acid
- ellagitannin
- emblicanin-a
- emblicanin-b
- ethylgallic acid (3-ethoxy-4,5-di-hydroxy benzoic acid)
- flavone glycosides
- flavonol glycosides
- gallic acid
- isostrictiniin
- luteolin
- pectin
- pedunculagin
- phenolic glycosides
- phyllaemblicin-a
- phyllaemblicin-b
- phyllaemblicin-c
- punigluconin
- punigluconoin
- quercetin,
- trigallayl glucose
- vitamin C (ascorbic acid)

15.4   ETHNOPHARMACOLOGY OF *EMBLICA OFFICINALIS*

Ethnopharmacology of *Emblica officinalis* includes[12,15,23]: laxative, erysipelas, stomachic, digestive, antipyretic, diuretic, ophthalmopathy, aphrodisiac, cephalalgia, and carminative.

Amla fruits have been used for thousands of years for the treatment of hyperglycemia, asthma, jaundice, bronchitis, heart issue, cephalalgia, ophthalmopathy, dyspepsia, edema, weakness, biliousness, colitis, tooting, hyperacidity, PU, erysipelas, skin ailments, sickness, irritations, pallor, gauntness, hepatopathy, haematogenetic, strangury, looseness of the bowels, hemorrhages, leucorrhea, menorrhagia, discontinuous fevers and greyness of hair.[12,15,23] Fruits of this plant are important sources of Asa. The leaves are used in aphrodisiac manifestations, fever, asthma, bronchitis and vomiting. The bark, roots and the ripe fruit are sharp in taste. The unripe fruit is used as a calming agent, laxative, and diuretic.[17,18]

15.5 ROLE OF *EMBLICA OFFICINALIS* FOR TREATMENT OF PEPTIC ULCER

The dominant chief place of phytochemicals has been their use to stop GI diseases.[20,21] The amla plant showed protective activity against acetic acid-induced ulcers in rats. Pharmacological, biochemical and histopathological studies indicate that the fruit extract has important anti-secretory, antiulcer and cyto-protective activities.[21–22,33,34] It exhibits MIC from 0.91 to 1.87 g/L.

In addition, ethanol fraction demonstrated GI security against NSAID-induced gastropathy. It causes up-regulation in anti-inflammatory cytokine (Fig. 15.2) equity.[27,28] The water extract of fruits in rats produced a noteworthy elevation in seepage of gastric mucous and hexosamines in indomethacin-making open afflicted part. Treatment with this plant extract against l-arginine-induced pancreatitis in rat displayed decrease in the lipase level. Histoarchitecture observations show remarkable reduction in inflammation.[25,35]

The plant extract containing rutin has pancreato-protective potential activity in cerulean-containing pancreatitis in rats.[36] The system is associated with acquiring higher quantity of serum lipase and amylase ratio, rebating in the levels of IL-1 and iL-18 collagen, caspase-1myeloperoxidase function, oxidative weight, and caspase-1m-RNA expression.[25]

15.6 SUMMARY

Experiments on the effects of Amla on some cancer cell-lines have demonstrated decisive results in animal models. It remains a species with very high potentiality and the great number of probable states for further observations. Ama has the potential to be a nontoxic anti-ulcer and chemoprotective agent.

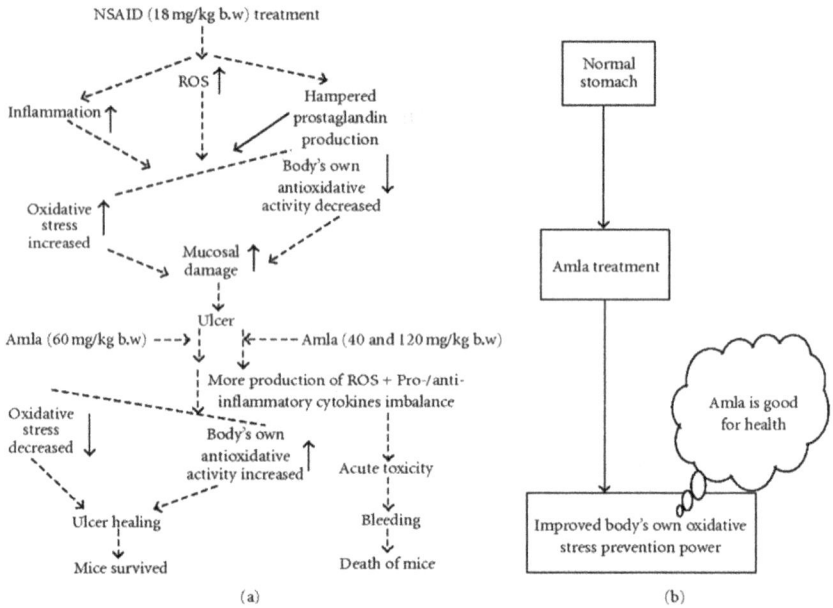

FIGURE 15.2   Mechanism of role of *Emblica officinalis* in peptic ulcer.

KEYWORDS

- clinical study
- *Emblica officinalis*
- muscarinic receptor
- peptic ulcer
- preclinical study

REFERENCES

1. Ahmad, I.; Mahmoud, Z.; Mohammad, F. Screening of Some Indian Medicinal Plants for Their Antimicrobial Properties. *J. Ethnopharmacol.* **1998**, *62* (2), 183–193.
2. Blaser, M. J. Gastric Campylobacter Organisms, Gastritis, and Peptic Ulcer Disease. *Gastroenterology* **1987**, *93* (2), 371–383.

3. Dasaroju, S.; Gottumukkala, K. M. Current Trends in The Research of *Emblica Officinalis* (Amla): A Pharmacological Perspective. *Int. J. Pharma. Sci. Rev. Res.* **2014,** *24* (2), 150–159.

4. Firuzi, O.; Lacanna, A.; Petrucci, R.; Marrosu, G.; Saso, L. Evaluation of The Antioxidant Activity of Flavonoids by Ferric Reducing Antioxidant Power Assay and Cyclic Voltammetry. *Biochem. Biophys. Acta* **2005,** *1721* (3), 174–184.

5. Graham, D. Y. Campylobacter Pylori and Peptic Ulcer Disease. *Gastroenterology* **1989,** *96* (2), 615–625.

6. Griffin, M. R.; Piper, J. M.; Daugherty, J. R.; Snowden, M.; Ray, W. A. Nonsteroidal Anti-Inflammatory Drug Use and Increased Risk for Peptic Ulcer Disease in Elderly Persons. *Ann. Intern. Med.* **1991,** *114* (4), 257–263.

7. Huang, J. Q.; Sridhar, S.; Hunt, R. H. Role of *Helicobacter Pylori* Infection and Non-Steroidal Anti-Inflammatory Drugs in Peptic-Ulcer Disease: Meta-Analysis. *Lancet* **2002,** *359* (3), 14–22.

8. Huang, T. K.; Ding, Z. Z.; Zhao, S. X. Modern Compendium of *Materia Medica. Beijing: Med. Sci. Technol.* **2001,** *6* (3), 1859–1860.

9. Ihantola, V. A.; Summanen, J. Anti-inflammatory Activity of Extracts from Leaves of *Phyllanthus Emblica. Planta Medica* **1997,** *63* (6), 518–524.

10. Kamboj, V. P. Herbal Medicine. *Current Science,* **2000,** *78* (1), 35–39.

11. Khan, K. H. Roles of *Emblica Officinalis* in Medicine: Review. *Bot. Res. Int.* **2009,** *2* (4), 218–228.

12. Kirtikar, K. R.; Basu, B. D. Indian Medicinal Plants. *Med. Plant* **1935,** *6* (2), 5–12.

13. Kuipers, E. J.; Thijs, J. C.; Festen, H. P. The Prevalence of *Helicobacter Pylori* in Peptic Ulcer Disease. *Aliment. Pharmacol.Therap.* **1995,** *9*, 59–69.

14. Kumar, K. S.; Bhowmik, D.; Dutta, A.; Yadav, A. P. Recent Trends in Potential Traditional Indian Herbs *Emblica officinalis* and its Medicinal Importance. *J. Pharmacognosy Phytochem.* **2012,** *1* (1), 18–28.

15. Malfertheiner, P.; Chan, F. K.; McColl, K. E. Peptic Ulcer Disease. *Lancet* **2009,** *374* (9699), 1449–1461.

16. Mirunalini, S.; Krishnaveni, M. Therapeutic Potential of *Phyllanthus Emblica* (amla): The Ayurvedic Wonder. *J. Basic Clin. Physiol. Pharmacol.* **2010,** *21* (1), 93–105.

17. Mishra, P.; Verma, M.; Mishra, V.; Mishra, S.; Rai, G. K. Studies on Development of Ready to Eat Amla (*Emblica officinalis*) Chutney and its Preservation by Using Class One Preservatives. *Am. J. Food Technol.* **2011,** *6*, 244–252.

18. Pal, D.; Ahuja, C.; Mukherjee, S. *Celsia coromandeliane* Vahl-A: New Biomarker with Immense Pharmaceutical Applications. *J. Drug Deliv. Therap.* **2019,** *9* (3), 1109–1115.

19. Pal, D.; Sahoo, M.; Mishra, A. K. Analgesic and Anticonvulsant Effects of Saponin Isolated from the Stems of *Opuntia Vulgaris* Mill in Mice. *Eur. Bull. Drug Res.* **2005,** *13*, 91–97.

20. Pal, D. K.; Dutta, S. Evaluation of the Antioxidant Activity of the Roots and Rhizomes of *Cyperus rotundus* L. *Ind. J. Pharma. Sci.* **2006,** *68*(2), 230–238.

21. Pal, D. K.; Mandal, M.; Senthilkumar, G. P.; Padhiari, A. Antibacterial Activity of *Cuscuta reflexa* Stem and *Corchorus olitorius* Seed. *Fitoterapia* **2006,** *77* (8), 589–591.

22. Palav, Y. K.; D'mello, P. M. Standardization of Selected Indian Medicinal Herbal Raw Materials Containing Polyphenols as Major Phytoconstituents. *Ind. J. Pharma. Sci.* **2006,** *68* (4), 12–17.

23. Paul, K. P.; Shaha, R. K. Nutrients, Vitamins and Minerals Content in Common Citrus Fruits in The Northern Region of Bangladesh. *Pak. J. Biol. Sci.* **2004,** *7* (2), 238–242.

24. Peterson, W. L. *Helicobacter Pylori* and Peptic Ulcer Disease. *New Engl. J. Med.* **1991,** *324* (15), 1043–1048.

25. Rahman, S.; Akbor, M. M.; Howlader, A.; Jabbar, A. Antimicrobial and Cytotoxic Activity of the Alkaloids of Amla (*Emblica Officinalis*). *Pak. J. Biol. Sci.* **2009,** *12* (16), 1152–1159.

26. Rawal, S.; Singh, P.; Gupta, A.; Mohanty, S. Dietary Intake of *Curcuma Longa* and *Emblica Officinalis* Increases Life Span in Drosophila Melanogaster. *Biomed Res. Int.* **2014,** *15* (6), 321–324.

27. Sarkhel, S.; Chakravarty, A. K.; Das, R.; Gomes, A. Snake Venom Neutralising Factor from the Root Extract of *Emblica Officinalis* Linn. *Orient. Pharm. Exp. Med.* **2011,** *11* (1), 25–33.

28. Scartezzini, P.; Speroni, E. Review on Some Plants of Indian Traditional Medicine with Antioxidant Activity. *J. Ethnopharmacol.* **2000,** *71* (1), 23–43.

29. Svedlund, J.; Sjödin, I.; Dotevall, G. GSRS: Clinical Rating Scale for Gastrointestinal Symptoms in Patients with Irritable Bowel Syndrome and Peptic Ulcer Disease. *Digest. Dis. Sci.* **1988,** *33* (2), 129–134.

30. Variya, B. C.; Bakrania, A. K.; Patel, S. S. *Emblica Officinalis* (Amla): Review for Its Phytochemistry, Ethno-Medicinal Uses and Medicinal Potentials with Respect to Molecular Mechanisms. *Pharmacol. Res.*, **2016,** *111*, 180–200.

31. Wagner, H. Phytomedicine Research in Germany. *Environ. Health Perspect.* **1999,** *107* (10), 779–781.

32. Wong, C. C.; Li, H. B.; Cheng, K. W.; Chen, F. A Systematic Survey of Antioxidant Activity of 30 Chinese Medicinal Plants Using the Ferric Reducing Antioxidant Power Assay. *Food Chem.* **2006,** *97* (4), 705–711.

33. Yadav, S. S.; Singh, M. K.; Singh, P. K.; Kumar, V. Traditional Knowledge to Clinical Trials: A Review on Therapeutic Actions of *Emblica officinalis*. *Biomed. Pharmacotherap.* **2017,** *93*, 1292–1302.

34. Yamada, T.; Searle, J. G.; Ahnen, D.; Aipers, D. H. *Helicobacter pylori* in peptic ulcer disease. *JAMA* **1994,** *272* (1), 65–69.

35. Yoshida, Y.; Niki, E. Antioxidant Effects of Phytosterols and Its Components. *J. Nutr. Sci. and Vitaminol.* **2003,** *49* (4), 277–280.

36. Zhang, Y.; Zhao, L.; Guo, X.; Li, C.; Li, H.; Lou, H.; Ren, D. Chemical Constituents from *Phyllanthus Emblica* and the Cytoprotective Effects on H_2O_2-Induced PC12 Cell Injuries. *Arch. Pharma. Res.* **2016,** *39* (9), 1202–1211.

CHAPTER 16

Therapeutic Properties of Fermented Foods and Beverages

S. SUPREETHA and NANDINI DUTTA

ABSTRACT

Indian traditional foods have good amounts of carbohydrates, protein, fats, vitamins, minerals and phytochemicals (from herbal plants) that make an important part of a balanced diet depending on various cultural factors of the diverse population. The traditional foods of India include usage of various ingredients that are mainly influenced by the ayurvedic interpretations aiming at creating equilibrium for mind, body and spirit. Fermentation is a popular technique used in traditional foods with many health benefits to enhance flavor, texture, appearance and digestibility of food, to increase the essential amino acids, fatty acids, vitamins and to reduce anti-nutrient factors with improved shelf-life. The therapeutic properties are mainly due to the presence of prebiotics, probiotics, bioactive microbial metabolites, bioavailable vitamins and minerals in the fermented food.

16.1 INTRODUCTION

India is a vast country with different religious and traditional practices where food plays a significant role in the cultural performance. Certain ethnic foods and beverages of India are known to have therapeutic properties, such as, protection against gastrointestinal diseases, prevention of cardiovascular, immune-responsive disorders, allergies, diabetes, and cancer.

Indian traditional fermented foods and beverages are classified based on the substrate involved in fermentation, method of preparation, region, and microorganism involved in fermentation. The major groups are based on fermentation of cereals, pulses, milk, fruits, vegetables, meat and fish. The therapeutic benefits obtained after consumption include: prevention against gastrointestinal diseases, cancer, hypertension, cardiovascular diseases, diabetes and allergic reactions by production of specific bioactive compounds during the fermentation. Due to the several health benefits, the market demand for fermented food and beverages is increasing enormously; hence, commercial production is being carried out with several efforts and being packed in suitable containers for efficient storage and distribution.

This chapter explores: (1) history of Indian traditional food and beverages; (2) role of starter culture in the development of characteristic changes in the food products; (3) different traditional Indian food and beverages with respect to substrate of fermentation and its therapeutic properties; and (4) innovations in production and packaging of traditional food and beverages.

16.2 HISTORY OF INDIAN TRADITIONAL FOOD AND BEVERAGES

The history of Indian food is traced back to Indus valley civilization of the Harappa and the Mohenjadaro before 3000 B.C.[96,161,162,184]. Indian cuisine is considered as one of the most diverse cuisines in the world due to diverse traditions and culture followed across the country.[161] For example: Evidence of preparation of *idli* is dated back to 1100 A.D.,[42] for which the method of preparation was described by Indian poet Chavundaraya in 1025 A.D.[52]; and the preparation of *idli* with rice, spices and semolina is mentioned in 1130 A.D. in a *Samskrita* book called *Manasollasa*.[142] The process of preparation of *dosa* is mentioned in the 6th century in the Tamil Sangam literature of ancient India.[151] Similarly, the history of *dhokla* and *khaman* dates back to 1066 A.D..[96] *Jalebi* is probably of the Persian or Arabic origin, introduced to India during Mughal era in 1450 A.D.[42]

The ethnic fermented food and beverages (*chilra, marchu, gundruk, sinki, goyang, selroti*, etc.) prepared from cereals, vegetables and meat have religious significance. They are prepared and distributed during Indian festivals, marriage ceremonies and social gatherings. The names of the different dishes are adopted from the local dialect and is derived either based on the raw material used or specially fabricated vessel used for preparation or by the method of preparation.[154,162,185] *Kinema*, a popular fermented soybean product of Sikkim and Darjeeling is known to be introduced to India during *Kirat* dynasty from 600 B.C. to 100 A.D.[168] *Kinema* is known to be originated from *limboo* language (*Kirat* dialect), which means the flavor obtained during fermentation.[162]

Use of fermented milk and milk products was widely accepted by ancient civilization in India, which is supported by several historical documents, such as: *Vedas.* Consumption of fermented milk and milk products has ethnic, social, religious and traditional importance, its dietary usage is mentioned in religious documents of 4000 B.C.[162] Wide use of *dahi,* butter milk and ghee are reported in 8000 B.C. during the period of Lord *Krishna* as an important part of a regular diet[92,112]; in *Vedas* and *Upanishads.*[184] The production of fermented foods and beverages is specific to different regions due to traditions followed, raw material available and local climatic conditions (Table 16.1).

TABLE 16.1 Classification of Region-Wise Traditional Foods and Beverages in India.

Region	Product with local name	Substrate	Therapeutic property
North	*Lassi, naan, tungtap, jamma*	Milk, wheat flour, meat	Anti-allergic, anti-oxidant, alleviates lactose intolerance.
South	*Idli, dosa, adai, vada, kanji*	Dehulled black gram, milled rice	Anti-diabetic, anti-thrombic.
East	*Misti doi, shidal*	Milk, fish	Prevents hepatic diseases, anti-oxidant.
West	*Dhokla, khaman, shrikhand*	Gram flour, milk	Anti-mutagenic, anti-hypertensive.
Northeast	*Kinema, tungrymbai, kargyong, gnuchi*	Soybean, meat, fish	Anti-allergic, prevents CVD.

Lassi and buttermilk are obtained as byproducts during preparation of butter or ghee; and both are popular non-alcoholic beverages in India. Fermented milk is also used in the preparation of different traditional sweets, such as, *shrikhand* prepared by concentrated fermented milk or *dahi* and consumed during festivals in Gujrat, Karnataka and Maharashtra, *misti doi* is prepared with sweetened fermented milk in West Bengal, *rabadi* is prepared with fermenting milk, cereals and pulses and millets as a thick slurry in North and Western parts of India. The fermented fish products have a key role in the social gatherings and religious occasions and are used as main dish in meals; for example: *tungtap, hentak and ngari* are unique and main fermented fish products in Himachal Pradesh.[165]

16.3   STARTER CULTURE USED AND THEIR ROLE IN FERMENTED FOOD AND BEVERAGES

The starter culture is the group of microorganisms that are involved in the fermentation of foods and food products. It aids in the conversion of complex sugars into simple sugars, acids and flavor compounds that can improve the appearance, texture, flavor, and taste of a food along with improved digestibility, nutrient profile, nutrient bioavailability and prolonged shelf-life of the product. The major group of microorganisms that are helpful in the fermentation are bacteria, yeast and mold. The predominant group of bacteria for fermentation is lactic acid bacteria (such as: *Lactococcus, Lactobacillus, Streptococcus, Pediococcus*, etc.), which can covert lactose to lactic acid; and Acetobacter species that oxidizes alcohol to acetic acid.[57,58]

Bacillus group includes *Bacillus licheniformis, B. pumilus and B. subtilis*, etc. that carries out alkaline fermentation. This group causes hydrolysis of protein and forms amino acids, peptides and ammonia that can elevate the alkalinity of the substrate (especially protein rich foods, such as: legumes and soybean) as a result of which growth of spoilage causing microorganisms is inhibited.[13] Yeast is involved in the fermentation by producing alcohol as the major product. *Saccharomyces* sp. and *Schizosaccharo myces* sp. are the main species that bring about fermentation. *S. boulderi* and *Sch. pombe* are dominant yeasts involved in the fermentation of traditional fermented beverages.[149] Different changes related to acid and flavor development, production of antimicrobial compounds that are related to change in texture and protein digestibility (Table 16.2) occur in the food products during fermentation.

16.4   INDIAN TRADITIONAL FERMENTED FOODS AND BEVERAGES

Fermentation is a traditional method of food preservation, which is one of the safest and economical process since ancient times.[19] During the process of fermentation, the complex large biomolecules are broken down into small simple biomolecules by the action of microorganisms. Fermentation process helps to increase the bioavailability of the nutrients especially essential fatty acids, essential amino acids and vitamins along with enhancement of aroma, flavor, texture and appearance of the food products (Table 16.2). It also helps to conserve the energy used for cooking and destroys the anti-nutrients present in the raw material thus resulting in a safer product.[68]

There are numerous substrates and microorganisms involved in fermentation. However, the process of fermentation can be classified on the major end-product produced, such as: lactic acid fermentation, alcoholic fermentation, alkali fermentation and acetic acid fermentation. Lactic acid fermentation is carried out in the fermented milk and milk products, meat sausage, *gundruk, sinki,* etc., by lactic acid bacteria (LAB), where lactose is converted to lactic acid. Similarly, alcohol fermentation is carried out in cereal - based alcoholic beverages (such as: *toddy* and *kanji)* by yeast with production of ethanol from sugars. Whereas, acetic acid bacteria convert ethanol into acetic acid in certain soybean fermented products during acetic acid fermentation; and alkaline fermentation is carried out under alkaline conditions in certain soybean products.[7]

16.4.1   Fermented Foods Based on Cereals

Cereal-based fermented foods are consumed as staple foods that contribute maximum to the energy intake.[46] In cereal based fermented food, the substrate used is primarily cereals, such as rice, raggi, oats and wheat, etc. Enhancement of flavor, texture with improved digestibility and prolonged shelf-life are the main changes resulting from cereal fermentation.[99] The examples of important cereal-based local foods and beverages in India are: *idli,*[1,53,90,125,148,150,153,175,179] *dosa,*[12,45,115,148,153] *uttapam* and *adai,*[19] *dhokla/ khaman,*[5,12,57,115] *vada, zutho* or *zhichu,*[27,84] *selroti,*[25,85,165,185] *seera,*[165] *Bhatti jaanr* and *nigaar,*[162,163,174] *bhatooru,*[16,97,154] *Naan,*[19] *chhang* or *lugri,*[154] *haria* or *harhia,*[25] *yu,*[25,144] etc.

Dosa is reported to cure rheumatism and neural disorders.[45] Due to fermentation of the substrates, the net protein utilization and biological value is reported to improve in the *dhokla.*[5] Due to low glycemic index, *dhokla* is advised for consumption by diabetic patients, it also has potential to reduce blood cholesterols thus reduces the risk of cardiovascular disorders. *Seera* is advised to be consumed especially by individuals suffering from jaundice or hepatitis. Since, *bhaati jaanr* has high calorific value and is inexpensive, it is mainly consumed by post-natal women and ailing old people to gain strength and energy. *Haria or*

TABLE 16.2 Changes Occurring in Traditional Food and Beverages during Fermentation.

Parameter	Characteristics	Changes occurring in products
Acid production	Acidity increases, pH reduces.	Development of acidic flavor and sour taste. Protein denaturation leads to gelation.[63]
Change in texture	Texture changes due to denaturation of proteins.	Saccharification of starch softens the texture. Denaturation of protein results in gelation with increase in viscosity. Production of carbon dioxide and other gases imparts air in cells forming spongy texture.[111]
Enhanced protein digestibility	Improved bioavailability of amino acids and protein. Enhanced nutrient profile and protein utilization.	Increase in peptides and amino acids. Formation of free asparagine, cystine and histidine. Fermented milk products have enhanced protein digestibility. In cereals and pulses, fermentation promotes release of protein from matrix by partial degradation.[38]
Flavor development	Improves flavor profile and aesthetic property.	Diacetyl, acetaldehyde, acetoin, pungent ammoniacal flavor compounds are released that impart characteristic flavor.[186]
Production of anti-microbial compounds	Production of secondary metabolites, e.g., organic acids, alcohol, hydrogen peroxide, carbon dioxide, diacetyl and bacteriocins.	Organic acids inhibit bacteria, yeast and mold. Hydrogen peroxide inhibits growth of microorganisms especially in raw milk. Diacetyl controls gram-negative bacteria, yeasts and molds.[26] Bacteriocins inhibit Gram-positive bacteria.[140]

harhia is an ethno-pharmacological beverage.[25] During fermentation, the starch hydrolyzing enzymes and oligosaccharides sugars can enhance the antioxidant property of the *haria*.[25]

16.4.2   Legume-Based Products

Legumes contains complex sugars, such as, oligosaccharides, oligo-fructo-saccharides and anti- nutrient factors, which lead to allergic reactions and disorders. Fermentation of legumes neutralizes anti-nutrient compounds and improves the nutrient bioavailability of the food. The examples of important legume-based (black gram, soybean, etc.) local foods and beverages in India are: *vada*,[137] *maseura* or *masyaura* or *dhalbodi* or *sandige*,[21,22] *wari*,[46,148] *jalebi*,[18,20,148] *aakhone* or *axone*,[84,166] *bekang*,[21,22,168] *hawaija*,[56,65,144,166] *kinema*,[136,160,162] *peruyaan*,[14,144] and *tungrymbai*.[21,22,56]

As a result of fermentation, increase in amino nitrogen, non-protein nitrogen, soluble protein, riboflavin and thiamine is observed in *maseura*.[22] The fermented *wari* is observed with increase in total acids, soluble nitrogen, thiamine, riboflavin and cyanocobalamin.[148] The fermentation of soybean in *bekang* possesses high degree of hydrophobicity indicating probiotic property.[21] *Bekang* is known to have antioxidant and free radical scavenging capacity.[22] Due to high specificity for the production of fibrin by *Bacillus* sp., *hawaija* is rich in dietary fiber,[144] thus it helps to reduce cholesterol and digestive diseases. Fermentation of soybeans with only *B. subtilis* reduces the fermentation time, enhances the amount of soluble protein and results in *kinema* having pleasant nutty flavor with highly sticky texture.[158] *Tungrymbai* is known to have high amount of polyglutamic acid due to *B. subtilis* and probiotic property due to *Ent. faecium*. *Tungrymbai* also possesses antioxidant and free radical scavenging properties.[22]

16.4.3   Dairy-Based Products

The fermented milk and milk products are obtained by the inoculation and souring of milk using starter culture. Different microorganisms involving the group of lactic acid bacteria, *Leuconostoc*, probiotic bacteria and yeast are employed in the production of different types of fermented dairy products. Fermentation of milk results in change in appearance, flavor, texture and nutritional profile. However, the crucial role of starter culture lies in the production of bioactive peptides, essential amino acids, essential fatty acids, antioxidant molecules, anti-allergic and anti-hypertensive compounds. The examples of important local foods and beverages in India based on dairy are: *dahi*,[28,105,163] *misto doi* or *payodhi* or *lal dahi* or *lal doi*,[28,39,121] *shrikhand* or *amarkhand*, [49,64,72] *rabadi*,[45,66] *Lassi* or butter milk,[101,113] *chhach* or *majjige* or *matha*,[152] *chhurpi* or *chhursingba* or *chhur chirpen* or *chhurpupu*,[28,144,164] *chhu* or *sheden*,[28] *phuli*,[32,144] and *somar*,[28,163].

Since, the glycaemic index of pearl millet is low, *rabadi* aids in controlling blood sugar levels especially in people suffering with non- insulin dependent diabetes mellitus. The phytic acid content is reduced after fermentation of *rabadi*.[45] Addition of pearl millet to *rabadi* increases the bioavailability of minerals, enhances total soluble sugar, starch and protein digestibility by removal of antinutrient factors.[66] *Lassi* is found to have stimulant and anti-spasmodic properties that can reduce headache and rheumatism.[113] *Lassi* is considered as probiotic. *Lassi* contains bioactive components, such as, amino acids, peptides, vitamins and minerals that have immense therapeutic and nutritional importance and is used extensively in treating diarrhea, dysentery, chronic specific and nonspecific colitis, piles and jaundice.[101] *Chhach* is characterized by mild acidic flavor and sour taste.[152] *Somar* is reported to increase appetite and cure digestive disorders.[28]

16.4.4   *Products Based on Vegetables and Fruits*

Vegetables and fruits are perishable as it begins to deteriorate soon after harvesting hence, to enhance the shelf-life it is preserved by fermentation, drying or canning. During fermentation, initially the heterofermentative salt resistant lactic acid bacteria (*Leuconostoc* sp. and *Lactobacillus brevis)* predominates followed by homofermentative species (*L. plantarum* and *Pediococcus* sp.) with increase in acidity the yeast cells increase. Fermentation produces characteristic aroma, flavor and texture in the product by the conversion of sugars into acid, carbon dioxide and other metabolites. Preservation of vegetables depends on the reduction of enzyme activity, inhibition of oxidative changes and inhibition of growth of pathogenic microorganisms.[169] The examples of important local foods and beverages in India based on fruits and vegetables are: *sinki*,[55,159,164,168] *anishi*,[7,169] *goyang*,[160,168] *gundruk*,[160–163,168] *inziangsang* or *ziangsang*,[163,168] *khalpi*,[161,163] *kanji*,[58,155,167] *toddy* or *tari*[27,58].

The lactic acid bacteria present in *gundruk* are reported to remove anti-nutritional factors[162] and exhibit anti-microbial properties.[168]

16.4.5   Products Based on Meat and Fish

Lactic acid fermentation is involved in the preservation of meat and fish products,[10,11] using organisms, such as: *Lb. plantarum, Ped. acidilactici* and *Ped. pentosaceus.* Due to enzymatic changes that takes place during fermentation, the myofibrillar and sarcoplasmic proteins breakdown, salt soluble myofibrillar proteins are gellified and provide firm consistency and texture to the product with development of flavor compounds by the lipolytic activity of LAB.[89] The ethnic fermented fish products in India are mainly prepared by drying and smoking; and these exhibit anti-diabetic, anti-cancerous, and anti-oxidant properties, etc. For example, *hentak* is consumed by women during their final stages of pregnancy and by patients recovering from sickness or injury.[136] The examples of important local foods and beverages in India based on meat and fish are: *jamma,*[100,118] *arjia,*[100] *chartayshya,*[100,118] *honoheingrain,*[18] *kargyong,*[118] *satchu,*[118,119,158] *suka ka masu,*[118,119] *suka ko maccha,*[174] *nhari,*[56,97,172] *hentak,*[136,171,172] *gnuchi,*[174] *karati* or *Bordia* or *Lashim,*[172] *shidal,*[61,93–95,144] *sidra,*[174] *sukuti,*[172] and *tungtap.*[123,124,171,173]

16.5   THERAPEUTIC PROPERTIES OF INDIAN TRADITIONAL FERMENTED FOODS AND BEVERAGES

Fermentation initially aimed at food preservation resulting from reduction in water activity, reduction in pH and formation of metabolites having inhibitory effect, such as: organic acids, bacteriocins and ethanol. Development in technology has laid down the understanding on improved nutritional value, removal of toxic compounds, inhibition of pathogens, enhanced organoleptic, rheological properties with prolonged shelf-life.[7]

The Indian traditional foods have several health benefits and therapeutic properties by providing essential nutrients, bioactive molecules and health promoting compounds. The functional compounds responsible for therapeutic properties can be chemical or biological in nature that include: dietary fiber, antioxidants, vitamins and minerals, oligosaccharides, lignins, essential fatty acids, flavonoids, miscellaneous phytochemicals, and lactic acid bacterial cultures that are present in cereals, legumes, milk and milk products, fruits and vegetables, nuts, spices, and meat/ fish products.[152]

Therapeutic benefits of fermented foods and beverages include: Alleviation of lactose intolerance, alleviation in gastrointestinal disorders and IBS symptoms, anti-allergenicity, anti-hypertensive, anti-mutagenic, anti-oxidant, anti-thrombic, improvement in immune system, management of body weight, prevention of cardiovascular and hepatic diseases, prevention of diabetes, reduction in blood pressure, reduction in cholesterol content, reduction in different types of cancer, reduction in inflammatory diseases, reduction in neurodegenerative disorders, reduction in oxidative stress, and strengthening of skeletal tissues.

16.5.1 Prevention of Gastrointestinal Disorders and Inflammatory Bowel Diseases (IBD)

The probiotic microorganisms present in the fermented foods inhibit pathogenic microorganisms and aids in alleviation of digestive disorders, such as: antibiotic-associated diarrhea, infantile and traveler's diarrhea, bloating and abdominal pain.[85] It is also reported to reduce the symptoms including bloating, stool frequency and occurrence of irritable bowel syndrome (IBS).[135] The starter culture of fermented products mainly contributes to the alteration of microbial ecosystem in the gastrointestinal tract.[85]

The lactic acid bacteria in fermented food reduces the symptoms of inflammatory bowel diseases (IBD),[141] paucities and ulcerative colitis,[104] enhances the intestinal mobility and reduces gastrointestinal tract pH that aids in relieving constipation.[133] Crohn's disease can be effectively prevented by the modification of intestinal microflora. Certain species of lactic acid bacteria (such as: *Lb. plantarum*, *Lb. rhamnosus*) and yeast (such as: *S. boulardii*) help to reduce diarrhea,[1,85,156] bloating, abdominal pain, flatulence and constipation in people suffering from IBS[82] and inflammatory disorders (such as: atopic dermatitis and IBD).[81]

16.5.2 Prevention of Hepatic Disease

Hepatic disease (also called hepatic encephalopathy) is a life - threatening situation of liver disease.[23] The probiotic microorganisms (such as: *Lb.*

acidophilus, Lb. plantarum, Bifidobacteria sp., *Lb. casei, Lb. delbrueckii var bulgaricus, St. thermophilus* and *Ent. faecum*) present in fermented food and milk products have the ability to disrupt the pathogenesis occurring in liver along with reducing the risk of bleeding by lowering the portal pressure due to the enzymatic action and metabolic products produced during fermentation.[141,145]

16.5.3 Protection from Allergic Reactions

The probiotic microorganisms improve the gut microflora in the body thus reducing certain infections and allergies of urogenital tract.[35] Fermented soya-products inhibit angiotensin I- converting enzyme that affects hypo-allergenicity and anti-allergic activity.[65] Heat inactivated probiotic strain of *Lactobacillus* exhibits antiallergic effect on ovalbumin sensitized reactions.[50] Probiotic microorganisms help in enhancing mucosal barrier, which functions to modulate and to reduce the allergic reactions by microbial stimulation of the immune system.[82] The exo-polysaccharide produced in the sourdough by fermentation with *Lb. animalis, Lb. reuteri* and *Lb. curvatus* acts as hydrocolloid and help in carrying out natural fermentation of gluten-free dough thus reducing the severity of celiac conditions.[131,132]

The casein complex formed during fermentation of milk increases lactose tolerance by reducing the allergic reactions in the gastro-intestinal digestion.[4] Fermented soybean exhibits anti-allergic effect against atopic dermatitis by decreasing the allergic responses, such as: ear thickness, dermis thickness, auricular lymph node and infiltering mast cells.[79] Fermented vegetables containing *Lactobacillus* reduce atopic dermatitis and food allergy.[182] The omega fatty acids in fermented milk and fish products reduce antiallergic effects including reduced sensitization to allergens and alleviation of symptoms of atopic dermatitis, eczema and asthma.[47]

16.5.4 Synthesis of Nutrients and Bioavailability

The nutritional quality of fermented food is comparatively high than that of unfermented food. The nutritional profile can be enhanced by nutrient synthesis, enhancement of bioavailability and by enzymatic breakdown of complex compounds by the starter culture. In the fermented food, the nutrient components in the cells as complex and indigestible compounds are liberated during the fermentation process especially in cereals, grains and seeds.

Physicochemical and enzymatic breakdown of cellulose, hemicellulose and other indigestible polymers are converted into simpler sugars and their derivatives. The nutrient quality and bioavailability and digestibility of cereals are reported to be enhanced by lactic acid bacteria and yeast fermentation. Thus, fermentation reduces the amount of antinutrient factors, such as phytic acid, saponins, tannins, proteinase inhibitors (such as: trypsin inhibitors and chymotrypsin inhibitors) leading to improved bioavailability of simple sugars, proteins and minerals (such as: iron, magnesium).[48]

The probiotic organisms in the fermented food can improve the bioavailability of the minerals by hydrolysis of phytates, biofortification of folates and detoxification of mycotoxins by binding to the surface of cell-wall of the yeast. Fermentation by yeast is reported to cause enrichment of food with prebiotics, such as: fructo-oligosaccharides.[86] It is reported to lower blood serum cholesterol by forming high density lipids[114]; and exhibits antioxidative, antimutagenic and antitumor properties[70].

The essential cofactor involved in the biosynthesis of nucleotides is folate or vitamin B9 that are crucial for cellular replication and growth. *S. cerevisiae* produces high amount of folate per weight and is regarded as the rich dietary source of native folate.[107] The mesophilic LAB cultures (such as: *Lactobacillus, Leuconostoc, Pediococcus, Carnobacterium, Enterococcus, Streptococcus, Oenococcus, Tetragenococcus, Vagococcus, and Weissella*[34]) especially *Lactococcus* spp. are able to produce vitamin-K by metabolization.[83] Fermentation also enhances the bioavailability of vitamin B12 10-folds that helps in the formation and functioning of nervous system and formation of blood cells.[188]

16.5.5   *Prevention of Cardiovascular Disease (CVD)*

Consumption of fiber rich food with low amount of fats especially saturated fat reduces the risk of CVD, and low intake of antioxidants and vitamins especially vitamin E also reduces the risk of CVD.[129,130] The lactic acid bacteria especially probiotic strains in fermented milk lowers the blood serum cholesterol from 3.0 to 1.5 g/L in hypercholesterolemic individuals.[2] Fermented grain products have high potential to reduce the

LDL and increase the HDL in blood serum, reduction of hypertension, obesity, inflammation, hyperhomo-cysteinemia, vascular reactivity and coronary heart disease (CHD), diabetes by reducing insulin resistance, enhances antioxidant property.[6,8]

Increase in nutrient bioavailability, improvement in digestibility and assimilation and reduction in cholesterol level of blood by inhibition of hydroxy-methylglutaryl coenzyme-A reductase, which is the key enzyme responsible for cholesterol biosynthesis during fermentation from linoleic acid and oleic acid,[130] is achieved by consumption of fermented soybean products.[78,79] The phytosterols produced during fermentation of *kinema* reduce cholesterol thereby reducing the risk of CVD.[65,136]

16.5.6 Anti-Mutagenic Property

It has been reported through animal studies that the lactic acid bacteria especially *Lactococcus acidophilus* in *dahi* and other fermented milk exhibit anti-mutagenic property either by preventing initiation of cancer or by suppressing the initiated cancer. The anti-mutagenic property has been reported due to changes caused in the fecal enzymes that are responsible for the cause of colon carcinogenesis, uptake of mutagenic compounds by cells and aids in reduction of mutagenesis due to chemical mutagens and helps to suppress the tumors by improving the immune system.[51]

16.5.7 Anti-Thrombic Property

Thrombosis is the condition of blood clot formation within a blood vessel that prevents normal flow of blood through the circulatory system. Blood clot in humans is carried out by more than 20 different enzymes, whereas plasmin is the only enzyme that interrupts the formation of blood clot.[88] Food products with high LDL content are known to cause clots and form plaques by deposition in blood vessels that blocks the blood supply and might lead to chest pain and heart attack; hence, consumption of fermented products reduces the accumulation of LDL in the blood vessels. Similarly, accumulation of fibrin in blood vessels reduces the flow of blood thereby increasing the viscosity of blood, which builds up the pressure in the vessels leading to myocardial infarction and other cardiovascular diseases.[88] Therefore to prevent thrombosis, consumption of fermented food as a source of fibrinolytic enzymes[145] or fibrinolytic enzymes isolated from starter culture used in fermented food is advised.[88,145]

16.5.8 Anti-Oxidant Property

The process of oxidation produces free radicals that damage the cell membrane, cell structures including cellular proteins, lipids and DNA. The free radicals can be neutralized to some extent by cellular phospholipids, further production of free radicals' overloads in the cells and causes certain diseases including cardiovascular disease, liver disease, oral cancer, esophageal cancer, gastric cancer and bowel cancer. Oxidation is accelerated by stress, cigarette smoking, alcohol consumption and exposure to pollution. The enzyme system, such as, catalase, glutathione peroxidase, superoxide dismutase and non-enzymatic antioxidants comprising of vitamin C, tocopherols, carotenoids and phenolic compounds help to prevent cells from oxidative damage.[57]

The fermented dairy products have high antioxidant activity due to release of bioactive peptides (such as: lactalbumin, lactoglobulin and caseins) as a result of proteolytic activity during the fermentation.[32,109,171] The antioxidant activity in the cultured dairy products is mainly dependent on the origin of milk, fat content of milk, presence and position of amino acids (especially tryptophan, tyrosine, and methionine) and microorganisms used for fermentation.[32] The antioxidant activity of fermented milk is also enhanced by the formation of conjugated linoleic acid (CLA) along with vitamin A and vitamin E during fermentation.[43] Biosynthesis of folates by starter microorganisms (especially *St. thermophilus*, *L. hirci-lactis* and *L. laudensis*[177]) involves antioxidant and free radical scavenging mechanisms.[76]

The high antioxidant activity of the sourdough-based bakery products is mainly due to formation of phenolic compounds, organic acids (ferulic acid), gamma amino butyric acid (GABA), and bioactive peptides. The total phenolic content is found to increase in wholegrain and barley by fermentation with lactic acid bacteria[49] (such as: *P. pentosaceus*, *Lb. paracasei*, *Lb. rhamnosus and S. cerevisiae*) in fermented grains.[29,127] The sourdough prepared using wheat, barley, chickpea, legume, rye and quinoa fermented with *Lb. brevis*, *Lb. plantarum*, *Lb. reuteri*, *Lb. rossiae*, *Lb. sanfranciscensis and Leu. mesenteroides* exhibits higher antioxidant property due to high GABA and small peptide contents.[41,89,128] The antioxidant activity in fruits and vegetables is mainly due to bioactive compounds from phenolics that are released after fermentation.[139]

Fermentation of meat and fish products releases bioactive peptides with antioxidant property.[183] Consumption of dry-cured meat products fermented with lactic acid bacteria results in formation of peptides with antiradical properties during gastrointestinal digestion.[60] The sausage fermented with *Bifidobacterium longum* exhibits lowest lipid oxidation, formation of high content of total unsaturated fatty acids (especially omega-3 and omega-6 fatty acids).[147] Hence, fermented food products can be used as a source of antioxidants and as an alternate to synthetic antioxidants.

16.5.9   Alleviation of Lactose Intolerance

The condition of inability to digest lactose in certain individuals is termed as lactose intolerance, which is mainly due to the deficiency in production of enzyme lactase or β- galactosidase. In individuals lacking sufficient production of lactase enzyme in the small intestine, consumption of lactose results in several abdominal symptoms, such as: diarrhea, bloating, abdominal pain and flatulence.[103] Milk inoculated with lactic acid bacteria (such as: *Lactococcus, Lactobacillus, Streptococcus, Pediococcus* and *Leuconostoc*) hydrolyses lactose to glucose and galactose during the process of fermentation; therefore, it reduces the symptoms of lactose indigestion and also helps to digest the milk sugar (lactose) by lactose intolerant person.[30]

16.5.10   Increase in Immunity

It is reported that consumption of fermented foods containing lactic acid bacteria or probiotic bacteria (especially: *Lb. bulgaricus, Lb. acidophilus, S. thermophilus* and *Bifi. bifidum*) inhibits the colonization and proliferation of pathogens or suppresses the effect of toxins released by them, hence, preventing the manifestation of infection.[102] Inhibition of proliferation of pathogenic organisms is the beneficial effect of lactic acid bacteria that are present in fermented or cultured milk products; and it is attributed to the production of antibacterial compounds from starter culture. Hence, consumption of live probiotic bacteria brings about immunomodulation in the body thereby enhancing the capacity of immune system.[35]

16.5.11 Antihypertensive Property

The peptides formed during fermentation due to enzymatic breakdown by metabolic enzymes or by proteinases of *Lactobacilli* are reported to have antihypertensive activity by lowering blood pressure.[54] The antihypertensive property is due to the inhibition of Angiotensin-Converting enzyme (ACE) that regulates the blood pressure through Renin-Angiotensin System (RAS). Lactic acid bacteria and certain strains of probiotic strains (such as: *L. lactis, Lb. plantarum*) are identified with antihypertensive effect.[14,15,128,129] The GABA produced by *St. salivarius* subsp. *thermophilus* also aids in antihypertensive benefits.[98]

Sourdough fermentation releases free amino acids and amino acid derivatives that impart flavor and taste to bakery products as a result of which the sodium content is reduced by reducing the amount of salt added in the bakery products, hence, functions as antihypertensive.[40] The proteolytic activity carried out by lactic acid bacteria during fermentation of sourdough transforms matrix proteins of cereal into bioactive peptides that are functional antihypertensive compounds.[108]

16.6 MARKET SIZE AND FORECAST GROWTH OF INDIAN TRADITIONAL FERMENTED FOOD AND BEVERAGES

The fermented food market is estimated to increase due to inclination of consumers towards the use of fermented foods with increase in health awareness. As fermented food plays an important role to maintain gastrointestinal health, to increase immunity and several health benefits, it is explored by consumers as prevention of several diseases related to digestive system, cardiovascular and defense mechanism.

To meet the existing and future consumer demand several technological and packaging innovations are being made for continuous production, easy storage and distribution with prolonged shelf-life. Owing to the increased demand for fermented foods and beverages, the market is estimated to increase at a rate of 4.98% through 2023. The growth in market for consumption of traditional food and beverages in India is increasing thus providing a promising processing line for manufacturers and suppliers.[189]

Although the production of traditional fermented food and beverages is majorly confined to domestic level, yet recent commercial production has paved the way for expansion of market. With wide spread benefits acquired by consuming traditional food products, the market growth is also foreseen in foreign regions thus emphasizing on the increased production.[189]

16.7 TECHNOLOGICAL ADVANCES IN PRODUCTION OF INDIAN TRADITIONAL FERMENTED FOODS AND BEVERAGES

The traditional fermented foods and beverages are mostly prepared at domestic level in small quantities or batches. Due to the benefits incurred by consumption of fermented food products and beverages, the demand for the ethnic fermented products are increasing constantly; hence to reach the market demand, commercial production has to be adopted.

Idli and *dosa* are incorporated with millets to enhance the dietary fiber and bioavailability of nutrients. Various spices and herbs can be added to improve the shelf-life of *idli* batter by antimicrobial property and to improve the nutritional and organoleptic properties.[45] Probiotic culture is also added to improve the nutritional and therapeutic properties of batter. Continuous *idli* and *dosa* batter are prepared by mechanized equipment with automated sensors and controls to monitor the soaking, grinding and fermenting parameters (such as: time, temperature, pressure and particle size). The fermented batter will be dispensed into the packaging pouch using gravity filler. *Idli* is prepared by mechanical filling of batter into suitable trays and cooking in preheated oven for specific period of time. Similarly, *vada* is prepared by dispensing the batter in the shape of rings into hot oil, where agitators flip the sides to allow uniform frying, and excess oil will be removed by scrubbers and finally *vada* is stacked on trays.

The antioxidant activity of fermented milk products is enhanced by subjecting milk to ultrasound treatment before fermentation, as ultrasonication increases lactose hydrolysis by carbohydrate metabolism, propagation ability of viable cells; thus releases more antioxidant components.[37] *Dahi* is incorporated with certain probiotic strains of bacteria to exhibit therapeutic properties.[136]

The fermented milk beverages are incorporated with dietary fiber to replace the fat content; similarly, soya solids are used along with milk solids in *misti doi*. Milk used for *dahi* or *misti doi* or *shrikhand* preparation is concentrated by vacuum concentration[77] or by membrane processing.[74] Butter milk is obtained from sweet cream,[64] condensed skim milk[73] is added to increase the total solids in the milk prior to the inoculation of starter to enhance the rheological properties. *Lassi*, buttermilk is sterilized using either batch sterilizer or continuous sterilizer or UHT treated followed by aseptic packaging to enhance the shelf-life.

Initially, only pork, beef and veal were used in the preparation of sausage, which recently includes camel meat, poultry meat, venison and mixed meat. The traditional casings made from animal intestine is being replaced by composite casing made with synthetic material or casein having good printability and heat saleability. The natural and edible casings can also be infused with different flavors to improve the palatability of the product, antimicrobial compounds to enhance the shelf-life along with the inhibition of pathogenic microorganisms.[3]

Liquid casing made from sodium alginate is applied especially on the surface of sausage intended for smoking. Sausages are incorporated with dietary fibers from wheat, oats, soya to replace the fat content and to aid in fiber fortification.[187] Humidity monitoring and controlling devices are used in the manufacture of dry sausages. They are included with probiotic bacteria that are protected by microencapsulation in alginate to maintain the viability against processing conditions.[10,92]

Proteolytic enzymes are being incorporated along with calpains, cathepsins and peptidases[177] during meat processing that produces peptides and free amino acids to provide antihypertensive, antioxidant and anti-microbial activities.[11] Due to adoption of continuous sausage production, there is a sharp increase in product integrity, particle definition, texture and yield with the help of vacuum pumps, inline grinding, automatic hanging devices and product flow controls.[3]

16.8　INNOVATIONS IN PACKAGING AND DISTRIBUTION OF INDIAN TRADITIONAL FERMENTED FOOD AND BEVERAGES

Packaging plays a major role for protection, storage and distribution of food products. They also aid in the preservation of food by preventing contamination and spoilage, and can be used as a marketing tool by using proper techniques and temporal dimension for providing identification, information and instruction.[91]

The *idli* or *dosa* batter is packed in high density polyethylene, low density polyethylene or high molecular poly propylene laminates coupled with modified atmosphere packaging (MAP). *Dhokla* is packed in polyethylene pouch, polypropylene or polystyrene cups and sealed with EVOH and cardboard laminated with aluminum foil. The fermented soybean products (such as: *kinema, tungrymbai, bekang*, etc.) are packed in polyethylene bags, LDPE pouches, polystyrene foam tubs. *Dahi* is packed in LDPE or HDPE foil, polystyrene or high intensity polystyrene cups, polypropylene cups sealed with aluminum foil-based peelable lids; whereas *misti doi* and *shrikhand* is packed in polystyrene or HIPS cups or polypropylene and polyethylene bags or cardboard boxes lined with glassine paper, although it is also distributed in earthen pots. *Lassi, buttermilk, chaach* or *majjige* is packed in LDPE pouch or PVC lined HDPE pouch, if pasteurized and laminated pouches are sterilized or UHT treated in case of Tetrapak.[136]

The fermented vegetables and fruits are usually packed in glass jars or laminated polyethylene pouch or metalized polyester pouches.

The fermented meat products are packed in synthetic casing made with casein or polyethylene and are vacuum sealed for prolonged storage. Fermented fish products are packaged in wooden boxes, glass jars, and polyethylene pouches. Intelligent packaging aids to detect and display the acidity, pH, gas content and enzyme concentration in the product can be mounted on the packaging material. The shelf-life and the aesthetic properties of the food products can be enhanced by infusion of antimicrobial agents, enzyme inhibitors, natural or synthetic microbial preservatives, buffers to maintain equilibrium and gas absorbers or emitters for O_2 and CO_2 scrubbing depending on the product requirement.[48]

16.9 SUMMARY

Traditional foods and beverages in India provide several health benefits and nutrition. Fermentation of different substrates yields product with differing sensory profile, nutritional quality and shelf-life. The starter culture involved in the fermentation brings the characteristic changes in the product (such as: acid production, gas formation, textural changes, etc.). Due to several health benefits resulting from the consumption of fermented foods, it is widely accepted by the consumers and demand for the same is increasing as a result of which efforts are being made for technical and packaging innovations.

KEYWORDS

- bioavailability
- fermentation
- food and beverages
- food processing
- Indian traditional food and beverages
- therapeutic properties

REFERENCES

1. Agarwal, K. N.; Bhasin, S. K. Feasibility Studies to Control Acute Diarrhoea in Children by Feeding Fermented Milk Preparations Actimel and Indian *Dahi*. *Eur. J. Clin. Nutr.* **2002**, *56*, 56–59.
2. Agerholm-Larsen, L.; Raben, A.; Haulrik, N.; Hansen, A. S.; Manders, M.; Astrup, A. Effect of 8 Week Intake of Probiotic Milk Products on Risk Factors for Cardiovascular Diseases. *Eur. J. Clin. Nutr.* **2000**, *54* (4), 288–292.
3. Akpan, I. P.; Hugo, C. J.; Hugo, A. Current Trends in Natural Preservatives for Fresh Sausage Products. *Trends Food Sci. Technol.* **2017**, *45* (1), 12–23.
4. Alessandri, C.; Sforza, S.; Palazzo, P.; Lambertini, F.; Paolella, S.; Zennaro, D. Tolerability of a Fully Matured Cheese in Cow's Milk Allergic Children: Biochemical, Immunochemical and Clinical Aspects. *Public Libr. Sci. One* **2012**, *7* (1), 40–42.
5. Aliya, S.; Geervani, P. An Assessment of the Protein Quality and Vitamin B Content of Commonly Used Fermented Products of Legumes and Millets. *J. Sci. Food Agric.* **1981**, *32* (8), 837–842.
6. Ameli, S.; Hultgårdh-Nilsson, A. Effect of Immunization with Homologous LDL and Oxidized LDL on Early Atherosclerosis in Hypercholesterolemic Rabbits. *Arteriosclerosis Thrombosis Vasc. Biol.* **1996**, *16* (8), 1074–1079.
7. Anal, A. K. Quality Ingredients and Safety Concerns for Traditional Fermented Foods and Beverages from Asia: A Review. *Fermentation* **2019**, *5* (1), 8–14.
8. Anderson, M.; Bermüdez-Humarán, L. G. Lactic Acid Bacteria as Live Vectors: Heterologous Protein Production and Delivery Systems. In *Biotechnology of Lactic Acid Bacteria Novel Applications*; Mozzi, F., Raya, R. R., Vignolo, G. M., Eds., Vol. 12; Blackwell Publishing: New Jersey, USA, 2010; pp 125–180.
9. Antunes, A. E. C.; Grael, E. T., Moreno, I. Selective Enumeration and Viability of *Bifidobacterium animalis* subsp. *Lactis* in a New Fermented Milk Product. *Braz. J. Microbiol.* **2007**, *38* (1), 173–177.
10. Arihara, K. Strategies for Designing Novel Functional Meat Products. *Meat Sci.* **2006**, *74* (1), 219–229.

11. Arihara, K.; Ohata, M. (Eds.) *Functional Meat Products*; Wiley-Blackwell: New Jersey, USA, 2010; pp 423–439.

12. Battacharya, S.; Bhat, K. K. Steady Shear Rheology of Rice - Black Gram Suspension and Suitability of Rheological Models. *J. Food Eng.* **1997**, *32* (2), 241–250.

13. Battcock, M.; Azam-Ali, S. *Fermented Fruits and Vegetables: A Global Perspective.* FAO Agricultural Services Bulletin; Food and Agriculture Organization of the United Nations: Rome, 2001; p 134.

14. Beltrán-Barrientos, L. M.; González-Córdova, A. F. Randomized Double-blind Controlled Clinical Trial of the Blood Pressure-lowering Effect of Fermented Milk with *Lactococcus lactis*: A Pilot Study. *J. Dairy Sci.* **2018**, *101*, 2819–2825.

15. Beltrán-Barrientos, L. M.; Hernández-Mendoza, A.; González-Córdova, A. F.; Astiazarán-García, H.; Esparza-Romero, J.; Vallejo-Córdoba, B. Mechanistic Pathways Underlying the Antihypertensive Effect of Fermented Milk with *Lactococcus lactis* NRRL B-50571 in Spontaneously Hypertensive Rats. *Nutrients* **2018**, *10*, 262–274.

16. Bhalla, T. C. Traditional foods and beverages of Himachal Pradesh. *Ind. J. Trad. Knowledge* **2007**, 17–24.

17. Çabuk, B.; Nosworthy, M. G. Effect of Fermentation on the Protein Digestibility and Levels of Non-Nutritive Compounds of Pea Protein Concentrate. *Food Technol. Biotechnol.* **2018**, *56* (2), 257–263.

18. Chakkaravarthi, A.; Kumar, H. P.; Suvendu, B. *Jilebi*: Effect of Moisture Content, Curd Addition and Fermentation Time on the Rheological Properties of Dispersions. *J. Food Sci. Technol.* **2009**, *46* (6), 543–548.

19. Chavan, J. K.; Kadam, S. S.; Beuchat, L. R. Nutritional Improvement of Cereals by Fermentation. *Crit. Rev. Food Sci. Nutr.* **1989**, *28* (5), 349–400.

20. Chelule, P. K.; Mokoena, M. P.; Gqaleni, N. Advantages of Traditional Lactic Acid Bacteria Fermentation of Food in Africa. *Curr. Res. Technol. Educ. Topics Appl. Microbiol. Microb. Biotechnol.* **2010**, *2*, 1160–1167.

21. Chettri, R.; Tamang, J. P. *Bacillus* species Isolated from Naturally Fermented Soybean Foods of India. *Int. J. Food Microbiol.* **2015**, *197*, 72–76.

22. Chettri, R.; Tamang, J. P. Functional Properties of Naturally Fermented Soybean Foods of India. *Int. J. Food Microb.* **2014**, *3* (3), 87–103.

23. Cunningham-Rundles, S.; Ahrne, S. Dunn. Probiotics and Immune Response. *Am. J. Gastroenterol.* **2000**, *95*, 22–25.

24. Cusano, E.; Simonato, B.; Consonni, R. Fermentation Process of Apple Juice Investigated by NMR Spectroscopy. *LWT Food Sci. Technol.* **2018**, *96*, 147–151.

25. Das, A.; Raychaudhuri, U.; Chakraborty, R. Cereal Based Functional Food of Indian Subcontinent: A Review. *J. Food Sci. Technol.* **2012**, *49* (6), 665–672.

26. de Bok, F. A.; Janssen, P. W. Volatile Compound Fingerprinting of Mixed-Culture Fermentations. *Appl. Environ. Microbiol.* **2011**, *77* (17), 6233–6239.

27. Deka S. C. Review on Fermented Foods and Beverages of the North-East India. *Int. Food Res. J.* **2012**, *19*, 377–392.

28. Dewan, S.; Tamang, J. P. Dominant Lactic Acid Bacteria and their Technological Properties Isolated from the Himalayan Ethnic Fermented Milk Products. *Antonie van Leeuwenhoek* **2007**, *92* (3), 343–352.

29. Dordević, T. M.; Šiler-Marinković, S. S.; Dimitrijević-Branković, S. I. Effect of Fermentation on Antioxidant Properties of Some Cereals and Pseudo Cereals. *Food Chem.* **2010**, *119*, 957–963.

30. Ebringer, L.; Ferenčík, M.; Krajčovič, J. Beneficial Health Effects of Milk and Fermented Dairy Products. *Folia Microbiol.* **2008**, *53* (5), 378–394.

31. Fardet, A.; Rock, E. *In vitro* and *in vivo* Antioxidant Potential of Milks, Yoghurts, Fermented Milks and Cheeses: Narrative Review of Evidence. *Nutr. Res. Rev.. Food Technol. Biotechnol.* **2018**, 56, 257–264.

32. Fardet, A.; Rock, E.; Rémésy, C. Is the *in-vitro* Antioxidant Potential of Whole-Grain Cereals and Cereal Products Well Reflected in-vivo? *J. Cereal Sci.* **2008**, *48* (2), 258–276.

33. Farnworth, E. R. T. (Eds.) *Handbook of Fermented Functional Foods*; CRC Press: Boca Raton, FL, 2018; pp 52–70.

34. Fu, X.; Harshman, S. G.; Shen, X. Multiple Vitamin K Forms Exist in Dairy Foods. *Curr. Dev. Nutr.* **2017**, *1* (6), 6–8.

35. Galdeano, C. M.; Perdigon, G. Probiotic Bacterium *Lactobacillus casei* Induces Activation of the Gut Mucosal Immune System through Innate Immunity. *Clin. Vaccine Immunol.* **2006**, *13*, 219–226.

36. Galli, V.; Mazzoli, L.; Luti, S. Effect of Selected Strains of Lactobacilli on the Antioxidant and Anti-inflammatory Properties of Sourdough. *Int. J. Food Microbiol.* **2018**, *286*, 55–65.

37. Gholamhosseinpour, A.; Hashemi, S. M. B. Ultrasound Pre- treatment of Fermented Milk Containing Probiotic *Lactobacillus plantarum* AF1: Carbohydrate Metabolism and Antioxidant Activity. *J. Food Process Eng.* **2019**, *42* (1), 12–30.

38. Ghosh, D.; Chattoraj, D. K.; Chattopadhyay, P. Studies on Changes in Microstructure and Proteolysis in Cow and Soy Milk Curd During Fermentation Using Lactic Cultures for Improving Protein Bioavailability. *J. Food Sci. Technol.* **2013**, *50*, 979–985.

39. Ghosh, J.; Rajorhia, G. S. Technology for Production of *Mishti Doi:* A Traditional Fermented Milk Product. *Ind. J. Diary Sci.* **2015**, *43* (2), 239–246.

40. Gobbetti, M.; De Angelis, M.; Di Cagno, R. Novel Insights on the Functional/ Nutritional Features of the Sourdough Fermentation. *Int. J. Food Microbiol.* **2018**, 4–12.

41. Gobbetti, M.; Rizzello, C. G.; Di Cagno, R.; De Angelis, M. How the Sourdough May Affect the Functional Features of Leavened Baked Goods. *Food Microbiol.* **2014**, *37*, 30–40.

42. Gode, P. K. Some Notes on the History of Indian Dietetics with Special Reference to the History of *Jalebi. New Ind. Antiques* **1943**, *6*, 169–181.

43. Grażyna, C.; Hanna, C.; Adam, A.; Magdalena, B. M. Natural Antioxidants in Milk and Dairy Products. *Int. J. Diary Technol.* **2017**, *70* (2), 165–178.

44. Gregory III, J. F. (Eds.). *Chemical and Nutritional Aspects of Folate Research: Analytical Procedures, Methods of Folate Synthesis, Stability and Bioavailability of Dietary Folates. Advances in Food and Nutrition Research Series*, Vol. 33; Academic Press: Cambridge, MA, 1989; pp 1–101.

45. Gupta, E.; Dubey, R. P. Formulation and Nutritional Composition of Value Added *Idli* Prepared Using Selected Dried Herbs. *Int. J. Curr. Res. Rev.* **2011**, *3* (10), 93–98.

46. Guyot, J. P. Cereal-Based Fermented Foods in Developing Countries: Ancient Foods for Modern Research. *Int. J. Food Sci. Technol.* **2012,** *47* (6), 1109–1114.
47. Han, S.; Kang, G.; Ko, Y.; Kang, H.; Moon, S.; Ann, Y.; E. Yoo. Fermented Fish Oil Suppresses T-Helper 1/2 Cell Response in a Mouse Model of Atopic Dermatitis via Generation of CD4+CD25+Foxp3+ T Cells. *BMC Immunol.* **2012,** *13,* 44–49.
48. Hasan, M. N.; Sultan, M. Z.; Mar-E-Um, M. Significance of Fermented Food in Nutrition and Food Science. *J. Sci. Res.* **2014,** *6* (2), 373–386.
49. Hole, A. S.; Rud, I.; Grimmer, S.; Sigl, S.; Narvhus, J.; Sahlstrøm, S. Improved Bioavailability of Dietary Phenolic Acids in Whole Grain Barley and Oat Groat Following Fermentation with Probiotic *Lactobacillus acidophilus*, *Lactobacillus johnsonii*, and *Lactobacillus reuteri*. *J. Agric. Food Chem.* **2012,** *60,* 6369–6375.
50. Hong, W.; Chen, Y. The Antiallergic Effect of Kefir *Lactobacilli*. *J. Food Sci.* **2010,** *75* (8), 244–253.
51. Hosono, A.; Kashina, T.; Kada, T. Antimutagenic Properties of Lactic Acid-Cultured Milk on Chemical and Fecal Mutagens. *J. Dairy Sci.* **1986,** *69* (9), 2237–2242.
52. Iyengar, S. H. *Lokopakara of Chavundarava* (Chavundarva of Lokopkar). *Madras–India: Orient. Manuscripts Libr.* **1950,** *2* (15), 20–26.
53. Iyer, B. K.; Singhal, R. S.; Ananthanarayan, L. Characterization and in Vitro Probiotic Evaluation of Lactic Acid Bacteria Isolated from *Idli* Batter. *J. Food Sci. Technol.* **2013,** *50,* 1114–1121.
54. Jauhiainen, T.; Korpela, R. Milk Peptides and Blood Pressure. *J. Nutr.* **2007,** *137,* 825–829.
55. Jeyaram, K.; Mohendro Singh, W. Molecular Identification of Dominant Microflora Associated with *Hawaijar*: A Traditional Fermented Soybean (*Glycine Max* (L.)) Food of Manipur, India. *Int. J. Food Microbiol.* **2008,** 22, 259–268.
56. Jeyaram, K.; Mohendro Singh, W. Molecular Identification of Dominant Microflora Associated with *Hawaijar*: Traditional Fermented Soybean (*Glycine max* L.) Food of Manipur, India. *Int. J. Food Microbiol.* **2008,** *122,* 259–268.
57. Joshi, S. C.; Jain, P. K. Review on Hypolipidemic and Antioxidant Potential of Some Medicinal Plants. *World J. Pharm. Pharma. Sci.* **2014,** *3,* 357–80.
58. Joshi, S.; Biswas, K. Antioxidants in Fermented Foods. Chapter 3; In *Health Benefits of Fermented Foods and Beverages*; Tamang, J. P., Ed.; CRC Press: Boca Raton – FL, 2015; pp 553–565.
59. Kadiri, O. Review on the Status of the Phenolic Compounds and Antioxidant Capacity of the Flour: Effects of Cereal Processing. *Int. J. Food Prop.* **2017,** *2* (1), 798–809.
60. Kaeska, P.; Stadnik, J. Stability of Antiradical Activity of Protein Extracts and Hydrolysates from Dry-Cured Pork Loins with Probiotic Strains of LAB. *Nutrients* **2018,** *10,* 521.
61. Kakati, B. K.; Goswami, U. C. Microorganisms and the Nutritive Value of Traditional Fermented Fish Products of Northeast India. *Global J. Biosci. Biotechnol.* **2013,** *2* (1), 124–127.
62. Kaprasob, R.; Kerdchoechuen, O. Changes in Physicochemical, Astringency, Volatile Compounds and Antioxidant Activity of Fresh and Concentrated Cashew Apple Juice Fermented with *Lactobacillus plantarum*. *J. Food Sci. Technol.* **2018,** *55,* 3979–3990.
63. Karovičová, J.; Kohajdová, Z. Lactic Acid Fermentation of Various Vegetable Juices. *Acta Aliment.* **2005,** *34* (3), 237–246.

64. Karthikeyan, S.; Desai, H. K.; Upadhyay, K. G. Storage Changes of *Shrikhand* as Influenced by Level of Total Solids in Sweet Cream Butter Milk. *Ind. J. Dairy Biotechnol. Sci.* **2001,** *12,* 38–44.

65. Keishing, S.; Banu, A. T. *Hawaijar*: Fermented Soya of Manipur, India. *IOSR-J. Environ. Sci. Toxicol. Food Technol.* **2013,** *4* (2), 29–33.

66. Khetarpaul, N.; Chauhan, B. M. Effects of Germination and Pure Culture Fermentation by Yeasts and *Lactobacilli* on Phytic Acid and Polyphenol Content of Pearl Millet. *J. Food Sci.* **1990,** *55* (4), 1180–1180.

67. Kingston, J. J.; Radhika, M.; Roshini, P. T. Molecular Characterization of Lactic Acid Bacteria Recovered from Natural Fermentation of Beet Root and Carrot Kanji. *Ind. J. Microbiol.* **2010,** *50,* 292–298.

68. Kitts, D. D.; Weiler, K. Bioactive Proteins and Peptides from Food Sources: Applications of Bioprocesses used in Isolation and Recovery. *Curr. Pharma. Design* **2003,** *9* (16), 1309–1323.

69. Klimek, M.; Wang, S.; Ogunkanmi, A. Safety and Efficacy of Red Yeast Rice (*Monascus Purpureus*) as an Alternative Therapy for Hyperlipidemia. *Pharm. Therap.* **2009,** *34* (6), 313–318.

70. Kogani, G.; Pajtinka, M. Yeast Cell Wall Polysaccharides as Antioxidants and Antimutagens: Can They Fight Cancer? *Neoplasma* **2008,** *55* (5), 387–392.

71. Kourelis, A.; Kotzamanidis, C. Preliminary Probiotic Selection of Dairy and Human Yeast Strains. *J. Biol. Res.* **2010,** *13,* 93–99.

72. Kulkarni, C.; Belsare, N.; Lele, A. Studies on *Shrikhand* Rheology. *J. Food Eng.* **2006,** *74* (2), 169–177.

73. Kumar, A.; Solanky, M. J.; Chauhan, A. K. Storage Related Lipolysis Changes in *Lassi. Ind. J. Diary Sci.* **2013,** *56,* 20–22.

74. Kumar, S.; Pal, D. Quality of Curd Manufactured from Buffalo Milk Concentrated by Reverse Osmosis. *Ind. J. Diary Sci.* **2014,** *47,* 766–769.

75. Kumura, H.; Tanoue, Y.; Tsukahara, M. Screening of Dairy Yeast Strains for Probiotic Applications. *J. Diary Sci.* **2004,** *87* (12), 4050–4056.

76. Laiño, J. E.; LeBlanc, J. G.; Savoy de Giori, G. Production of Natural Folates by Lactic Acid Bacteria Starter Cultures Isolated from Artisanal Argentinean Yogurts. *Can. J. Microbiol.* **2012,** *58,* 581–588.

77. Lata, M.; Balasubramanyam, B. V.; Rao, K. J. Suitability of Concentrated Milk for *Dahi* Preparation. *Ind. J. Diary Sci.* **2003,** *56,* 359–362.

78. Lee, C. H. Creative Fermentation Technology for the Future. *J. Food Sci.* **2004,** *69,* 33–34.

79. Lee, H. R.; Cho, S. D.; Lee, W. K. Digestive Recovery of Sulfur-Methyl-L-Methionine and its Bio-Accessibility in *Kimchi* Cabbages Using a Simulated *In vitro* Digestion Model System. *J. Sci. Food Agric.* **2014,** *94,* 109–112.

80. Li, Z.; Teng, J.; Lyu, Y.; Hu, X.; Zhao, Y.; Wang, M. Enhanced Antioxidant Activity for Apple Juice Fermented with *Lactobacillus plantarum* ATCC14917. *Molecules* **2019,** *24,* 51–55.

81. Lim, S. M. Microbiological, Physicochemical and Antioxidant Properties of Plain Yogurt and Soy Yogurt. *Korean J. Microbiol.* **2013,** *49,* 403–414.

82. Macfarlane, G. T.; Cummings, J. H. Probiotics, Infection and Immunity. *Curr. Opin. Infect. Dis.* **2002,** *15* (5), 501–506.

83. Manoury, E., Jourdon, K., Boyaval, P. Quantitative Measurement of Vitamin K2 (Menaquinones) in Various Fermented Dairy Products Using a Reliable High-Performance Liquid Chromatography Method. *J. Diary Sci.* **2013,** *96* (3), 1335–1346.

84. Mao, A. A.; Odyuo, N. Traditional Fermented Foods of the *Naga* Tribes of North-eastern, India. *Ind. J. Trad. Knowledge* **2007,** *6* (1), 37–41.

85. Marteau, P.; Seksik, P.; Jian, R. Probiotics and Intestinal Health Effects: A Clinical Perspective. *Br. J. Nutr.* **2002,** *88* (S1), 51–57.

86. Maugeri, F.; Hernalsteens, S. Screening of Yeast Strains for Transfructosylating Activity. *J. Mol. Cataly. B Enzymatic* **2007,** *49* (4), 43–49.

87. Medrano, M.; Pérez, P. F.; Abraham, A. G. Kefiran Antagonizes Cytopathic Effects of *Bacillus Cereus* Extracellular Factors. *Int. J. Food Microbiol.* **2008,** *122* (2), 1–7.

88. Mine, Y.; Wong, A. H. Fibrinolytic Enzymes in Asian Traditional Fermented Foods. *Food Res. Int.* **2005,** *38,* 243–250.

89. Montemurro, M.; Pontonio, E.; Gobbetti, M.; Rizzello, C. G. Investigation of the Nutritional, Functional and Technological Effects of the Sourdough Fermentation of Sprouted Flours. *Int. J. Food Microbiol.* **2018,** *20* (5), 2–8.

90. Mukherjee, S. K.; Albury, M. N.; Pederson, C. S. Role of *Leuconostoc mesenteroides* in Leavening the Batter of *Idli*: Fermented Food of India. *Appl. Microbiol.* **1965,** *13,* 227–231.

91. Mustafa, M.; Nagalingam, S.; Tye, J.; Shafii, A. H.; Dolah, J. Looking Back to the Past: Revival of Traditional Food Packaging. *J. Food Sci. Technol.* **2009,** *18,* 4–18.

92. Muthukumarasamy, P.; Holley, R. A. Microbiological and Sensory Quality of Dry Fermented Sausages Containing Alginate Microencapsulated *Lactobacillus reuteri. Int. J. Food Microbiol.* **2006,** *111,* 164–169.

93. Muzaddadi, A. U. Minimization of Fermentation Period of *Shidal* from Barbs (*Puntius* spp.). *Fishery Technol.* **2015,** *52,* 34–41.

94. Muzaddadi, A. U.; Basu, S. Accelerated Process for Fermented Fish *(Seedal)* Production in Northeast Region of India. *Ind. J. Animal Sci.* **2012,** *82* (2), 98–106.

95. Muzaddadi, A. U.; Basu, S. *Seedal*: Indigenous Fermented Fishery Product of North-East India. *Fish. Chimes* **2003,** *23* (1), 30–32.

96. Nair, B. M.; Prajapati, J. B. The History of Fermented Foods. In *Handbook of Fermented Functional Foods*; CRC Press: Boca Raton, FL, 2003; pp 17–42.

97. Nehal, N. Knowledge of Traditional Fermented Food Products Harbored by the Tribal Folks of the Indian Himalayan Belt. *Int. J. Agric. Food Sci. Technol.* 2013, *4,* 401–414.

98. Nejati, F.; Rizzello, C. G. Manufacture of a Functional Fermented Milk Enriched of Angiotensin-I Converting Enzyme (ACE)-Inhibitory Peptides and -Amino Butyric Acid (GABA). *LWT Food Sci. Technol.* **2013,** *51,* 183–189.

99. Nout, M. R. Rich Nutrition from the Poorest–Cereal Fermentations in Africa and Asia. *Food Microbiol.* **2009,** *26* (7), 685–692.

100. Oki, K.; Rai, A. K.; Sato, S.; Watanabe, K.; Tamang, J. P. Lactic Acid Bacteria Isolated from Ethnic Preserved Meat Products of the Western Himalayas. *Food Microbiol.* **2011,** *28* (1), 1308–1315.

101. Padghan, P. V.; Mann, B.; Sharma, R.; Kumar, A. Studies on bio-functional activity of traditional Lassi, *J. Diary Sci.* **2015,** *30,* 14.

102. Panesar, P. S.; Marwaha, S. S. Biotechnology in Agriculture and Food Processing: Opportunities and Challenges. In *Food Processing: Biotechnological* Applications;

Gandhi, D. N., Marwaha, S. S., Arora, J. K., Eds.; Asiatech Publishers Inc.: New Delhi, 2013; pp 209–220.

103. Panesar, P. S.; Panesar, R.; Singh, R. S.; Kennedy, J. F.; Kumar, H. Microbial production, Immobilization and Applications of β-D-galactosidase. *J. Chem. Technol. Biotechnol. Int. Res. Process Environ. Clean Technol.* **2006,** *81* (4), 530–543.

104. Parvez, S.; Malik, K. A.; Ah Kang, S.; Kim, H. Y. Probiotics and Their Fermented Food Products are Beneficial for Health. *J. Appl. Microbiol.* **2006,** *100* (6), 1171–1185.

105. Patil, M. M.; Pal, A.; Anand, T.; Ramana, K. V. Isolation and Characterization of Lactic Acid Bacteria from Curd and Cucumber. *Ind. J. Biotechnol.* **2010,** *9*, 166–172.

106. Patring, J. D.; Hjortmo, S. B.; Jastrebova, J. A.; Svensson, U. K.; Andlid, T. A.; Jägerstad, I. M. Characterization and Quantification of Folates Produced by Yeast Strains Isolated from *Kefir* Granules. *Eur. Food Res. Technol.* **2006,** *223* (5), 633–637.

107. Patring, J. D.; Jastrebova, J. A.; Hjortmo, S. B. Development of a Simplified Method for the Determination of Folates in Baker's Yeast by HPLC with Ultraviolet and Fluorescence Detection. *J. Agric. Food Chem.* **2005,** *53* (7), 2406–2411.

108. Peñas, E.; Diana, M.; Frias, J.; Quílez, J.; Martínez-Villaluenga, C. Multistrategic Approach in the Development of Sourdough Bread Targeted Towards Blood Pressure Reduction. *Plant Foods Human Nutr.* **2015,** *70*, 97–103.

109. Pessione, E.; Cirrincione, S. Bioactive Molecules Released in Food by Lactic Acid Bacteria: Encrypted Peptides and Biogenic Amines. *Front. Microbiol.* **2016,** *7*, 876.

110. Potter, N. N.; Hotchkiss J. H. (Eds.). *Food Science*; CBS Publishers and Distributors: New Delhi, 2006; pp 264–277.

111. Poutanen, K.; Flander, L.; Katina, K. Sourdough and Cereal Fermentation in a Nutritional Perspective. *Food Microbiol.* **2009,** *26* (7), 693–699.

112. Prakash, O. Food and Drinks in Ancient India. *Ind. J. Trad. Knowledge* **1961,** 14–25.

113. Prasad, R. K.; Singh, S. K. Fermented Indigenous Indian Dairy Products: Standards, Nutrition, Technological Significance and Opportunities for its Processing. *J. Pure Appl. Microbiol.* **2017,** *11* (2), 1199–1213.

114. Psomas, E. I.; Fletouris, D. J.; Litopoulou-Tzanetaki, E.; Tzanetakis, N. Assimilation of Cholesterol by Yeast Strains Isolated from Infant Faeces and Feta Cheese. *J. Diary Sci.* **2003,** *86* (11), 3416–3422.

115. Purushothaman, D.; Dhanapal, N.; Rangaswami, G. Microbiology and Biochemistry of *Idli* Fermentation. *Symp. Indigen. Ferment. Food Bangkok, Thailand* **1977,** *1977*, 30–35.

116. Qian, B.; Xing, M.; Cui, L.; Deng, Y.; Xu, Y.; Huang, M.; Zhang, S. Antioxidant, Antihypertensive and Immunomodulatory Activities of Peptide Fractions from Fermented Skim Milk with *Lactobacillus delbrueckii* ssp. *bulgaricus*. *J. Dairy Res.* **2011,** *78*, 72–79.

117. Radhakrishnamurty, R.; Desikachar, H. S.; Srinivasan, M.; Subrahmanyan, V. Studies on *Idli* Fermentation, Part II: Relative Participation of Black Gram Flour and Rice Semolina in the Fermentation. *J. Sci. Indus. Res.* **1961,** *20*, 342–345.

118. Rai, A. K.; Tamang, J. P.; Palni, U. Microbiological Studies of Ethnic Meat Products of the Eastern Himalayas. *Meat Sci.* **2010,** *85*, 560–567.

119. Rai, A. K.; Tamang, J. P.; Palni, U. Nutritional Value of Lesser-Known Ethnic Meat Products of the Himalayas. *J. Hill Res.* **2010,** *23* (12), 22–25.

120. Rai, R.; Kharel, N.; Tamang, J. P. HACCP Model of *Kinema*: Fermented Soybean Food. *J. Sci. Indus. Res.* **2014**, *73*, 588–592.
121. Raju, P. N.; Pal, D. The Physicochemical, Sensory and Textural Properties of *Misti Dahi* Prepared from Reduced Fat Buffalo Milk. *Food Bioproc. Technol.* **2009**, *2* (1), 101–108.
122. Ramana, B. L. V. *Standardization of a Method of Manufacture of Lassi with Enhanced Shelf Stability.* M.Sc. Thesis; NDRI Deemed University, Karnal, India, 1994; p 118.
123. Rapsang, G. F.; Joshi, S. R. Bacterial Diversity Associated with *Tungtap*, an Ethnic Traditionally Fermented Fish Product of Meghalaya. *Ind. J. Trad. Knowledge* **2012**, *11*, 134–138.
124. Rapsang, G. F.; Kumar, R.; Joshi, S. R. Identification of *Lactobacillus Puhozihii* from *Tungtap*: A Traditionally Fermented Fish Food and Analysis of its Bacteriocin genic Potential. *Afr. J. Biotechnol.* **2011**, *10*, 12237–12243.
125. Reddy, N. R.; Sathe, S. K.; Pierson, M. D.; Salunkhe, D. K. *Idli* - Indian Fermented Food: A Review. *J. Food Qual.* **1982**, *5*, 89–101.
126. Rios-Corripio, G.; Guerrero-Beltrán, J. Á. Antioxidant and Physicochemical Characteristics of Unfermented and Fermented Pomegranate (*Punica granatum L.*) Beverages. *J. Food Sci. Technol.* **2019**, *56*, 132–139.
127. Rocchetti, G.; Miragoli, F.; Zacconi, C.; Lucini, L.; Rebecchi, A. Impact of Cooking and Fermentation by Lactic Acid Bacteria on Phenolic Profile of Quinoa and Buckwheat Seeds. *Food Res. Int.* **2019**, *119*, 886–894.
128. Rodríguez, L. R.; Pingitore, E. V. Biodiversity and Technological- Functional Potential of Lactic Acid Bacteria Isolated from Spontaneously Fermented Quinoa Sourdoughs. *J. Appl. Microbiol.* **2016**, *120*, 1289–1301.
129. Rodríguez-Figueroa, J. C. Antihypertensive and Hypolipidemic Effect of Milk Fermented by Specific *Lactococcus lactis* Strains. *J. Diary Sci.* **2013**, *96* (7), 4094–4099.
130. Rodríguez-Figueroa, J. C.; González-Córdova, A. F. Hypotensive and Heart Rate-lowering Effects in Rats Receiving Milk Fermented by Specific *Lactococcus lactis* Strains. *Br. J. Nutr.* **2013**, *109*, 827–833.
131. Rühmkorf, C.; Jungkunz, S.; Wagner, M. Optimization of Homo-exopolysaccharide Formation by *Lactobacilli* in Gluten-free Sourdough. *Food Microbiol.* **2012**, *32*, 286–294.
132. Rühmkorf, C.; Rübsam, H.; Becker, T.; Bork, C. Effect of Structurally Different Microbial Homoexo polysaccharides on the Quality of Gluten-Free Bread. *Eur. Food Res. Technol.* **2012**, *235* (1), 139–146.
133. Sanders, M. E.; Klaenhammer, T. R. Review: The Scientific Basis of *Lactobacillus acidophilus* NCFM Functionality as a Probiotic. *J. Diary Sci.* **2001**, *84* (2), 319–331.
134. Sankaran, R. (Eds.) Fermented Foods of the Indian Subcontinent. In *Microbiology of Fermented Foods*; Springer: Boston, MA, 1998; pp 753–789.
135. Şanlier, N.; Gökcen, B. B.; Sezgin, A. C. Health Benefits of Fermented Foods. *Crit. Rev. Food Sci. Nutr.* **2019**, *59* (3), 506–527.
136. Sarkar, S. Innovations in Indian Fermented Milk Products: Review. *Food Biotechnol.* **2008**, *22* (1), 78–97.
137. Sathe, G. B.; Mandal, S. Fermented Products of India and its Implication: A Review. *Asian J. Dairy Food Res.* **2016**, *35* (1), 26–32.

138. Sen, N. P.; Miles, W. F.; Donaldson, B.; Panalaks, T.; Iyengar, J. R. Formation of Nitrosamines in a Meat Curing Mixture. *Nature* **1973,** *245* (5), 104–105.

139. Septembre-Malaterre, A.; Remize, F.; Poucheret, P. Fruits and Vegetables, as a Source of Nutritional Compounds and Phytochemicals: Changes in Bioactive Compounds during Lactic Fermentation. *Food Res. Int.* **2018,** *104,* 86–99.

140. Settanni, L.; Corsetti, A. Application of Bacteriocins in Vegetable Food Bio-preservation. *Int. J. Food Microbiol.* **2008,** *121* (2), 123–138.

141. Shanahan, F. Inflammatory Bowel Disease: Immunodiagnostics, Immunotherapeutics and Ecotherapeutics. *Gastroenterology* **2001,** *120,* 622–635.

142. Shrigondekar, G. K. *Manasollasa* of King Somesvara. *Gaekwad's Orient. Ser.* **1939,** *84* (1), 21–23.

143. Shukla, S.; Park, J.; Park, J. H.; Lee, J. S.; Kim, M. Development of Lotus Root Fermented Sugar Syrup as a Functional Food Supplement/Condiment and Evaluation of its Physicochemical, Nutritional and Microbiological Properties. *J. Food Sci. Technol.* **2018,** *55,* 619–629.

144. Singh, T. A.; Devi, K. R.; Ahmed, G.; Jeyaram, K. Microbial and Endogenous Origin of Fibrinolytic Activity in Traditional Fermented Foods of Northeast India. *Food Res. Int.* **2014,** *55,* 356–362.

145. Solga, S. F. Probiotics can Treat Hepatic Encephalopathy. *Med. Hypotheses* **2003,** *61,* 307–313.

146. Solieri, L.; Rutella, G. S.; Tagliazucchi, D. Impact of Non-Starter *Lactobacilli* on Release of Oki Bovine Milk Fermentation. *Food Microbiol.* **2015,** *51,* 108–116.

147. Song, M. Y.; Vanba, H.; Park, W. S. Quality Characteristics of Functional Fermented Sausages Added with Encapsulated Probiotic *Bifidobacterium longum* KACC 91563. *Korean J. Food Sci. Animal Resour.* **2018,** *38,* 981–994.

148. Soni, S.; Sandhu, D.; Vilkhu, K. Studies on *Dosa* and Indigenous Indian Fermented Food: Some Biochemical Changes Accompanying Fermentation. *Food Microbiol.* **1991,** *2,* 175–181.

149. Spano, G.; Capozzi, V. Food Microbial Biodiversity and Microbes of Protected Origin. *Front. Microbiol.* **2011,** *2* (1), 237–245.

150. Sridevi, J.; Halami, P. M.; Vijayendra, S. V. N. Selection of Starter Cultures for *Idli* Batter Fermentation and Their Effect on Quality of *Idli. J. Food Sci. Technol.* **2010,** *47* (5), 557–563.

151. Srinivasa, P. T. I. Pre-Aryan Tamil culture. *Madras (India): Univ. Madras* **1930,** *1930,* 8–36.

152. Srinivasan, K. Traditional Indian Functional Foods. *Funct. Foods East Nutraceutical Sci. Technol. Ser.* **2010,** *10,* 51–76.

153. Steinkraus, K. (Eds.). Handbook of Indigenous Fermented Foods. Chapter 2. In *Indigenous Fermented Foods Involving an Acid Fermentation: Preserving and Enhancing Organoleptic and Nutritional Qualities of Fresh Foods*; Steinkraus, K., Ed.; CRC Press: Boca Raton, FL, 2018; pp 111–349.

154. Sundar, S.; Jha, T. K.; Thakur, C. P.; Bhattsingh, S. K.; Rai, M. Oral Multitone for the Treatment of Indian Visceral Leishmaniasis. *Trans. R. Soc. Trop. Med. Hygiene* **2006,** *100* (1), 26–33.

155. Sura, K.; Garg, S.; Garg, F. C. Microbiological and Biochemical Changes During Fermentation of *Kanji. J. Food Sci. Technol.* **2001,** *38,* 165–167.

156. Szajewska, H.; Skórka, A.; Ruszczyński, M.; Gieruszczak-Białek, D. Meta-Analysis: *Lactobacillus* GG for Treating Acute Diarrhea in Children. *Aliment. Pharmacol. Therap.* **2007,** *25* (8), 871–881.

157. Tamang, B.; Tamang, J. P. Role of Lactic Acid Bacteria and Their Functional Properties in *Goyang*: Fermented Leafy Vegetable Product of *Sherpas*. *J. Hill Res.* **2007,** *20* (2), 53–61.

158. Tamang, B.; Tamang, J. P. Traditional Knowledge of Bio-Preservation of Perishable Vegetables and Bamboo Shoots in Northeast India as Food Resources. *Ind. J. Trad. Knowledge* **2009,** *8,* 81–95.

159. Tamang, J. P. *Sinki*: Traditional Lactic Acid Fermented Radish Tap Root Product. *J. Gen. Appl. Microbiol.* **1993,** *39,* 395–408.

160. Tamang, J. P.; Dewan, S.; Tamang, B. Lactic Acid Bacteria in *Hamei* and *Marcha* of North East India. *Ind. J. Microbiol.* **2007,** *47* (2), 119–125.

161. Tamang, J. P.; Kailasapathy, K. (Eds.). *Fermented Foods and Beverages of the World*; CRC Press: Boca Raton, FL, 2010; p 820.

162. Tamang, J. P.; Samuel, D. Dietary Cultures and Antiquity of Fermented Foods and Beverages. *Ferment. Foods Bever. World* **2010,** *2010,* 1–40.

163. Tamang, J. P.; Tamang, B.; Schillinger, U. Identification of Predominant Lactic Acid Bacteria Isolated from Traditionally Fermented Vegetable Products of the Eastern Himalayas. *Int. J. Food Microbiol.* **2005,** *105* (3), 347–356.

164. Tamang, J. P.; Tamang, N.; Thapa, S. Microorganisms and Nutritional Value of Ethnic Fermented Foods and Alcoholic Beverages of North East India. *Ethnic Ferment. Foods Alcohol. Bever. Asia* **2012,** *20,* 4–12.

165. Tamang, J. P.; Thapa, N.; Bhalla, T. C. Ethnic Fermented Foods and Beverages of India. *Ethnic Ferment. Foods Alcohol. Bever. Asia* **2016,** *24,* 17–72.

166. Tamang, J. P.; Thapa, N.; Tamang, B.; Rai, A.; Chettri, R. Microorganisms in Fermented Foods and Beverages. *Health Benefits Ferment. Foods Bever.* **2015,** 1–110.

167. Tamang, J.; Kim, B.; Song, D. S.; Lim, Y. T. Modulation of Th1/Th2 Balance by *Lactobacillus* Strains Isolated from *Kimchi* via Stimulation of Macrophage Cell Line J774A.1 *In vitro*. *J. Food Sci.* **2011,** *76* (2), H55–H61.

168. Tamang, J. P. (Eds.). *Himalayan Fermented Foods: Microbiology, Nutrition and Ethnic Values*; CRC Press: New Delhi, 2009; pp 38–56.

169. Tamang, J. P.; Tamang, B.; Schillinger, U.; Franz, C. M. Identification of Predominant Lactic Acid Bacteria Isolated from Traditionally Fermented Vegetable Products of the Eastern Himalayas. *Int. J. Food Microbiol.* **2005,** *105,* 347–356.

170. Tavakoli, M.; Habibi Najafi, M. B.; Mohebbi, M. Effect of the Milk Fat Content and Starter Culture Selection on Proteolysis and Antioxidant Activity of Probiotic Yogurt. *Heliyon* **2019,** *5,* 4–9.

171. Thapa, N. *Studies on Microbial Diversity Associated with Some Fish Products of the Eastern Himalayas*. PhD Thesis; North Bengal University, India, 2002; p 189.

172. Thapa, N.; Pal, J.; Tamang, J. P. Microbial Diversity in *Ngari, Hentak* and *Tungtap*: Fermented Fish Products of North East India. *World J. Microbiol. Biotechnol.* **2004,** *20,* 599–607.

173. Thapa, S.; Tamang, J. P. Product characterization of *Kodo ko Jaanr*: Fermented Finger Millet Beverage of the Himalayas. *Food Microbiol.* **2004,** *21,* 617–622.

174. Thapa, S.; Tamang, J. P. Microbiological and Physicochemical Changes during Fermentation of *Kodo Ko Jaanr*: Traditional Alcoholic Beverage of the Darjeeling Hills and Sikkim. *Ind. J. Microbiol.* **2006,** *46* (4), 333–341.

175. Thyagaraja, N.; Hosono, A. Binding Properties of Lactic Acid Bacteria from *Idly* Towards Food-Borne Mutagens. *Food Chem. Toxicol.* **1994,** *32* (9), 805–809.

176. Tidona, F.; Meucci, A.; Povolo, M.; Pelizzola, V. Applicability of *Lactococcus hircilactis* and *Lactococcus laudensis* as Dairy Cultures. *Int. J. Food Microbiol.* **2018,** *271*, 1–7.

177. Toldra, F.; Aristoy, M. C.; Flores, M. Contribution of Muscle Aminopeptidases to Flavor Development in Dry-Cured Ham. *Food Res. Int.* **2000,** *33*, 181–185.

178. Vasudha, S.; Mishra, H. N. Non- Dairy Probiotic Beverages. *Int. Food Res. J.* **2013,** *20* (1), 8–15.

179. Venkatasubbaiah, P.; Dwarakanath, C. T.; Sreenivasamurthy, V. Microbiological and Physicochemical Changes in *Idli* Batter during Fermentation. *J. Food Sci. Technol.* **1984,** *21*, 59–62.

180. Villalva, M. F. A.; González-Aguilar, G. Bioprocessing of Wheat (*Triticum. aestivum cv. Kronstad*) Bran from Northwest Mexico: Effects on Ferulic Acid Bioaccessibility in Breads. *CyTA J. Food* **2018,** *16*, 570–579.

181. Won, T. J.; Kim, B.; Lim, Y. T.; Song, D. S. Oral Administration of *Lactobacillus* Strains from Kimchi Inhibits Atopic Dermatitis in NC/Nga Mice. *J. Appl. Microbiol.* **2011,** *110* (5), 1195–1202.

182. Xing, L.; Liu, R.; Cao, S.; Zhang,W.; Guanghong, Z. Meat Protein-based Bioactive Peptides and their Potential Functional Activity: Review. *International J. Food Sci. Technol.* **2019,** *2019*, 22–34.

183. Yang, X.; Zhou, J.; Fan, L.; Qin, Z.; Chen, Q.; Zhao, L. Antioxidant Properties of a Vegetable - Fruit Beverage Fermented with two *Lactobacillus plantarum* Strains. *Food Sci. Biotechnol.* **2018,** *27*, 1719–1726.

184. Yegna-Narayan, A. K. Dairying in Ancient India. *Ind. Dairyman* **1953,** *5*, 77–83.

185. Yonzan, H.; Tamang, J. P. Traditional Processing of *Selroti*: Cereal Based Ethnic Fermented Food of the Nepalis. *Ind. J. Trad. Knowledge* **2009,** *8* (1), 110–114.

186. Zareba, D.; Ziarno, M.; Obiedzinski, M. Volatile Profile of Non-Fermented Milk and Milk Fermented by *Bifidobacterium animalis* subsp. *lactis*. *Int. J. Food Prop.* **2012,** *15* (5), 1010–1021.

187. Zhang, W.; Xiao, S.; Samaraweera, H.; Lee, E. J.; Ahn, D. U. Improving Functional Value of Meat Products. *Meat Sci.* **2010,** *86*, article ID: 15e31.

188. Zironi, E.; Gazzotti, T.; Barbarossa, A. Determination of Vitamin B12 in Dairy Products by Ultra Performance Liquid Chromatography-Tandem Mass Spectrometry. *Ital. J. Food Safe.* **2014,** *3*, 4513–4518.

189. Zhanl, W. A: Indian Food Industry Report, 2019; p 84; https://indiamicrofinance. com/indian-food-industry-report-2019-pdf.html; Accessed on January 5, **2020.**

Index

For Product Safety Concerns and Information please contact our EU
representative GPSR@taylorandfrancis.com
Taylor & Francis Verlag GmbH, Kaufingerstraße 24, 80331 München, Germany

www.ingramcontent.com/pod-product-compliance
Lightning Source LLC
Chambersburg PA
CBHW060344220326
41598CB00023B/2798